T0331800

FUTURE DEVELOPMENTS IN BLOOD BANKING

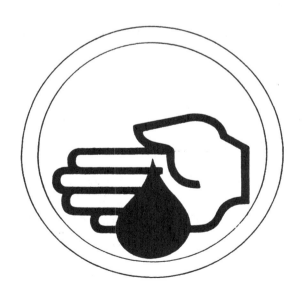

DEVELOPMENTS IN HEMATOLOGY AND IMMUNOLOGY

Lijnen, H.R., Collen, D. and Verstraete, M., eds: Synthetic Substrates in Clinical Blood Coagulation Assays. 1980. ISBN 90-247-2409-0

Smit Sibinga, C.Th., Das, P.C. and Forfar, J.O., eds: Paediatrics and Blood Transfusion. 1982. ISBN 90-247-2619-0

Fabris, N., ed: Immunology and Ageing. 1982. ISBN 90-247-2640-9

Hornstra, G.: Dietary Fats, Prostanoids and Arterial Thrombosis. 1982. ISBN 90-247-2667-0

Smit Sibinga, C.Th., Das, P.C. and Loghem, van J.J., eds: Blood Transfusion and Problems of Bleeding. 1982. ISBN 90-247-3058-9

Dormandy, J., ed: Red Cell Deformability and Filterability. 1983. ISBN 0-89838-578-4

Smit Sibinga, C.Th., Das, P.C. and Taswell, H.F., eds: Quality Assurance in Blood Banking and Its Clinical Impact. 1984. ISBN 0-89838-618-7

Besselaar, A.M.H.P. van den, Gralnick, H.R. and Lewis, S.M., eds: Thromboplastin Calibration and Oral Anticoagulant Control. 1984. ISBN 0-89838-637-3

Fondu, P. and Thijs, O., eds: Haemostatic Failure in Liver Disease. 1984. ISBN 0-89838-640-3

Smit Sibinga, C.Th., Das, P.C. and Opelz, G., eds: Transplantation and Blood Transfusion. 1984. ISBN 0-89838-686-1

Schmid-Schönbein, H., Wurzinger, L.J. and Zimmerman, R.E., eds: Enzyme Activation in Blood-Perfused Artificial Organs. 1985. ISBN 0-89838-704-3

Dormandy, J., ed: Blood Filtration and Blood Cell Deformability. 1985. ISBN 0-89838-714-0

Smit Sibinga, C.Th., Das, P.C. and Seidl, S., eds: Plasma Fractionation and Blood Transfusion. 1985. ISBN 0-89838-761-2

Dawids, S. and Bantjes, A., eds: Blood Compatible Materials and their Testing. 1986. ISBN 0-89838-813-9

Smit Sibinga, C.Th., Das, P.C. and Greenwalt, T.J., eds: Future Developments in Blood Banking. 1986. ISBN 0-89838-824-4

Future Developments in Blood Banking

Proceedings of the Tenth Annual Symposium on Blood Transfusion,
Groningen 1985, organized by the Red Cross Blood Bank Groningen-Drenthe

edited by

C.Th. SMIT SIBINGA and P.C. DAS

Red Cross Blood Bank Groningen-Drenthe
The Netherlands

T.J. GREENWALT

Paul I. Hoxworth Blood Center, Cincinnati, Ohio, U.S.A.

1986 **MARTINUS NIJHOFF PUBLISHING**
a member of the KLUWER ACADEMIC PUBLISHERS GROUP
BOSTON / DORDRECHT / LANCASTER

Distributors

for the United States and Canada: Kluwer Academic Publishers, 101 Philip Drive, Assinippi Park, Norwell, MA 02061, USA
for the UK and Ireland: Kluwer Academic Publishers, MTP Press Limited, Falcon House, Queen Square, Lancaster LA1 1RN, UK
for all other countries: Kluwer Academic Publishers Group, Distribution Center, P.O. Box 322, 3300 AH Dordrecht, The Netherlands

Library of Congress Cataloging in Publication Data

```
Symposium on Blood Transfusion (10th : 1985 :
    Groningen, Netherlands)
    Future developments in blood banking.

    (Developments in hematology and immunology)
    1. Blood banks--Congresses.  I. Smit Sibinga, C. Th.
II. Das, P. C.  III. Greenwalt, Tibor Jack, 1914-
IV. Stichting Rode Krius Bloedbank Groningen/Drente.
V. Title.  VI. Series.  [DNLM: 1. Blood Banks--
congresses.  W1 DE997VZK / WH 460 S9896 1985f]
RM172.S96  1985        362.1'784          86-16439
ISBN 0-89838-824-4
```

ISBN 0-89838-824-4 (this volume)
ISBN 90-247-2432-5 (series)

Copyright

PRINTED IN THE NETHERLANDS

TRAVENOL

Acknowledgement

This publication has been made possible through the support of Travenol, which is gratefully acknowledged.

CONTENTS

III. Laboratory aspects

IV. Clincial aspects

MODERATORS AND SPEAKERS

Moderators

T.J. Greenwalt	– Paul I. Hoxworth Blood Center, Cincinnati OH, USA
C.Th. Smit Sibinga	– Red Cross Blood Bank Groningen-Drenthe, Groningen, NL
C.F. Högman	– The Blood Centre University Hospital, Uppsala, S
P.C. Das	– Red Cross Blood Bank Groningen-Drenthe, Groningen, NL
H.F. Polesky	– The War Memorial Blood Bank, Minneapolis, MN, USA
R.L. McShine	– Red Cross Blood Bank Groningen-Drenthe, Groningen, NL
M.R. Halie	– Division of Hematology, University Hospital Groningen, Groningen, NL

Speakers

F.A. Ala	– Regional Blood Transfusion Centre, Birmingham, UK
J.M. Anthony	– Travenol Laboratories, Deerfield, IL, USA
J.C. Bakker	– Central Laboratory of the Dutch Red Cross, Amsterdam, NL
A.E.G. Kr. von dem Borne	– Central Laboratory of the Dutch Red Cross, Amsterdam, NL
C. Coffe	– Regional Blood Transfusion Service, Besançon, F
P.C. Das	– Red Cross Blood Bank Groningen-Drenthe, Groningen, NL
G.M. Fahy	– American Red Cross, Blood Services Laboratories, Bethesda, MD, USA
L.I. Friedman	– American Red Cross, Blood Services Laboratories, Bethesda, MD, USA
T.J. Greenwalt	– Paul I. Hoxworth Blood Center, Cincinnati OH, USA
C.F. Högman	– The Blood Centre University Hospital, Uppsala, S
D.W. Huestis	– The University of Arizona, Tucson, AZ, USA
B.A. Jameson	– Max von Pettenkofer-Institut, München, FRG

R.E. Klein — American Red Cross Blood Services, Winston Salem, NC, USA

K. Koerner — Blood Transfusion Services Baden-Würtemberg, Ulm, FRG

L.C. Lasky — Veterans Adminsitration Medical Center, Minneapolis, MN, USA

S.L. Lentz — Minneapolis, MN, USA

A. Maas — Red Cross Blood Bank Groningen-Drenthe, Groningen, NL

K. Mayer — Sloan-Kettering Cancer Center, New York, NY, USA

R.L. McShine — Red Cross Blood Bank Groningen-Drenthe, Groningen, NL

L. Noel — Regional Blood Transfusion Service, Versailles, F

F.V. Plapp — Community Blood Center of Greater Kansas City, Kansas City, MI, USA

H.K. Prins — Central Laboratory of the Dutch Red Cross, Amsterdam, NL

J.M. Sangster — London, UK

R.K.B. Schuurman — Eurotransplant, Leiden, NL

P.S. Skinner — Ulrich Schnoor GmbH, Neumünster, FRG

C.Th. Smit Sibinga — Red Cross Blood Bank Groningen-Drenthe, Groningen, NL

H.A.W. van Vianen — Geographical Institute University of Groningen, Groningen, NL

K. Wallevik — Blood Bank and Blood Grouping Laboratory, Århus, DK

Encapsulation of hemoglobin in liposomes making longer sojourn in the circulation possible seems more attractive because it also reduces the likelihood of renal damage. There has also been much discussion of using perfluorocarbons for O_2 and CO_2 transport. I do not believe that they will ever replace donor blood. But suitable analogues and improved emulsifiers which will make it possible to store perflurocarbon emulsions at room temperature, will make these products useful for getting oxygen to tissue crevices inaccessible to erythrocytes. Very much further in the future I can envision a form of *blood banking gardening*. There is hope that it will be possible to isolate dedicated precursors of red cells, leukocytes and even platelets from the bone marrow and in some instances from the peripheral blood and to grow them in culture by methods that will make it possible to harvest the desired formed elements. I will let your imagination run with that idea.

The control of disease transmission by blood products must be given high priority in the future. It is likely that a practical method for detecting the antigens of the HTLV-III virions will be developed within the next 5 years. There is much work already underway to achieve this as well as the development of a vaccine. In the future we should be able to convince the funding agencies to give the problem of non-A non-B hepatitis a higher priority. I feel confident that within the next 5 years specific tests of the non-A non-B virus group will become available. The development of a vaccine should follow. The cytomegalovirus problem will draw more and more attention as we increase the number of organ (including bone marrow) transplantations and in the increasing use of blood products for managing premature infants. The present methods of screening donors are not completely satisfactory. It will become possible for us to pinpoint more accurately those donors whose blood actually contains the virus. A test for IgM anti-CMV antibodies will prove to be more useful for identifying the much smaller percentage of donors who should not be used for transfusing immunocompromised patients. Production of factor VIII and factor IX concentrates by DNA recombinant techniques will eliminate the remaining hazard of transmitting viral hepatitis with the presently available heated products. There have been some difficulties in producing the factor VIII material, but I am reasonably certain the product will become available within 3 to 5 years. Unfortunately the market is so limited for factor IX that development of this product factor by recombinant methodology will probably not occur unless it is subsidized.

I believe that we have not come to the end of the list of viruses and prions which can be transmitted by blood products. New problems are bound to occur in the future e.g., HTLV-I, multiple sclerosis, Alzheimer's disease. In the meantime if we solve the problems associated with AIDS and hepatitis it is most likely that our surgical colleagues will relax their concern about the use of blood and will cause new problems of supply.

We are already in the midst of changes in laboratory procedures. Monoclonal reagents will replace all the antibodies which are now used for processing donor blood, crossmatching and essentially all serological procedures. Solid phase methods will replace our presently used techniques. The large automated machines we now use for performing the serological tests for processing blood will be replaced by microtiter solid phase techniques with automated reading and positive sample identification. The signals will be fed directly into the computerized laboratory stream. Computers will co-ordinate all the steps used in donor history taking, laboratory testing, labelling, issuance of blood products, inventory control and ultimately will be used in closing the now open loop of identity between the crossmatched unit and the patient designated to receive it. The massive amounts of paperwork which are now involved will largely be eliminated.

The serious problem of graft versus host disease in bone marrow transplantation will be eliminated by obtaining better matching between the organ donor and the recipient using selected DNA probes. T-cell depletion techniques will be simplified. Within the next 10 years non-related marrow donors will be used fairly frequently and international computer-linked files will be developed. Techniques will be found for increasing the yield of pluripotent cells from the peripheral blood of selected donors. This may make possible the reconstitution of patients using frozen stored pluripotent cells harvested by selective apheresis. Thus marrow transplantation will not have to be restricted to the 25 to 30% of patients who happen to be fortunate enough to have a matching living related donor. Successful management of many malignancies will be made possible by the use of autologous bone marrow transplants. The present worry about reimplanting contaminating tumor cells will be eliminated by the use of specific monoclonal antibodies tagged with ricin and other cell toxins targeted to destroy the undesirable residual tumor cells while sparing the needed pluripotent precursors.

The range of hemapheresis products useful for the management of patients will be increased and improved. Essentially pure concentrates of single donor platelets without any contaminating leukocytes and pure concentrates of lymphocytes and subsets of lymphocytes will become available for use as indicated. Hollow fiber and membrane techniques will make rapid plasmapheresis for obtaining plasma for fractionation and other purposes simple and routine. Patients not qualified to give whole blood will be selectively used as plasma donors. Clarification of the indications for therapeutic hemapheresis will gradually evolve. Membrane cascade filtration systems will replace more cumbersome methods for removing lipids, biologic and exogenous toxic materials making it possible to return to the patient not only the formed elements but also the purified plasma. Thus the need for using plasma derivatives and other solutions will be eliminated. Specific columns will be used for selectively removing undesirable plasma components. Examples of such systems include activated charcoal, Staphylococcus protein A and monoclonal antibody columns.

Further education of physicians in transfusion medicine is absolutely essential. Within the next 5 to 10 years present efforts to introduce more opportunities for instruction in transfusion medicine will be introduced into the curricula of medical schools, training programs for house staff and the continuing education of physicians. Excellent computer assisted instruction programs for these purposes will be developed. They will be so flexible and adaptable that they should have international utility. Transfusion medicine will continue to receive recognition from the professions and the public. Specialists in transfusion medicine will regularly be used as consultants.

Funding agencies will ultimately recognize the importance of research and development in transfusion medicine and the proportion of research money earmarked for such purposes will be increased.

I suggest that 15 years from now, on the occasion of the silver anniversary Groningen symposium, the predictions of *Nostradamus* be reviewed to test their accuracy using the retrospectroscope.

T.J. Greenwalt, MD
Chairman

I. Community aspects

CHANGING DEMOGRAPHIC ASPECTS

H.A.W. van Vianen

According to a definition of the United Nations demography is: 'The scientific study of human populations with respect to their size, their structure and their development'. This development is the outcome of continuous processes that affect a population: mortality, fertility and mobility (or migration).

In the last century the populations of what are now called the developed countries passed through the various stages of demographic transition, which represents a shift from high mortality/high fertility to low mortality/low fertility. Although these developments had important consequences for population size and population structure, mortality and fertility levels were such that population growth continued until quite recently. The aging of the population was compensated by a proportional growth of the younger age groups.

In the last decades however fertility did fall below the level that is needed to guarantee replacement and most developed countries are confronted with the prospect of a stagnating or even declining population, where the proportion of elder people rose rapidly. This 'greying' of the population gives rise to some concern in particular with respect to the growing costs of old age security.

These demographic developments will have consequences for the health care system and in particular for transfusion medicine because the blood-giving and the blood-using segments of the population are affected in different ways [1].

Unfortunately a thorough demographic study of donor or recipient populations has not been published yet and the available data are not adequate to construct the necessary demographic measures. Therefore this paper will be restricted to a broad sketch of the population developments and their consequences for blood banking. Most data pertain to the Netherlands but the inferences can be generalized for most developed countries.

When discussing the mortality decline it is more appropriate to talk of an epidemiological revolution. In figure 1 a graph is presented depicting the distribution of deaths by age for two different female cohorts. The first distribution concerns the actual mortality experience of Dutch women born in 1871 [2]. The distribution has two major peaks, the first, the highest, relates to the mortality risks of infancy and early childhood, the second peak is situated around age 80. The second distribution represents the mortality experience to be expected for women born in 1980 if mortality risks, currently observed in the Netherlands, should apply during their lifetime [3].

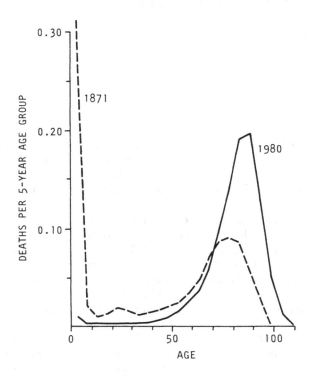

Figure 1. Distribution of deaths by age for women born in the Netherlands in 1871 and 1980.

Only a slight peak at infancy remains, related to perinatal mortality. Mortality has shifted almost completely to very high ages and is peaked around age 85.

This dramatic change has been accomplished primarily by a nearly complete eradication of infectious diseases as a major cause of death. People now generally live to much higher ages, but the virtual disappearance of infectious disease has led to a consequent rise of degenerative and wasting diseases as a major health problem. Aging is accompanied by a rapid rise of chronic morbidity and disability. Figure 2 depicts the mortality survival curve and hypothetical curves representing the probabilities of surviving to a given age without progressive degenerative disease or disability [4]. (There have been some studies to these morbidity/disability curves but, as far as the author knows, not in the Netherlands).

The gap between mortality and morbidity/disability widens with age until at the highest ages it closes again due to the extinct of the cohort. However, the proportion of disabled persons rises continuously with age. It can be assumed safely that the health situation of these elder persons is a major determinant for the demand for blood. Data on blood recipients by age are not readily available, but as a proxy the hospitalization rates presented in

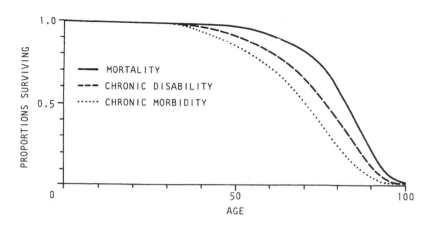

Figure 2. Observed mortality and hypothetical morbidity and disability survival curves for females in the Netherlands in 1980. (Source: WHO, 1984)

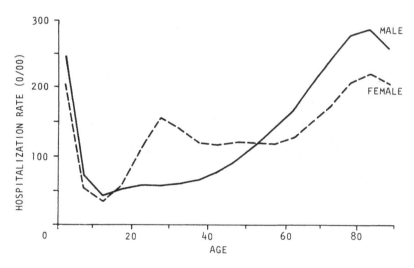

Figure 3. Hospitalization rates by age and sex in the Netherlands in 1981 – 1982. (Source: CBS, 1985)

figure 3 [5] can be used. The high rates at young ages, related to birth in a hospital, tonsilectomies, etc. and the high rates for young women related to partus, sterilization, etc. are not interesting for this purpose, because transfusion will probably play a minor role. In order to get a rough estimate of the consequences of future demographic developments the hospitalization rates by age and sex as observed in 1981 – 1982 were applied to the actual population of 1980 and the low variant of the population projections for 2000 and 2020 [6]. Only the population aged 40 and over was considered.

4

This exercise leads to a rise in demand of 35% in the year 2000 and of 65% in 2020. The procedure is questionable of course, but gives an estimate of the right order of magnitude of the demographic effects of aging.

The increase in demand for blood and blood products will be much higher because technological innovations have been a consistent trend historically and can be anticipated in the future. Another source of rising demands can be found in the growing disadvantages of men over women. In figure 4 the relative decline of mortality risks by age and sex between 1950 and 1980 are presented [7]. There is a spectacular decline of mortality for infants and young children. For women mortality declined at all ages but for men the picture is much less favourable. Between 55 and 75 years mortality risks now are about 20% *higher* than in 1950. Much of this increase is related to diseases of the heart and the vascular system. A continuing pressure on the health system with an accompanying demand for surgery to remedy this situation is likely.

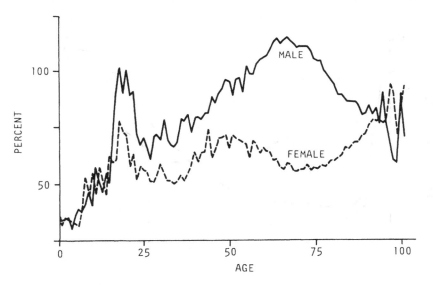

Figure 4. Age specific mortality in 1980 as a percentage of mortality in 1950 in the Netherlands. (Source: CBS, 1985)

Although fertility decline in the developed countries started around 1870, fertility dropped under the replacement level in the beginning of the 1970s and consequently the 'baby boom' generations will be around 30 years of age by the year 2000. As many donors belong to this age bracket a growing pressure upon the blood supply system may be expected from the turn of the century onwards.

In order to estimate the order of magnitude, data concerning the dynamics of a donor population are needed. Unfortunately all studies reporting demographic data contain figures on the number of donors by age and sex only. It is impossible to infer from these data how much of the observed differences between age groups are the result of varying recruitment policies in the past or the result of continuous processes of entry into and exit from the population. As a proxy the age and sex distribution of donors registered at the 'Bloedbank Groningen-Drenthe' were used (C.Th. Smit Sibinga: personal communication). Most reported age distributions of voluntary blood services have roughly the same characteristics: the majority of donors are male, participation rates for men remain high from 20 to 50 years, for women participation rates fall off rapidly after age 30 [8]. It was further assumed that men donate blood more often than women in a ratio of 3 to 2.

Applying these figures to the Dutch population forecasts leads to the surprising result that the supply of blood will be 17% and 4% higher in 2000 and 2020 respectively as compared to 1980.

However a few comments are in order. The Blood Bank Groningen-Drenthe is characterized by a rather large participation rate of donors in the age group 30 – 50 years, which age group is not so heavily affected by demographic developments in the period under consideration. Commercial blood banks generally recruit from younger age groups and in that case demographic impacts are less favourable.

Blood transfusion is a technique using biological materials and therefore creates new opportunities for the transmission of microorganisms. Although a number of diseases that can be transmitted are identified (e.g. hepatitis and recently AIDS) it is probable that new transfusion transmissable diseases will appear, leading to further reductions of the donor population. High mobility of the population (tourism, immigration) and changing life styles may enhance the introduction of new organisms.

Further, changes in the population caused by migration need to be considered. The distribution of blood groups in migrant populations may be different and rare bloodgroups or blood diseases like thalassemia and sickle cell anemia are introduced. However, more important is the part of the immigrant population that has a different cultural background from the resident population. A background from which the voluntary donation of blood may not carry the same value as in our society. The growth of the share of immigrants and their descendents in the younger age groups can lead to additional pressures on the recruitment of donors.

Discussion

The main findings of this exercise are presented in figure 5.
- Due to demographic developments the demand for blood will increase continuously with 35% and 65% in 2000 and 2020 respectively. The actual demand will be much larger due to new indications for blood products and additional pressures from the high incidence of heart and vascular diseases in men.

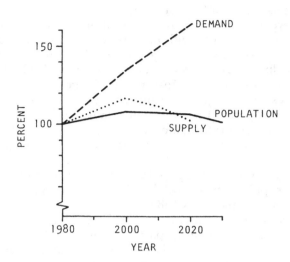

Figure 5. Estimates of the demographic effects on demand and supply of blood and blood products in the Netherlands.

– The supply of blood does not change very much in the period under consideration, there may even be a slight increase by the year 2000. However, the identification of new transfusion transmissable diseases and changes in the ethnic composition of the population may lead to substantial reductions in the age groups eligible for blood donation.

A segment of the recipient population consuming a very large amount of blood products, the hemophiliacs, are not taken into account in the foregoing because no reliable demographic data could be traced.

All forecasts contain some 'ceteris paribus' clause. Recent advances in biotechnology have raised the prospect that alternative sources for some blood products may be available by the end of the 1980s [9] If this might prove correct most of my speculations will be irrelevant.

References

1. Peetoom F, Gaynor SM. The future blood supply system in the USA: a prognosis. In: Smit Sibinga CTh, Das PC, Seidl S, eds. Plasma Fractionation and Blood Transfusion. Martinus Nijhoff Publ., Boston, 1985:3 – 8.
2. CBS. Generatie sterftetafels voor Nederland. Staatsuitgeverij, 's-Gravenhage 1975.
3. Storm H, van Dipten J. Overlevingstafels voor Nederland 1982/83 en 1983. Maandstatistiek van de bevolking 1985;33:44 – 64.
4. World Health Organization. The uses of epidemiology in the study of the elderly. Technical Report Series 706, Geneva 1984.

5. CBS. Diagnosestatistiek ziekenhuizen 1981 – 1982. Staatsuitgeverij, 's-Gravenhage 1985.
6. CBS. Prognose van de bevolking van Nederland na 1980. Staatsuitgeverij, 's-Gravenhage 1984.
7. Anonymous. Maten voor de mannelijke oversterfte. Maandstatistiek Bevolking 1985;33:10 – 1.
8. Bazuin H. Sociale kenmerken en motivatie van bloeddonors. Master thesis. Vakgroep medische sociologie. RUG en Stichting Rode Kruis Bloedbank Groningen-Drenthe, Groningen 1978.
9. Office of Technology Assessment. Blood Policy and Technology. Washington 1985.

CHANGING EMPHASIS IN COLLECTION PROCEDURES

C.F. Högman

Introduction

Two main factors determine the collection procedures:
1. the availability of 'safe' blood donors, and
2. the need of the different constituents of human blood for therapeutical and diagnostic purposes.

Mobile blood collection is a useful way to make it easy for motivated people to donate blood. It has the disadvantage, with presently available techniques, that the time between collection and component separation cannot conveniently be made as short as in a stationary blood bank. Furthermore, the limited space available in mobile blood collection has restricted the choice of collection procedure.

Anticoagulants

One of the major problems which is involved in the collection and storage of blood is the fact that very large quantities are sometimes transfused to a recipient within a short period of time. Ideally, therefore, storage conditions should be such that the blood maintains its therapeutical effects unchanged. At least the requirement must be fulfilled that any decomposed parts of the blood and metabolites formed during storage shall not cause harmful effects, and the chemicals shall not be toxic in the amounts used.

This leaves us to chose between heparin and sodium citrate. Other anti-coagulants such as EDTA or sodium oxalate will be far less acceptable.

Heparin prevents clotting by strongly potentiating the plasma anti-thrombin, thereby inhibiting several coagulation enzymes. It leaves the concentration of Ca^{2+} intact which increases the stability of the factor VIII complex at $+4°C$ [1]. However, it is not suitable for long-term refrigerated storage of blood. After a massive transfusion it can cause disturbances of the recipient's coagulation system due to the relatively long in vivo half-life of 40 – 80 minutes.

Sodium citrate acts by chelating Ca^{2+}. It is stable in refrigerated storage of blood and is very rapidly metabolized in the liver of the recipient following transfusion. Under special conditions, such as very massive transfusion or insufficient liver function of the recipient, decreased ionized calcium concentration may occur. Removal of Ca^{2+} from the stored plasma has marked destabilizing effect on the factor VIII complex at refrigerator storage.

Anticoagulation versus preservation

Whole blood which is anticoagulated with citrate or heparin can be kept at refrigerator temperature for a limited period of time only, before the blood glucose has been consumed by the metabolizing blood cells. In order to maintain red cell viability for some weeks extra glucose has to be added and further improvement can be achieved with inorganic phosphate and purines such as adenine. ACD and CPD with or without additives intended to counteract the loss of adenine groups in the red cells, thus represent a combination of anticoagulant and red cell preservative.

The pH effects in stored blood

Originally the acid pH of ACD solution was aimed at allowing the citrate-glucose solution to be sterilized by heat without caramelization of the glucose. Still this is an important function of the content of citric acid. From a metabolic point of view cooling to $+4°C$ would make non-acidified blood alkaline, increasing pH by about 0.5 pH units. This strongly inhibits glycolysis and ATP formation.

The acidity of the anticoagulants thus serves the purpose of bringing pH to a normal level at the beginning of storage by which the relation between ATP and the other adenine nucleotides, ADP and AMP, can be maintained. If the concentration of AMP increases which happens later during storage, there is an accelerated loss of adenine groups due to deamination of AMP. This loss can be counteracted by addition of adenine to the storage medium by which AMP can be synthetized. The decreased pH of the collected blood also serves the purpose of allowing an even resuspension after sedimentation of the platelets by centrifugation. In this environment the platelets are rendered temporarily less reactive than at physiological pH levels.

The break-down of glucose during storage results in an increased concentration of lactate and a decreasing pH. The pH of fresh CPD blood is about 7.6 at $+4°C$ (7.1 when measured at $+37°C$). After one week it has decreased by about 0.2 pH units. The metabolic activity of the red cells is about four times larger during the first storage week than during the fifth week. Therefore, the pH decreases less rapidly after some weeks of storage, less ATP is formed and consequently the adenylate energy charge is no longer kept at the normal level.

The decreasing pH has a profound effect on the glycerate 2,3-bisphosphate (previously called 2,3-disphosphoglycerate). After collection in ACD the $2,3-P_2$-glycerate is maintained at a normal level for about 5 days only, in CPD for about 10 days. A complete depletion is usually seen after 3 weeks, at least when the blood has been exposed to separation into components which often delays cooling to the storage temperature. The breakdown of $2,3-P_2$-glycerate results in an increase in the concentration of organic phosphate from initially 1.2 to 1.8 mmol. Transfused red cells resynthetize their $2,3-P_2$-glycerate in the circulation but full restoration may not occur until after 24 h or more.

Quality criteria and possibilities of improvement

Let us try to define certain quality criteria and then see what can be done to improve the quality.

Plasma

Citrate, as it is in the ACD and CPD anticoagulants, gives good or reasonably good stability for most of the plasma proteins except factor VIII. Its rapid removal from the circulation by metabolization in the liver gives it an advantage over heparin when massive volumes of plasma are transfused. Heparin on the other hand has a definite advantage over citrate by stabilizing factor VIII. Thus in an additive system where plasma is used exclusively for fractionation we may consider using heparin. Such a system has recently been described, allowing an improved yield of factor VIII in the end product, if the fractionation procedure is changed accordingly [2]. The blood is collected in a heparin solution, plasma is expressed to a satellite bag, and then CPD or CPD adenine solution is drained into the erythrocyte unit.

Whenever plasma is to be used for transfusion purposes citrate still is number one, but we may consider to reduce the concentration to 10-15 mmol/l instead of the present 20. This will reduce citrate toxicity in massive transfusions and improve the stability of factor VIII [3]. Such a change puts emphasis on good collection techniques including sufficient mixing of the blood with the anticoagulant. This, however, is a requirement which should be met even with present techniques of anticoagulation.

Red cells

Many studies have shown a correlation between erythrocyte adenosinetriphosphate (ATP) and posttransfusion survival. It seems likely that maintenance of the total nucleotide content rather than a high energy level is important [4]. Loss of nucleotides can be compensated for by addition of adenine. This substance shall preferably be submitted to the cells via an additive system and not via the anticoagulant, thereby reducing the amount of unused adenine which is transfused to the recipient. Several such systems have been described. The SAG system in which the red cells are collected in CPD and subsequently suspended in an unbuffered solution of sodium chloride, adenine and glucose, is the most simple one. It has shown its usefulness in large clinical applications but should not be used when a maximum volume of plasma is harvested [5]. Then the SAGM or Sagman system [6] is to be preferred because the addition of mannitol prevents hemolysis which may otherwise occur at the end of storage. It is usually used for 35-42 days storage of red cells.

In the circle pack system [7], the red cells are collected in a modified CPD-solution with double the normal amount of glucose. The red cells are suspended in a phosphate buffered solution containing sodium chloride and a low concentration of glucose and adenine. The red cells receive sufficient glucose via the anticoagulant but the plasma will thus contain a double concentration of glucose. The adenine content is suboptimal and the red cells should probably not be stored more than 28-35 days at most. Nutricel® is a similar system containing the same dose of adenine as the SAG/Sagman systems. The 2,3-P_2-glycerate is better maintained in these systems than in the SAG/Sagman systems. The red cells can be stored for 35-42 days. In USA the Adsol® system is now used at a great extent. It is very similar to Sagman; collection is made in CPD but the resuspension medium contains double the amount of glucose, 50% more adenine and 25% more mannitol. It is registered for 49-day storage but recent studies indicate that 35-42 days is likely to be a more satisfactory shelf life [8]. All the additive systems require the red cells to be stored in bags made of PVC plasticized by DEHP. This plasticizer incorporates itself in the red cell membrane which is thereby stabilized. Improvement of red cell shape and posttransfusion survival has been demonstrated [9].

During storage the red cell morphology is grossly changed from the normal discocyte shape to different varieties of echinocytes and spherocytes. The change is reversible in vivo and in vitro. However, the spiculated red cell will lose part of its membrane due to microvesiculation. Not until recently this has been properly quantitated, showing that the formation of microvesicles increases with storage time [10]. Apparently the membrane loss is irreversible. Therefore, further improvements of the maintenance of red cell morphology may be a means for reducing microvesiculation and thereby improving preservation.

As has been mentioned above the formation of lactate during storage causes a successive decrease in pH. By the use of an ion exchanger the pH can be made to decrease less rapidly. In this way 2,3-P_2-glycerate can be maintained normal for a longer period of time [11]. Other means of maintaining 2,3-P_2-glycerate are addition of dihydroxyacetone, ascorbate-phosphate or phospho-enol-pyruvate. All these substances seem to be virtually non-toxic, but their poor stability at autoclaving causes problems.

By suspending red cells in a hypotonic solution containing ammonium chloride, adenine, glucose, citrate, phosphate and mannitol, storage at 24°C for 100 days seems to be possible [12]. The ATP levels rose to twice normal and the in vivo viability was about 80%. However, the cells will have to be washed before transfusion.

Platelets

Platelets do not tolerate storage in the cold; they then rapidly lose their normal survival property. At room temperature storage, platelet viability is maintained much better. However, a major problem has been a rapidly decreasing pH, particularly in units with a high yield of platelets (above 80×10^9 per unit). At a pH below 6.2 an irreversible damage occurs. The pH decrease depends on accumulation of lactate when the platelets use anaerobic glycosis for their ATP production. In the presence of sufficient oxygen the much more effective ATP synthesis via oxydative phosphorylation can be used which prolongs the in vitro storage time. The introduction of new types of plastic, PL-742, CLX, PL-1240, has been an important step to improve platelet preservation. There is, however, a loss of capacity to function and survival during the 5-7 days now maximally applied. Some platelet units show considerable release of intracellular constituents, such as alpha-granules. There is a risk of damaging the platelets by too tough centrifugation or inappropriate mixing during storage. The pH sometimes rises to levels above 7.3 which has been paralleled by abnormal shape [13] and microvesiculation.

Another disadvantage is in the loss of plasma when platelet concentrates are prepared; both that used for suspension of the platelets and that trapped in the red cell unit. It would be much more suitable to have a system, like that used for red cells, by which platelets could be suspended in a synthetic storage medium in which they could also be transfused. There is good hope for such systems in the future, since relatively simple buffer solutions with glucose seem to give the platelets sufficient support [14].

Preparation by apheresis

Plasma donation using plasmapheresis is used extensively to supply raw material for plasma fractionation. In this way the interval between donation and freezing of the separated plasma can be made so short that virtually no deterioration of factor VIII occurs. So far 4% citrate, ACD or CPD solutions have been used almost exclusively for the purpose since heparin has caused difficulties in the fractionation to high purity factor VIII concentrates. It is disturbing, however, that the yield of factor VIII in the final product has been mostly below 20%. This is in contrast to freeze dried cryoprecipitate preparations where the yield can be at least two or three times higher. The high purity factor VIII concentrates have the advantage over cryoprecipitate that they can be LAV/HTLV-III inactivated by heat treatment. Research in progress indicates that heparin as primary anticoagulant may be a way to improve the final yield even in the high purity preparations [15].

Manual, double plasmapheresis which has been the method mostly used, is now being replaced by machines in many blood centers, either using centrifugation, filtration or a combination of both. Shortened donor time, reduced demand of staff and improved safety are the major advantages, increased cost the major disadvantage.

Cytapheresis techniques for preparing platelets and white cells with improved immunological compatibility are well established procedures. More effective and less complicated machines are to be expected.

A cautious look towards the future

Blood component therapy has come to stay. It is important, however, that both blood bankers and clinicians learn how to use the components in the most effective and economic way. Emphasis on education is then important.

The great majority of patients in need of a transfusion require red cells, not plasma which can be saved for fractionation. If the stability of factor VIII could be improved, e.g. by reducing the citrate concentration or using heparin, it would be easier to obtain high quality components from mobile collections.

The use of red cell units with very little remaining plasma means that the normal *blood-group identical* transfusion can be replaced by a *blood-group compatible* red cell transfusion. This means that only four blood groups need to be kept in stock: Rh-positive and Rh-negative untis of type O and A. Type O is then used for B recipients and type A for AB recipients.

The type B and AB donors can be used preferably as plasma donors. Some of the presently available machines can be used in mobile units. Female donors, irrespective of blood type, with hemoglobin levels in the lower range would also be suitable for plasma donation rather than donation of a normal unit of whole blood.

Removal of white cells and platelets is already a standard procedure in many European blood banks. New improved techniques to remove buffy coat in combination with filtration will make the red cell unit both unreactive in patients with leukocyte antibodies and non immunogenic.

Platelet concentrates should be much more effectively depleted of white cells than is normally done to-day. In this way we can expect that the immunogenicity will be strongly reduced, causing less refractoriness. A combination of presently available centrifugation and filtration techniques can be expected to do the job.

The possibility that factor VIII will be supplied to the hemophiliacs via DNA hybridization technique will strongly reduce the need of plasma. Then the emphasis will be put on the proper supply of red cells, platelets and plasma, the latter to provide other plasma proteins than factor VIII.

Conclusions

The additive system approach is likely to replace whole blood and traditional red cell concentrates.

In the next few years different ways will probably be tested to improve the yields and providing the patients with safer and more effective blood products.

References

1. Rock GA, Cruickshank WH, Tackaberry ES, Palmer DS. Improved yields of Factor VIII from heparinized plasma. Vox Sang 1979;36:294-300.
2. Smit Sibinga CTh, Welbergen H, Das PC, Griffin B. High-yield method of production of freeze-dried factor VIII by blood banks. Lancet 1981;ii:449-50.
3. Farrugin A, Prowse C. Factor VIII stability in unfrozen plasma: effect of anticoagulant. Abstract British Blood Transfusion Society, 2nd Meeting, Manchester 1984.
4. Högman CF, de Verdier C-H, Ericson Å, Hedlund K, Sandhagen B. Studies on the mechanism of human red cell loss of viability during storage at 24°C in vitro. I. Cell shape and total adenylate concentration as determinant factors for posttransfusion survival. Vox Sang 1985;48:257-68.
5. Högman CF, Hedlunk K, Sahleström Y. Red cell preservation in protein-poor media. III. Protection against in vitro hemolysis. Vox Sang 1981;41:274-81.
6. Högman CF, Åkerblom O, Hedlund K, Rosén I, Wiklund L. Red cell suspensions in SAGM medium. Further experience of in vivo survival of red cells, clinical usefulness and plasma-saving effects. Vox Sang 1983;45:217-23.
7. Lovric AV, Prince B, Bryant J. Packed red cell transfusions: improved survival, quality and storage. Vox Sang 1977;33:346-52.
8. Valeri CR, Pivacek LE, Dennis RC, Palter M, Yeston N. 24-hour posttransfusion survival of human red cells after 4°C storage in Adsol for 39 to 49 days. Transfusion 1984;25:477 (abstract).
9. Au Buchon JP, Davey RJ, Estep T, Miripol J. Effect of the plasticizer di-2-ethylhexylphtalate on survival of stored red cells. Transfusion 1984;24:422 (abstract).
10. Greenwalt TJ, Bryan DJ, Dumaswala UJ. Erythrocyte membrane vesiculation and changes in membrane composition during storage in citrate-phosphate-dextrose-adenine 1. Vox Sang 1984;47:261-70.
11. Harmening Pittiglio D, Dawson RB. Supplementation of CPD adenine with phosphate anion exchange resins. A preliminary report. Abstr 18th Congr Int Soc Blood Transfusion. Karger Basel, 1984:184.
12. Meryman GA, Hornblower M, Syring R. Prolonged storage of red cells at 4°C. Abstr 18th Congr Int Soc Blood Transfusion. Karger Basel, 1984:171.
13. Fratantoni JC, Sturdivant B, Poindexter BJ. Aberrant morphology of platelets stored in five day containers. Thrombosis Research 1984;33:607-15.
14. Adams GA, Swenson SD, Rock G. Environmental factors in the storage of platelet concentrates. II. Plasma-free medium. Abstr 18th Congr Int Soc Blood Transfusion. Karger Basel, 1984:124.
15. Smit Sibinga CTh, Uithof J, McShine RL, Waltje J, Das PC. Advances in purification of heparin high yield factor VIII concentrate. Transfusion 1985;25:467 (abstract).

HTLV-III/LAV: THE ROLE OF MOLECULAR BIOLOGY IN VIRAL DETECTION AND PREVENTION

B.A. Jameson*, S. Modrow*, L. Gürtler*, J. Eberle*, H. Gelderblom**, D. Wernicke-Jameson*, K. von der Helm*, F. Deinhardt*, H. Wolf*

Introduction

The causative agent of the acquired immune deficiency syndrome (AIDS) appears to be a retrovirus designated either as human T lymphotropic virus (HTLV-III) [1] or lymphadenopathy-associated virus (LAV) [2]. Several isolates of this virus have recently been cloned and sequenced [3 – 5]. Thus the complete genomic sequence is known as well as the deduced amino acid sequence. The genetic map of HTLV-III is analogous to that of the other replication-competent retroviral genomes. Phylogenetically, the virus is a type C retrovirus and appears to belong to the lentiviridae subfamily [6,7].

HTLV-III causes severe and often fatal complications; its uncontrolled spread represents a major health concern. The high mortality rate associated with HTLV-III infections is primarily due to opportunistic infections and, in many ways, is reminiscent of the effects seen in cats infected with feline leukemia virus (FeLV) [8,9]. In addition to AIDS, HTLV-III has been associated with a variety of clinical syndromes, ranging from encephalopathies to inapparent persisting infections. Although the virus is most commonly spread from homosexual contacts, heterosexual contacts and contact with virus-containing blood products, such as clotting factors which have not been heat inactivated, can result in viral infections. Neonatal infections have also been observed as a result of maternal transmission [10].

Current diagnostic procedures rely on a patients' seroconversion as an index of viral infection. The enzyme-linked immunosorbent assay (ELISA) is the most widely used primary screening procedure to detect anti-viral antibodies. However, the use of only a single test, such as the ELISA, can lead to false positive or false negative results. The ELISA in combination with an immunofluorescence assay and immunoblots has proven to be a reliably effective system for the detection of anti-HTLV-III antibodies.

At present, there are no proven chemotherapeutic reagents for the treatment of AIDS. Although the development of such reagents are of extreme importance, the ultimate control and potential eradication of HTLV-III can only be achieved through immunoprophylactic measures.

Here we report evidence for an increasing prevalence of HTLV-III infections among hemophiliacs and other risk groups and have also found a possible inverse correlation between anti-HTLV-III core protein antibodies in infected individuals and the onset of AIDS. Additionally, we show the

* Max von Pettenkofer Institute, Un. of Munich, Munich FRG.
** Robert Koch Institute, Berlin FRG.

results of a technique, utilizing synthetic peptides, intended to aid in the identification of viral antigenic determinants capable of eliciting neutralizing antibodies.

Results and discussion

Patient sera, taken from individuals with hemophilia A and B, were screened for the presence of HTLV-III antibodies either immediately after being drawn or from sera which had been stored for up to seven years (table 1). All serum samples were screened for antibodies with both the ELISA and immunofluorescense assay. Seroconversion was first noted in 1980 and the percentage of seropositive hemophiliacs has continued to increase with each subsequent year. It is interesting to note that all of the individuals whose sera reacted positively with the HTLV-III antigen had previously been treated with blood clotting factors which had not been heat or chemically inactivated. Conversely, none of the hemophiliacs who had received only inactivated coagulation factors were antibody positive (W. Schramm, B. Kraus et al., unpubl. results).

Table 1. Prevalence of antibodies against HTLV-III proteins in hemophilia patients. The numbers are stated as positive/total number (%).

Year	Anti-HTLV-III
1978	0/ 8 –
1979	0/ 27 –
1980	1/ 22 (5%)
1981	4/ 37 (11%)
1982	15/ 64 (23%)
1983	35/ 96 (36%)
1984	57/132 (43%)
1985	36/ 75 (50%)

As of the time of this report, only five out of the 143 HTLV-III antibody positive hemophiliacs have shown signs of a lymphadenopathy syndrome (LAS) or AIDS-related complex (ARC). Three of these patients showed clinical symptoms within a year after seroconversion, while the clinical status of the other two patients changed within two years of conversion. None of the patients screened in our survey has yet to develop AIDS.

Serum samples from hemophiliacs who converted to anti-HTLV-III positive in the ELISA were concomitantly able to recognize virus envelope proteins (p110, 76, gp64, p30) and core proteins (p24 and p16) in western blots (fig. 1). Thus it would appear that from the onset of infection these individuals circulate sufficient disrupted virus to elicit an immune response to the HTLV-III core proteins. This seems to be true in general for asymptomatic carriers of the virus regardless of their particular risk group. We have

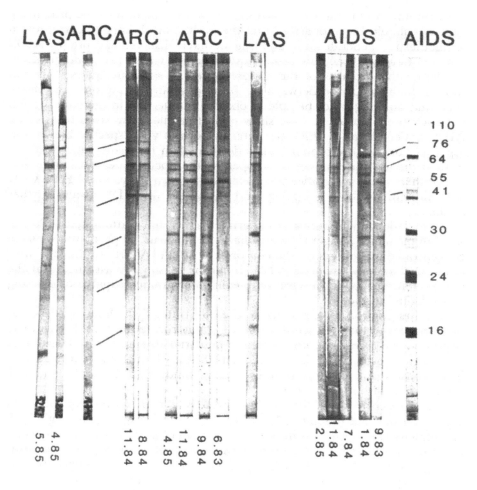

Figure 1. The pattern of anti-HTLV-III from four hemophiliacs is shown compared to the pattern of two homosexual AIDS patients. On the bottom of the strips the month and year of the blood drawing is given. In the two patients, who now have a lymphadenopathy syndrome, prominent bands against most of the viral proteins may be seen. In two of the ARC patients' sera a faint but steadily increasing staining intensity of the bands does indicate rising amounts of anti-HTLV-III, whereas in the third p30 and gp41 are stained, but not the core proteins p16 and p24. The following-up of the first AIDS patient in this figure shows a steady decline in the anti-HTLV-III level, especially of the p16 and p24, additionally the p30. Despite high antibody titers against all viral proteins, the second AIDS patient died of acute cryptococcosis and thus is a clear exception from this hypothetical finding of the correlation of the amount of anti-core antibodies and prognosis.

noticed that AIDS patients, in contrast to the asymptomatic carriers, generally show a tendency toward a diminished or non-existent antibody response towards the core proteins (fig. 1 and data not shown). Although our sampling size is limited, this observation may be of possible prognostic value. It should be emphasized that the decline or absence of core protein antibodies is a generalization and that we have observed exceptions. AIDS patients frequently exhibit acute superinfection which can synergistically accelerate the progress of the disease state. In some instances, this can shorten the time period between the onset of clinical symptoms and death such that one might not be able to observe the decline in the core protein antibody titers. In figure 1 we show typical profiles of western blots using AIDS patient sera in which the intensity of the virus-specific bands and especially of the core protein bands decline when the acute superinfection in their disease state cannot be stopped by therapeutic measures. Whether or not there exists a significant correlation between the reduced HTLV-III core protein antibody response and the onset of AIDS awaits further studies.

In an independent series of experiments, we have attempted to locate some of the major antigenic determinants of the virus. In particular we have concentrated our efforts on the env protein of HTLV-III. In analogy with other viral systems, such as FeLV, it can be reasonably assumed that the env protein harbours the viral antigenic determinants capable of eliciting neutralizing antibodies.

As a first approach we decided to use the strategy which has successfully been employed for the identification of poliovirus epitopes [11]. Synthetic peptides were produced from regions of potential antigenicity and used both as structural probes and as immunogens to test whether antibodies elicited in response to intact virus were capable of binding to the probe and vice versa.

It has recently been shown that there is a high correlation between segmental thermal mobility (flexibility) of a protein and major regions of antigenicity [12 – 14]. This implies that regions of a protein which are likely to occur on the surface of a protein and are involved in a predicted beta-turn, have the greatest likelyhood of naturally being recognized by the immune system. Consequently, we have analyzed the predicted envelop amino acid sequence [4] for regions of surface probability using the computer program described by Emini et al. [15] and for probable secondary structures according to the rules of Chou and Fasman [16]. Based on these computer predictions, two sites were chosen from which to synthesize peptides (peptide No. 1: amino acids 408 – 425 S – T – K – G – S – N – N – T – E – G – S – D – T and peptide No. 2: amino acids 477 – 491 P – G – G – G – D – M – R – N – W – R – S – E – L). These peptides were synthesized via standard solid phase synthesis techniques. An amino terminal lysine was attached to the sequence to facilitate the diimide-mediated coupling of a dipalmitic acid. The palmitic acid was added to enhance the peptides' immunogenicity and was used in place of a carrier protein.

The peptides were analyzed for their ability to fold such that they resembled surface components of the intact HTLV-III using specific antisera

Table 2.

Sera	Anti-HTLV-III antibodies	Anti-T-cell (H9) antibodies	Dot blot		ELISA	
			pept.1	pept.2	pept.1	
9955	–	–	–	–		n.d.
9661	–	–	–	–	–	(0.227)
9591	–	–	+	+	–	(0.265)
9679	–	–	–	–	–	(0.416)
9922	–	–	–	–		n.d.
9849	–	–	–	–		n.d.
9843	–	–	+ / –	–		n.d.
9958	–	–	–	–		n.d.
9926	–	–	+	+		n.d.
9517	–	–	–	+ / –	–	(0.300)
9427	–	+	+	+	+	(0.474)
9626	–	+	–	–	+	(0.488)
9435	–	+	+	+	+	(0.991)
9426*	–	+	+ +	+ +	+ +	(+ 2.0)
9609	–	+	–	–	–	(0.277)
9644	+	+	+	+	+	(0.871)
9923	+	–	+	+		n.d.
9778	+	–	+	+	+	(0.467)
9407	+	–	+	+	+ / –	(0.447)
9957	+	–	–	–		n.d.
9528	+	–	+ / –	–		n.d.
9420	+	–	+	+	–	(0.280)
9702	+	–	+	+	+	(0.467)
9700	+	–	+	+	+ / –	(0.452)
9703	+	–	+	+	–	(0.366)
9452	+	–	+	+	+	(0.522)
9455	+	–	–	–	–	(0.305)
9701	+	–	+	+	+	(0.773)
9704	+	–	+	+	–	(0.472)
9904	+	–	+	+		n.d.

* This sera possibly contains HLA class II antibodies according to our western blots.

from HTLV-III infected individuals. The results of this experiment are shown in table 2. The dot blot assays were performed using 1 microgram of synthetic peptide/dot bound to a nitrocellulose membrane. After washing and blocking the membrane with swine skin gelatin, various human patient sera was allowed to incubate with the peptide. The blots were again washed and blocked and the results were visualized after the addition of a donkey-anti-human peroxidase conjugated second antibody. The ELISA results were obtained in a similar fashion, except that 15 micrograms of peptide were cross-linked/well onto a 96 well microtiter plate via glutaraldehyde.

Our results indicate that both peptide sequences are part of an immuno-logically active region of the HTLV-III env protein. Of the serum samples

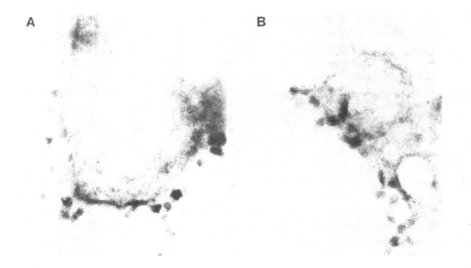

Figure 2. A. Immunoelectron micrograph (IEM) of HTLV-III infected H9-HT cells after incubations with a control rabbits preimmune serum and anti-rabbit IgG-ferritin conjugate. B. Essentially the same as A, except that the same control rabbits blood was taken five weeks after a single inoculation of 1 i.u. of heat inactivated HTLV-III.

which, in clinical tests, were shown to be HTLV-III specific, 80% reacted positively with both synthetic peptides. Such was not the case when the same sera were tested against a synthetic peptide derived from an immunorecessive region of poliovirus (data not shown). Unexpectedly, there was also an apparent cross-reaction with a protein(s) from the host T cell (H9 cell line). The cross-reaction was seen with both of the env-specific peptides. It is, therefore, unlikely, that the cross-reaction is simply a random artefact due to the peptides' amino acid composition. Based on these results, we consider it likely that the protein regions encoding these two peptides represent a major antigenic determinant(s) on the envelope protein of the virus.

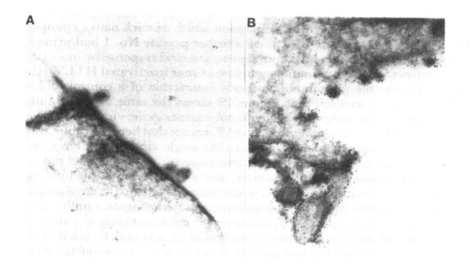

Figure 3. A. IEM of HTLV-III infected H9-HT cells after incubations with preimmune sera of rabbit No. 2 and anti-rabbit IgG-ferritin conjugate. B. Essentially the same as A, except that rabbit No. 2 was repeatedly inoculated with 400 micrograms/inoculation of peptide No. 1 prior to a single boost with HTLV-III as described in fig. 2B. The serum used here was taken five weeks after the viral boost.

To further characterize the env regions represented by peptides No. 1 and No. 2, the peptides were used to inoculate rabbits. All rabbits produced a strong anti-peptide antibody response. Anti-peptide No. 2 antibodies reacted positively in the anti-HTLV-III ELISA test, however, these sera also reacted positively with uninfected T cells. This result was consistent with the results obtained by the peptide binding assays outlined above. The antibodies produced in response to peptide No. 1, on the other hand, failed to reliably recognize HTLV-III antigen in the ELISA. Although both peptides stem from regions on the env protein likely to be surface exposed and predicted to occur in a region of beta-turn, peptide No. 1 has a predicted glycosylation site in its sequence whereas peptide No. 2 does not. This could account for the differences seen between the two anti-peptide sera.

One inherent problem of using peptide immunogens has been that the immune system often recognizes conformations of the peptide which only slightly resemble that of the target antigen. The result is that the anti-peptide antibodies bind poorly or not at all to the native antigen. In many instances there exist minor conformations of the peptide which resemble the native antigen. There can exist an immunological memory of these minor conformations such that the system is 'primed' for a circulating antibody response [17]. A single, subimmunogenic dose of intact antigen is sufficient to evoke this secondary response. The phenomenon of 'peptide-priming' has been successfully employed with several different viral systems, including FeLV, to induce monospecific sera and, thus facilitated the identification of neutralization antigenic sites [15,18 – 21].

The dot blot assay and the ELISA shown above indicate that peptide No. 1 is capable of assuming structures in solution which mimick native epitopes of HTLV-III. Consequently, we asked whether peptide No. 1 had primed the rabbits' immune system for a subsequent antiviral response by inoculating the animals with a subimmunogenic dose of heat inactivated HTLV-III. Figure 2A shows the preimmune antibody interaction of a control rabbit with HTLV-III infected H9 cells; figure 2B shows the same animal's antibody interaction five weeks after a single subimmunogenic viral boost. The same experiment is shown in figure 3A and B, except that here the rabbit was primed with the synthetic peptide prior to the single viral boost. Thus, we present here clear evidence that the subimmunogenic viral boost did not itself elicit a detectable anti-viral response, nor was there any virus binding activity present in preimmune sera. The immune response to the env-specific conformations of peptide No. 1 was apparently amplified upon a limited exposure to the intact virus (Fig. 3B). Upon closer examination it was observed that many of the peptide-primed antibodies in addition to binding to obviously budding particles, had also bound to region of the cellular membrane where there was no apparent budding of virus. Consequently, the same antibodies were checked against uninfected cells and were found to bind in the same manner as observed in the infected cells. Again this result was consistent with the data obtained from the peptide-binding assays as well as the results seen with the anti-peptide No. 2 antibodies. Although one cannot conclusively rule out the possibility that both synthetic peptides contain amino acid sequences which randomly mimick cell proteins on the membrane of H9 cells, this does seem unlikely. Assuming that an antibody recognizes an epitope consisting of a continuous stretch of six amino acids, the chance probability of both peptides randomly cross-reacting with the host cell membrane is $1:12^{20}$. One should seriously consider the possibility that the gp64 env protein of the HTLV-III bears a non-random structural similarity with a membrane surface protein of T cells and, further, that this similarity serves a vital function in the life cycle of the virus. Currently experiments are underway to test whether or not the antibodies produced in response to the peptides No. 1 and No. 2 are capable of neutralizing infectious HTLV-III. Additionally, we are attempting to further characterize the nature of this host cell cross-reactivity.

Conclusions

As mentioned above, the increasing prevalence of HTLV-III infections among hemophiliacs is most likely due to incomplete or lack of inactivation of blood clotting factors. The universal adoption of more stringent inactivation procedures should alleviate the major source of infection within this risk group.

Here we report the identification of a major antigenic determinant of the HTLV-III env protein. We observed a cross-reactivity with two separate env specific peptides with anti-T cell antibodies as well as cross-reactivity between anti-peptide antibodies and T cells. Although these results represent preliminary findings, they are sufficient to warrant extreme caution among those researchers involved in producing any potential vaccine against HTLV-III. One must avoid the possibility of an autoimmune response as a result of the vaccine itself.

References

1. Gallo RC, Salahuddin SZ, Popovic M et al. Frequent detection and isolation of cytopathic retroviruses (HTLV-III) from patients with AIDS and at risk for AIDS. Science 1984;224:500 – 4.
2. Barré-Sinoussi F, Chermann JC, Rey F et al. Isolation of a T-lymphotropic retrovirus from a patient at risk for acquired immune deficiency syndrome (AIDS). Science 1983;220:868 – 972.
3. Wain-Hobson S, Sonigo P, Danos O et al. Nucleotide sequences of the AIDS virus LAV. Cell 1985;40:9 – 17.
4. Ratner L, Haseltine W, Patarca R et al. Complete nucleotide sequence of the AIDS virus, HTLV-III. Nature 1985;313:227 – 33.
5. Sanchez-Pescador R, Power MD, Barr PJ et al. Nucleotide sequence and expression of an AIDS-associated retrovirus (ARV-2). Science 1985;227:484 – 92.
6. Sonigo P, Alizon M, Staskus K et al. Nucleotide sequence of the Visna lentivirus: Relationship to the AIDS virus. Cell 1985;42:369 – 82.
7. Chiu I, Yaniv A, Dahlberg JE et al. Nucleotide sequence evidence for the relationship of AIDS retrovirus to lentiviruses. Nature 1985;317:366 – 8.
8. Essex M, Sliski A, Jakowski R, Cotter S, Hardy WD. Immunosurveillance of naturally occurring feline leukemia. Science 1975;190:790 – 2.
9. Hardy WD. the virology, immunology and epidemiology of the feline leukemia virus. In: Hardy WD, Essex M, McClelland AJ eds. Feline Leukemia Virus. Elsevier Biomedical Press, 1980;10:33 – 78.
10. Wong-Staal F and Gallo RC. Human T-lymphotropic retroviruses. Nature 1985;317:395 – 403.
11. Jameson BA, Diamond D, Wimmer E, Nomoto A, Crainic R. Characterization of poliovirus antibody-dependent neutralization. In: Labsystem Research, Comps. Synthetic peptides in biology and medicine. Elsevier Biomedical Press, 1985.
12. Westhof E, Altschuh D, Moras D et al. Correlation between segmental mobility and the location of antigenic determinants in proteins. Nature 1984;311:123 – 6.
13. Tainer JA, Getzhoff ED, Alexander H et al. The reactivity of anti-peptide anti-

bodies is a function of the atomic mobility of sites in a protein. Nature 1984; 312:127 – 34.

14. Schulze-Gahmen U, Prinz H, Glatter U, Beyreuther K. Towards assignment of secondary structures by anti-peptide antibodies. Specificity of the immune response to a beta-turn. EMBO J 1985;4:1731 – 7.

15. Emini EA, Hughes JV, Perlow DS, Boger J. Induction of hepatitis A virus-neutralizing antibody by a virus-specific synthetic peptide. J Virol 1985;55: 836 – 9.

16. Chou PY, Fasman GD. Protein folding. Adv Enzymol 1978;47:46 – 148.

17. Emini EA, Jameson BA, Wimmer E. Priming for an induction of anti-poliovirus neutralizing antibodies by synthetic peptides. Nature 1983;304: 699 – 702.

18. Nunberg JH, Gilbert JH, Rodgers G, Snead RM, Nitecki DE, Winston S. Location of a determinant of virus neutralization on feline leukemia virus envelope protein gp70. In: Lerner RA, Chanock RM, Brown F, eds. Vaccines 85. Cold Spring Harbor Press, 1985;221 – 6.

19. Jameson BA, Bonin J, Wimmer E, Kew O. Natural variant of the Sabin type 1 vaccine strain of poliovirus and correlation with a poliovirus neutralization site. Virol 1985;143:337 – 41.

20. Jameson BA, Bonin J, Murray M, Kew O, Wimmer E. Peptide-induced neutralizing antibodies to poliovirus. In: Lerner RA, Chanock RM, Brown F, eds. Vaccines 85. Cold Spring Harbor Press, 1985:191 – 8.

21. Francis MJ, Fry CM, Rowlands DJ et al. Priming with peptides of foot-and-mouth disease virus. In: Lerner RA, Chanock RM and Brown F, eds. Vaccines 85. Cold Spring Harbor Press, 1985:203 – 10.

LEGAL ASPECTS OF BLOOD BANKING: AN AMERICAN PERSPECTIVE

S.L. Lentz, H.F. Polesky

Introduction

This paper seeks to provide a legal context within which to view recent developments and future challenges in blood banking. Legal and regulatory systems exist to further two principal goals in relation to blood banking. One is that of assuring that a safe and adequate supply of blood and blood components is available. The other is that of ensuring that both donors and recipients are treated in accord with state-of-the-art professional standards, without negligence, and with respect for their rights as patients.

While these goals may be international, legal systems are not. Unlike scientific standards, legal and regulatory structures do not, for the most part, cross national boundaries [1]. Thus, this paper will focus principally upon the legal and regulatory system of one country, the United States of America, in order to discuss in depth one nation's legal response to recent medical and societal developments affecting blood banking. Aside from the authors' familiarity with the American system, we believe that some emerging trends and problems may be most visible there. We do, however, start with the caveat that the American system represents but one approach to regulation of blood banking.

In the United States, Red Cross and independent community blood centers and hospitals collect virtually the entire whole-blood supply. In 1984, 12 million donors provided 12 million units of whole blood. At present, voluntary, unpaid donors are the norm at these blood centers; virtually none of the major blood centers now purchase whole-blood donations [2].

A pharmaceutical or plasma sector has also developed in the United States to meet the need for components derived from blood. Since the whole blood drawn is not adequate to supply this need, much of the plasma comes from plasmapheresis, with paid donors supplying a significant proportion of the plasma drawn. The tension between the voluntary whole blood system and the paid plasma system continues to form a theme in both societal and legal considerations of the blood supply.

In addition to ensuring an adequate supply of blood and components and to resolving the question of payment for donation, American blood banking has had to confront questions of safety in transfusion as related to transfusion-transmitted disease. Until recently, concerns about transfusion-transmitted disease focused upon hepatitis, a subject of significant litigation. Within the last three years, however, concern has shifted to newly emerging problems of transfusion-transmitted acquired immune deficiency syndrome (AIDS), which have just begun to create repercussions within the legal system. Other recent concerns with legal or regulatory ramifications include cost and usage, control and appropriate protection for donors.

The regulatory system

In a sense, it is inaccurate to speak of a regulatory system for American blood banking. In fact, there are multiple regulatory systems. The national government has a principal role in regulation. Pursuant to the United States Public Health Service Act [3], the Food and Drug Administration has major responsibility for regulation of blood banking, while other federal agencies play a minor role. Under the American federal system, however, state and local governments also have authority to regulate. A third layer of quasi-regulatory activity is provided by professional organizations, principally the American Association of Blood Banks, and their accrediting standards.

One basis for governmental regulation of blood is by analogy to regulation of drugs. Like all drugs, blood must meet standards relating to safety, potency, efficacy and labeling. A second basis for regulating blood banking practices is the concern for the quality of care provided to patients whose services are paid for by governmental funds.

The federal government regulates blood banks by requiring that any establishment drawing and processing blood for use in interstate commerce must have a license. In addition, each type of component produced must also be licensed. The specific regulations for these licenses are in the Code of Federal Regulations, 21 C.F.R. Parts 600 – 700. Currently, the Office of Biologics Research and Review (OBRR) of the Food and Drug Administration (FDA) administers these regulations. In practice, an establishment wishing to be licensed must provide OBRR with evidence that it has adequate and appropriate space and will meet 'good manufacturing practices'. Standard operating procedures (SOPs) must assure donor safety, use of approved collection methods, appropriate testing and proper labeling and storage. The SOPs for a specific component also include the methods for quality control. In addition to review of documentation and date, the OBRR conducts periodic (usually every 2 yars) inspections of licensed facilities. Unfortunately these inspections are often done by FDA field personnel who have little or no special training in blood banking.

The Health Care Financing Agency (HCFA) and the Centers for Disease Control, which have responsibility for hospitals participating in the Medicare/Medicaid programs and independent laboratories, regulate services provided to patients, such as prenatal diagnostic testing and compatibility testing. In general these agencies set requirements for personnel doing testing, evaluate participation in proficiency testing programs and monitor quality control practices. These programs involve a periodic inspection, which may be contracted to a state health department or delegated to a professional organization whose inspections are deemed equivalent, such as the Joint Commission on Accreditation of Hospitals (JCAH) and the College of American Pathologists (CAP). The latter approach is an example of the way in which professional organizations can sometimes undertake a regulatory responsibility [4].

State and local authorities may also regulate various aspects of blood banking. New York City, for example, requires that blood be retested for HBsAg, unless the original testing was done in a facility directed by an individual licensed by the City. In a very recent decision, *Hillsborough County* v. *Automated Medical Laboratories, Inc.* [5], the United States Supreme Court held that state and local regulatory power is not preempted by existing federal regulations. In this case a plasma center challenged local regulations requiring special health evaluation of plasma donors. The center attempted to argue that the federal donor requirements occupied the field. However, the Court rejected this argument as well as the argument that a single regulatory policy was necessary to protect the national blood supply. In ruling that the County of Hillsborough could enforce its local ordinances, the Supreme Court thus upheld the authority of state and local governments to regulate blood banking practices.

The process of establishing government regulations may be cumbersome and slow to respond to changes in practice or technology. New or modified regulations must go through several layers of bureaucracy as well as draft publication and public review before becoming effective. In contrast, standards established by voluntary professional groups such as AABB and CAP, as well as their inspection and accreditation checklists, are frequently reviewed and changed to reflect current knowledge and state-of-the-art practices.

An example of the contrast between governmental and voluntary approaches is afforded by the federal requirement that all donor units must undergo with a serologic test for syphilis [6]. Since syphilis is not a hazard to recipients, the AABB Standard eliminated this requirement several years ago. On the other hand, at present there is not yet a specific federal requirement for the anti-HTLV-III testing, but rather only a set of guidelines. In contrast, as of July 1, 1985 this testing was required by AABB.

The AABB *Standards for Blood Banks and Transfusion Services*, now in its eleventh edition, is the source document from which most blood banks derive their Standard Operating Procedures. The process of writing standards is one in which expert concensus is blended with data to provide minimum essentials for all aspects of transfusion practice from the donor to the recipient. Many other organizations, including the FDA, the CAP and the JCAH, recognize the AABB Standards as authoritative. The AABB and CAP inspection programs are carried out by professionals who are in active practice. As a result, the inspection process is an educational experience as well as a review of the methods and procedures in use.

One area not addressed by the AABB Standards is that relating to the auditing of transfusion practices by the ordering physician. This important topic is dealt with by the JCAH, which requires 'the evaluation of the appropriateness of all transfusions, including the use of whole blood and blood components' [7].

Medico-legal issues

Regulatory systems seek to promote compliance with state-of-the-art standards and thus avoid harm to donor and recipients. Despite effective regulation and quality control, however, injuries and accidents inevitably occur. For the individual who has been injured in the donation or transfusion process, a lawsuit for damages may be the most effective means of redress.

Under the American legal system, every accident or injury relating to transfusion does not result in legal liability. There are many potential causes of injury, from errors in drawing or labeling to provision of the wrong unit for transfusion, unwarranted transfusion or the use of contaminated blood. Although a person who suffers injury as a result may attempt to obtain compensation from the person or institution responsible, the American legal system does not attach liability in every instance. Except in limited circumstances where liability may be imposed without extensive proof of a lack of due care, the injured person must ordinarily show negligent acts or omissions in order to recover.

Negligent acts or omissions with respect to the donor, although rare, can lead to liability just as can a negligent transfusion. Negligence involves the creation of a foreseeable and unreasonable risk of harm. To recover, the injured donor or recipient must show that a duty of care was owed to him and that the duty was breached, with resultant harm to him. Because a lack of care can be difficult to demonstrate in some instances, particularly those involving hepatitis, some American courts for a brief period allowed recovery under theories of warranty liability or strict product liability; these theories did not require proof of negligence. Although negligence is again the basic legal theory, emerging medico-legal problems created by AIDS have renewed questions of whether American courts will adopt more expansive approaches to recovery.

Apart from negligence, the concept of informed consent can be a significant factor in determining liabilities related to the transfusion process. A physician who does not secure consent before drawing or transfusing blood may be subject to civil liability for battery. More recently, American courts have required that consent by 'informed': in other words, that it be knowledgeably given by a competent individual who has been told of potential risks.

Like negligence, the concept of informed consent is relevant not only in the donation stage but also with respect to recipients of transfusion. The legal question here becomes most critical in the case of patients who refuse a life-sustaining transfusion; in the United States, that refusal is frequently based on religious grounds and the courts, while not uniform, have increasingly honored these refusals.

A converse and newly emerging issue is that of the patients's right to treatment, including access to rare donors or to information about them. This controversy also raises issues of the donor's rights to privacy and confidentiality, a legal issue again prominent in recent concerns about AIDS.

The remainder of this paper discusses issues of negligence, strict liability, consent and confidentiality as they arise in the donation and transfusion process; it also ventures some thoughts on how the American legal system may react to issues raised by transfusion-transmitted AIDS. We do, however, want to note that case law developments, as well as statutes, vary from state to state. (Most cases in this area are decided by the state, rather than the federal, courts.) In addition, particularly in the American common law system, the law is always in flux. Thus our intent is simply to highlight critical issues and areas of legal concern.

A note on the American legal system

The United States has a dual system of courts: federal courts, which decide primarily matters of federal law, and state courts, which decide all other matters. Within each system there are both trial courts and one or more levels of appellate courts. Most lawsuits for negligence or malpractice are tried in state courts.

Given the common law heritage, a court deciding a case involving, for example, a claim of negligence in transfusion must look to a number of sources. Relevant legal sources may include the United States Constitution, state and federal statutes, state and federal administrative regulations, and case law. The last category means relevant judicial precedent as decided in reported cases (primarily appellate cases) in that jurisdiction. Under the American system, most lawsuits for negligence are tried before a jury: the judge instructs the jury on the law, but the jury decides the facts.

When faced with a claim of professional negligence or malpractice, the court will instruct the jury that the burden is on the complaining party or plaintiff to prove its case by a preponderance of evidence. To establish the duty of care owing, the plaintiff may point to a number of sources, including statutes and administrative regulations, standards promulgated by professional organizations such as the AABB, and practices in the relevant professional community. The last will usually be presented by means of testimony from an expert witness.

The blood donation

Consent, confidentially and care are hallmarks of the blood bank's obligation toward the donor. Although lawsuits by donors are relatively rare, failure to respect any of these obligations may expose the blood center to potential liability.

Before drawing blood, the blood bank must secure the donor's informed consent. This involves considerably more than a signature on a form. Rather, it means that the donor must be informed of the risks involved and make a voluntary and competent decision to face them. Although informed consent is a common law concept, it has also been incorporated into professional regulatory standards. For instance, the AABB provides that the 'consent of the prospective donor must be obtained in writing after the procedure is explained in terms the donor can understand and after the donor has an opportunity to ask questions and refuse consent' [8].

The nature of the information to be provided to the donor may vary with the type of donation at issue. For example, applicable regulations require additional information regarding risks of a hemolytic reaction to be given in the case of plasmapheresis donors [9].

The obligation to secure informed consent is but one aspect of the blood bank's obligation of care toward the donor. Once the donor provides informed consent, he still retains the right to sue if negligent acts by the blood bank result in harming him.

Blood banks and hospitals have sometimes tried to protect themselves from the potential of liability to the donor by obtaining not just the standard consent but also a signature on a form purporting to release the institution from any liability. American courts have not looked upon these releases favorably. In a number of cases, courts have held such releases invalid and ruled that blood banks and hospitals cannot be exempted from the obligation to use due care.

For example, the recent case of *Smith* v. *Hospital Authority of Walker* [10] concerned the validity of a release the plaintiff signed before donating blood. The document purported to absolve the hospital and its personnel of liability. Following the donation and allegedly as a result of negligence in the phlebotomy, the plaintiff suffered serious nerve injury in his arm. The court held that the release's exculpatory clause was void because it violated public policy (even though not any particular statute). The principles the court used would likely be applied to any release purporting to shield a blood bank from all negligence liability.

As part of their obligations of due care to the donor, blood banks also have an initial duty to screen and examine donors to make sure they are suitable candidates to give blood. A recent New York case illustrates this obligation. The donor claimed she told the screening nurse that she was anemic and had recently given birth. Nevertheless, the defendant drew her blood; she subsequently became very ill. The court in *Bowman* v *American National Red Cross* [11] found for the plaintiff on the basis of evidence that the screening was carelessly performed.

Of course, the obligation to use due care in testing and screening the donor is an obligation also owed to the recipient of the transfusion. Current concerns about transfusion-transmitted AIDS highlights the importance of this issue; and further ramifications of this duty with respect to AIDS are discussed in greater details in subsequent sections of this paper.

In addition to the duties to secure informed consent and to use due care, blood banks also have obligations of privacy and confidentiality with respect to donors. These obligations are not yet fully defined in American law, but they may grow out of the physician-patient relationship, state date privacy statutes, or constitutional and common law rights to privacy. Thus, in *Head* v. *Colloton* [12], a recent Iowa case, hospital records regarding the typing of a potential donor were held to be confidential information, exempt from disclosure under the state's public records statute.

Similarly, in a 1985 Florida case that is still on appeal, the court held that the records of 51 volunteer donors did not have to be produced [13]. The case involved a lawsuit for injuries from a car accident by a plaintiff who received transfusions and subsequently developed AIDS. Although the plaintiff sought the records in an effort to prove aggravated damages, neither the blood center nor the donors were parties to the lawsuit. In declining to order production of the records, the court found that the privacy of the donors – and the disincentive to voluntary donation that would result from revealing names and records – outweighed the plaintiff's proof needs.

Several states have passed or considered legislation protecting the confidentiality of donor records, particularly with regard to LAV/HTLV-III test results. Undoubtedly, issues of confidentiality and privacy, including matters of donor questioning and test result reporting, will receive increased legal attention in the near future.

Blood transfusion and hemotherapy

As in the case of donation, informed consent is an initial issue in transfusion. Although the basic law of informed consent is well established, it is not always clear just what risks and alternatives a physician needs to discuss with the patient in specific circumstances. Both the risk of hepatitis and, more recently, the risk of AIDS, have highlighted the importance of obtaining informed consent specifically for transfusion; these risks also highlight the importance of not administering unwarranted transfusions or failing to utilize appropriate alternatives. Careful explanation of possible consequences is not a legal bar to suit. However, as a practical matter, explanation and documentation of that explanation may provide the best defense to later claims.

Even though the transfusion recipient has given consent, he does retain the right to sue if negligence connected with the transfusion results in injury to him. Mislabeling of a unit of blood, administration of a unit to the wrong patient, errors in crossmatching, or unwarranted transfusion may all be the result of negligence.

Negligence means a departure from ordinary standards of care. In general, the plaintiff has to show four elements: duty, breach of duty, causation and damages. Ordinarily, the health care professionals and institutions involved will be required to exercise the degree of skill and care exercised by others in similar circumstances. In most cases, the plaintiff will be required to point to some specific evidence of negligent acts.

One approach taken by some plaintiffs is to claim a negligent failure to screen donors adequately. For example, the plaintiff in *Tufaro* v. *Methodist Hospital* [14], who contracted malaria, argued that the blood bank was negligent in screening prospective donors. (Similar claims may be anticipated in cases of transfusion-transmitted AIDS.) In deciding for the defendant, the court emphasized that the blood bank had utilized the donor-screening guidelines of the AABB. Here, as in a number of other cases, use of standard professional practices defeated claims of negligence.

Decisions have varied when claims of negligence, primarily in older cases, have been premised on the use of paid donors. Although courts have reached differing results on this issue, most have given at least some weight to a heightened incidence of hepatitis among paid donors. (Again, similar claims may be attempted in AIDS cases.) Courts have also reached varying results when claims have been based upon a hospital's failure to retest blood supplied by a commercial blood bank [15].

Other cases have considered mechanical errors in the transfusion process, alleged transfusion of too much or too little blood or the unavailability or outdating of blood [16]. Standards of care relevant to any negligence or malpractice transfusion-transmitted diseases, principally hepatitis, may not be able to point to any specific act of negligence. The greatest care taken during blood donation cannot eliminate all risks. While federal regulations require testing of donated blood for hepatitis, the laboratory tests, even when carefully performed, do not screen out all infectious donors. Similarly, routine questioning of potential donors is not absolutely effective, since they may not know they have a disease or may wish to hide it.

As a result, persons who contracted hepatitis from transfusion and wanted to sue for damages began to explore alternative legal theories. Starting about thirty years ago, transfusion recipients who suffered hepatitis sought to advance 'warranty liability' and 'strict liability' as bases for recovery. The former is a theory under American commercial statutes that says goods should be fit for the ordinary purposes for which they are sold and allows recovery for defective goods without proof of negligence. The latter is a common law theory that makes the seller of a defective, unreasonably dangerous product liable for harm to the user. Like warranty liability, it allows recovery without proof of negligence, but it requries no contract between buyer and seller.

Although a few American courts initially accepted one or another of these theories, that acceptance was short-lived. The law again in almost all American states required a showing of negligence to recover for transfusion-transmitted disease [17]. In some states the courts held that the provision of blood was a service rather than a sale; other courts concluded that blood was, like certain drugs, an unavoidably unsafe product. These courts then reasoned that because its benefits outweigh its risks, blood is excepted from strict liability. In other states, legislatures passed statutes to the same effect.

Although this issue was thus effectively resolved several years ago, it may reemerge in the context of lawsuits over transfusion-transmitted AIDS. Aside from this possibility, negligence – a lack of due care – remains the basic legal theory governing recovery for harm from transfusion in the American courts.

Access to and refusal of transfusion

Questions regarding hospitals' and physicians' duties to treat are particularly thorny issues. Claims may concern patients' rights to have access to rare forms of treatment or, conversely, their rights to refuse transfusion. The cases frequently pose not only legal issues but also difficult ethical questions.

American law ordinarily does not recognize a duty to initiate medical assistance or treatment. However, once a physician or hospital has undertaken treatment, there may be a duty to continue or not to abandon treatment. Concepts of negligence may also have bearing on this issue, as for example, in circumstances where a hospital fails to have a reasonably adequate supply of blood on hand to meet foreseeable patient needs.

One recent case has for the first time addressed the question of a patient's right to have access to a rare donor. In *Head* v. *Colloton* [12] a leukemia victim attempted to require a hospital to disclose the identity of a potential bone marrow donor who fit his histocompatibility profile and whose name was in the hospital's registry. Although the plaintiff learned that the potential donor existed, he did not know her identity and thus could not approach her directly; she had already refused a request to donate from the hospital. The court held against the plaintiff, ruling that the donor registry data were confidential under state law and that a donor is also in effect a patient entitled to reasonable expectations of privacy. The court thus found privacy rights to outweigh the plaintiff's need for treatment.

The courts have given substantially more consideration to cases involving refusal of transfusion than to cases about access to treatment. Many of these cases have arisen because the denomination of Jehovah's Witnesses views the transfusion of blood into the body as absolutely prohibited by its theology.

We have already discussed the importance of informed consent as a preface to transfusion. When a Jehovah's Witness refuses to consent, the health care provider faces the problem of reconciling respect for the patient's rights with his own desire to act in the patient's best interest and to avoid potential civil or criminal liability.

Many Jehovah's Witness cases have reached the courts. Children present the easier case: power to consent to medical procedures for a minor usually belongs to the parent. When the parent refuses consent, courts have generally been willing to order transfusion [18]. Certainly, this result is consistent when the child's life is at stake.

Adults have presented courts with more complex problems, given the usual rule that a competent adult has the right to give or refuse consent. The cases are far from uniform in their results, although some trends are beginning to emerge.

Some courts have been willing to by-pass the usual rules regarding consent by devising various rationales to override the patient's refusal. On the other hand, many courts have respected a competent adult's refusal, particularly if no dependent children were involved and the hospital was relieved of potential liabilities for failure to treat.

For example, in the case of *Application of President and Directors of Georgetwon College* [19], the court ordered transfusion of an adult Jehovah's Witness who was in imminent danger of death. The court emphasized the patient's desire to live, her status as the parent of a young child, and the hospital's possible exposure to civil or criminal liability. In almost circular fashion, the court concluded that the patient was not competent to make the treatment decision.

Since that 1964 decision, however, courts have indicated a growing willingness to respect patients' rights to refuse transfusion. Among the countervailing interests courts consider are those in preserving life, preventing suicide, safeguarding the integrity of the medical profession, and protecting innocent third parties, i.e. dependent children. However, in recent cases, only the last interest has with any consistency outweighed the competent adult's right to decline treatment.

In a number of cases, this respect for patient's rights has prevailed even when the likely result was death. For example, the case of *In re Osborne* [20] involved a mentally competent adult who believed he would be deprived of everlasting life if he received even an involuntary transfusion. He signed a statement releasing the hospital from liability for his death, and he made provisions for his family's future. Under these circumstances, the court found no basis to override his decision.

While there has been a general trend toward respecting patient's rights, several recent cases have muddied the waters somewhat: in one instance, relatives of a patient who declined transfusion and executed a release nonetheless recovered damages for negligence [21]. Thus, in most circumstances involving a patient refusing treatment, the safest course is probably to seek appropriate judicial resolution.

Into the future: Legal issues posed by transfusion-transmitted AIDS

Since its recognition less than five years ago, acquired immune deficiency syndrome has rapidly emerged as one of the most critical public health problems in the United States and, indeed, in the eyes of many members of the public, as the most critical. Transfusion was identified as a source of transmission of AIDS only a few years ago; legal issues regarding transfusion and AIDS are therefore only beginning to be heard in the courts. Since very little case or statutory law yet exists, the discussion that follows simply attempts to identify emerging issues and to offer some thoughts on possible judicial and legislative responses.

Issues related to potential liability of a blood bank for transfusion-transmitted AIDS include a number of concerns. How intensive and how detailed should questioning and screening of prospective donors be? Should persons be questioned explicitly about homosexual activity or simply be encouraged to defer themselves? How and to whom should a prospective donor's HTLV-III positive status be reported? What steps should be taken to ensure that confidentiality of this sensitive information is respected? What duty, if any, does a blood bank have to notify recipients of prior transfusions from a donor who, upon later testing, is identified as HTLV-III positive or from a donor who is subsequently diagnosed as having AIDS?

As we have noted above, questioning and screening of donors have important ramifications both for donors themselves and for transfusion recipients; failure to screen adequately can be a basis for negligence liability. Several years ago, when transmissibility of AIDS through transfusion and the heightened incidence among homosexuals were only beginning to be suspected, blood banks may have been somewhat more circumspect in their screening. This caution was in part related to the fact that barring all homosexuals, for example, might arguably have conflicted with state or local anti-discrimination statutes. At present, however, federal guidelines require deferral of any male who has had homosexual contact since 1977. (It might be noted that this standard, like the HTLV-III test, is still expressed as a guideline rather than a mandate, although it is effectively implemented nationwide.)

There remains some controversy about whether blood centers should employ direct questioning or simply provide the information and request potential donors in high-risk groups to defer themselves. A recent article in the *Journal of the American Medical Association* unequivocally recommends the former course. As the authors of that article note, 'even with the discovery of the causative agent of AIDS and the development of tests to detect the AIDS agent, historical questions may still be important, unless the new test is 100% sensitive and specific' [22].

While this issue remains undecided, it is certainly clear that failure to perform laboratory screening measures from the time that a test was available, or failure to perform the tests carefully, provides a basis for negligence liability. Just what standards might be applied to cases arising in the interim – when the association was known but the test not yet available – remains to be seen; however, it might be argued that thorough donor questioning and screening were even more critical during that period.

The availability of a laboratory test to screen for HTLV-III has created several problems even while it alleviated other major concerns. The availability of the test has raised significant issues about safeguarding the privacy and confidentiality of those with positive results and protecting them from unwarranted discrimination, while at the same time satisfying legitimate public health needs. Legislative responses to date have been very mixed and have run the gamut from mandatory reporting in one state (Colorado) to provisions forbidding the reporting of any results without the express written consent of the donor.

California and Wisconsin, for example, have passed laws designed to protect the confidentiality of test results and to prevent their use by employers and insurers [23]. On the other hand, a September 1985 decision by the American military to utilize the test on recruits and recent litigation resulting from efforts of some school systems to deny admission to children with positive tests exemplify recent efforts toward public identification and exclusion. Additional legislation is likely to be forthcoming as more states seek to reconcile the competing concerns.

A recent article in the *New York Times* summarized the privacy issues as follows:

> "Civil liberties advocates say the personal trauma of individuals exposed to the AIDS virus is intensified by fears that their test results will be disclosed and that harsh restrictions will be placed on their lives. If the uses of the test are not tightly controlled, some argue, the rights of hundreds of thousands of people may be endangered and a class of outcasts created for no good medical reasons. They say it is not difficult to imagine a move toward widespread mandatory blood screening and that those with positive tests results could face discrimination in jobs, schools or housing...
>
> Determining the blood test's proper role is especially complicated because most of those infected with the virus to date are homosexuals, a group that has suffered a legacy of discrimination." [23]

Apart from the potential liability of blood centers engaged in testing, a host of questions also faces hospitals and physicians providing transfusion services. A major issue for the physician involves the concept of informed consent. Does the physician have a duty to include information about the risk of AIDS in order to secure effective informed consent for transfusion? Some commentators have argued that he does indeed:

> "If one assumes that a physician is not negligent in giving the transfusion, the greatest legal danger is giving a patient blood without warning of the possible consequences; in fact, this is the critical issue in a recently filed AIDS suit." [22]

Other AIDS-related issues for doctors and hospitals that cary legal ramifications include the role of autologous or directed donations and the extent of the duty to inform patients who previously received transfusions from a donor who, upon later testing, is identified as HTLV-III positive or from a donor who is subsequently diagnosed as having AIDS. Along with blood centers, hospitals and physicians may also have to re-visit, in light of AIDS, their legal obligations to afford their employees a reasonably safe working environment.

Another issue that has begun to be raised is the question of what, if any, liability might be imposed upon a blood donor for transmission of AIDS. In at least one state, legislation was proposed that would have imposed criminal penalties for transmission of AIDS. To our knowledge, no judicial decision to date has imposed any liability, civil or criminal, upon a donor for adverse consequences of the donation. Although the likelihood of such a result may be remote, the consequences of any imposed or threatened penalties on donors might well be disastrous in a system almost wholly dependent upon the voluntary generosity of blood donors.

A final legal issue that has emerged in the wake of concern over transfusion-transmitted AIDS is the question whether strict liability might be re-imposed upon blood suppliers [24]. Several lawsuits recently filed by victims of transfusion-transmitted AIDS have attempted to argue that strict liability should apply, given the serious consequences of AIDS. However, the language of applicable statutes and judicial decisions would seem to leave little room for differentiating AIDS from other transfusion-transmitted diseases. Moreover, if a hospital or blood center does not properly use the testing and screening mechanisms available, it clearly remains subject to negligence liability.

Conclusion

The legal questions raised by transfusion-transmitted AIDS closely parallel the social and ethical concerns it has created. Our paper has attempted to outline the legal and regulatory framework affecting blood banking in the United States, in order to provide some insight into one nation's legal responses to recent medical and societal developments affecting blood banking. We do not possess a crystal ball that will enable us to predict judicial and legislative responses to all the newly emerging questions related to AIDS. We can only hope that at least the American courts will continue to exhibit respect for important individual rights and to balance concern for privacy and confidentiality of donors and patients with any legitimate public health needs.

References

1. It should, however, be noted that foreign establishments producing blood products for import and products imported into the United States are subject to federal licensure requirements. *See e.g.*, 21 C.F.R. Sec. 601.31.
2. Drake AW, Finkelstein SN, Sapolsky HM. The American blood supply. Cambridge: MIT Press, 1982.
3. 42 U.S.C. Sec. 262.
4. Hoppe Pa, Tourault MA. Quality control and regulatory requirements. In: Pittiglio D, ed. Modern blood banking and transfusion practices, Philadelphia. F.A. Davis Co. 1983:283 – 322.
5. – U.S. – , 105 S. Ct. 2371 (1985).
6. *See e.g.*, 21 C.F.R. Sec. 640.5 (1985).
7. JCAH, Accreditation Manual for Hospitals, 1985:112 – 4.
8. AABB Standards, Arlington U.S, 1984:B1.310.
9. *See* 21 C.F.R. Sec. 640.61 (1985).
10. 160 Ga.App. 387, 287 S.E. 2d 715 (1982).
11. 39 Misc. 2d 799, 241 N.Y.S. 2d 971 (Sup.Ct. 1963).
12. 331 N.W. 2d 870 (Iowa 1983).
13. *South Florida Blood Services Inc.* v. *Rasmussen*, – So. 2d – (Fla.App. 1985).
14. 368 So. 2d 1219 (La. Ct. App. 1979).
15. *See Sawyer* v. *Methodist Hospital*, 525 F. 2d 1102 (6th Cir. 1975); *Samuels* v. *Health and Hosp. Corp. of N.Y.*, 591 F. 2d 195 (2d Cir. 1979); *Gilmore* v. *St. Anthony Hospital*, 598 P. 2d 1200 (Okla. 1979).
16. Lentz SL, Polesky HF. Legal guidelines for blood banking and transfusion. II. Medical Laboratory Observer, 1984;Nov:83 – 92.
17. Lentz SL, Polesky HF. Legal guidelines for blood banking and transfusion. I. Medical Laboratory Observer, 1984;Oct:30 – 4.

18. Lentz SL. Refusal of treatment. In: AABB, Legal issues in transfusion medicine: Managing risk in a changing environment. Washington, DC 1985:83 – 97.
19. 331 F. 2d 1000 (D.C. Cir.), *cert. denied* 377 U.S. 985 (1964).
20. 294 A. 2d 372 (D.C. 1972).
21. *Shorter* v. *Drury*, 695 P. 2d 116 (Wash. 1985).
22. Miller PJ, O'Connell J, Leipold A, Wenzel RP. Potential liability for transfusion-associated AIDS. JAMA 1985;253:3419 – 24.
23. Eckholm E. Screening of blood for AIDS raises civil liberties issues. New York Times 1985;Sept 30:1(col.2), 9(col.1).
24. Bielan JM. Bad blood. Cal Lawyer 1985;Vol 5 No 4:29 – 32.

DISCUSSION

Moderators: T.J. Greenwalt and C.Th. Smit Sibinga

T.J. Greenwalt (Cincinnati): Dr. van Vianen, do you think that the converging incidence of risks between males and females in the older age group is due to the very bad smoking habits that the females – at least in our country – have picked up. Lung cancer has outstripped breast cancer as the major type of cancer in females.

H.A.W. van Vianen (Groningen): I know of these developments. Mortality risks for women have been declining for at least thirty years generally. However, there is clear evidence that mortality due to some specific causes, in particular lung cancer, is rapidly increasing. In fact, the age adjusted death rate for respiratory cancer doubled in the last fifteen years. The relation between tobacco addiction and lung cancer is well established and due to the long 'incubation period' and very limited success of medical intervention a substantive further rise can be expected.*

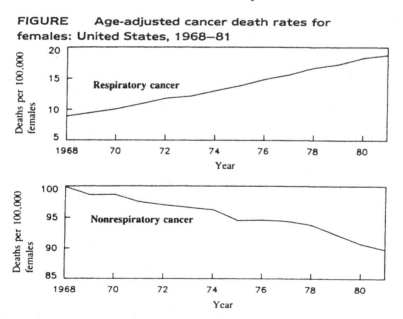

FIGURE   Age-adjusted cancer death rates for females: United States, 1968–81

Figure 1. Age-adjusted cancer death rates for females: United States, 1968 – 1981.

* Ravenholt RT. Addiction mortality in the United States 1980: Tobacco, Alcohol and other substances. Popul Dev Rev 1984;10:697 – 724.

H.F. Polesky (Minneapolis): Dr. Jameson, I want to comment about p24. We have to be very careful with regard to western blot results. Like the ELISA test it has a great number of methodologic factors. It may be the stain. We have used an alkaline phosphatase method. I noticed no p18, which we have seen fairly frequently. I wonder if you might just comment on the band at 18 which seems to occur. We see more often p24 without gp41 than the other, so there are some problems.

B.A. Jameson (München): The p18 is usually present. We do not detect it on our immunoblots, because it usually goes right through our paper.

H.F. Polesky: So, that is a methodologic difference.

B.A. Jameson: Right. I would like to make one other comment. We see a diminishing response against the core protein, but it is not completely absent. It does not contradict the Abbott results.

C.Th. Smit Sibinga (Groningen): That is true. Because it was shown that, specifically in the early ARC cases, the same pattern is actually showing up.

H.F. Polesky: I wonder if Dr. Högman would comment briefly about the controversy that has arisen over measurement of cell survival versus blood volume and which is the best way to approach this issue.

C.F. Högman (Uppsala): I would rather prefer not to comment on it, because I find it very intriguing and difficult to understand.

Just to explain, the majority of workers in the field using the chromium labelling technique of red cells stored for some time in vitro, have found a certain survival of the red cells which does not agree with the observations made in Dr. Valeri's laboratory. Dr. Valeri found less good red cell survival. I think there are some technical differences between Dr. Valeri's investigations and others. One thing which was claimed by Dr. Valeri was that he is doing a double-label technique, measuring thereby the red cell volume of the recipient. What he really finds is an initial removal of red cells within the first five minutes, which all the others will miss. It is difficult to understand why so much would really be removed so quickly, because not very much of the blood is going trough the spleen in the first five minutes. This would indicate, then, that the removal is taking place at some other sites, than in the spleen.

Some of the other workers actually have also used double-label technique and have found good correlation between the single and double chromium labelling technique. One single thing we could point to is the fact that Dr. Valeri does not wash his cells.

W.G. van Aken (Amsterdam): Mrs. Lentz, there is a governmental trend in a number of countries to organize consensus meetings on strategies and on treatment. Recently, in the United States, there has been such a meeting on the usage of FFP (fresh frozen plasma). In this country, we have also organized this type of meeting. My question is: How do lawyers look at the status of those meetings, and especially on reports and advices which come out of these consensus meetings. Are the statements which are made at those meetings representing a common opinion? Do they have a special position when lawyers discuss liability and negligence?

S.L. Lentz (Minneapolis): I cannot answer your question in the context of what happens in every country, since it is obviously different in the United States and probably in other countries that have a similar common law system.

What is said at, or what comes out of, a consensus meeting would have no greater weight than any other sources of professional opinion, than standards of regulatory organizations or voluntary organizations, or statutes. In fact, at least in the United States, creative lawyers will try to find whatever kind of professional opinion that will support the particular point of view they want to address. In the United States at least, all sorts of expert testimony can be placed in evidence in a trial, and lawyers will try whatever strategies they can to get the professional viewpoints favourable to them before the court.

T.J. Greenwalt: May I raise another question? Perhaps I am wrong, or inaccurate, but our legal system differs a little in that we have a system of contigency fees, which encourage frivolous lawsuits.

S.L. Lentz: It is true in the United States that lawyers bringing civil lawsuits for damages frequently undertake to do it with the understanding that they will be paid only if they recover a monetary award for their client. That system does not exist in all countries. For example, in Great Britain by way of contrast: Whichever party wins, the losing party is frequently required to pay the winning party's attorney's fees and that does not occur in the United States in most instances. I am not sure, however, that it can be safely said that the system of contigent fees necessarily encourages more ligitation. The alternative argument is that many people who otherwise could not get compensation for an injury that they have suffered, have a chance to get into court. Beyond that the threat of a lawsuit for malpractice or negligence is one way of keeping the medical profession straight. That is not an acceptable argument from the medical profession's viewpoint, but that is at least one legal perspective.

C. Th. Smit Sibinga: An issue actually, in the United States, is the ongoing debate on dedicated donations now that AIDS has hit blood banks as well. In our country, there is a law under construction regulating blood transfusion and amazingly enough, blood donors donating for cytapheresis and those donating autologously on good clinical grounds will be excluded from our regulations in the proposed law. These two issues do relate. Could you comment in terms of liability?

S.L. Lentz: At a meeting in the United States just about a month ago, which was the first national conference on legal aspects of transfusion, there were some very strong statements against the practice of directed donation, on the ground that that may in fact be less safe in the long run than any voluntary non-directed donor system. So, I am not sure that it makes sense to put that into a separate category, or even to make special provisions that permit such a system.

II. Production aspects

PERSPECTIVES OF THE FUTURE IN DEVELOPING COUNTRIES

F.A. Ala

Introduction

Many of the so-called developing countries have, in their hey day, made major contributions to the foundations of modern biomedical science. For instance, amongst the Islamic nations, the early instruction of medicine, surgical practice, and the study of anatomy in 14th and 15th Century Iran, Turkey and Egypt demonstrates considerable intellectual ferment and learning.

The extraordinary advances of medicine in Europe over the past 100 years, however, left these countries behind. Despite their recent efforts to establish modern medical care, it is the laboratory sciences and blood transfusion that have been most particularly neglected and poorly developed.

Although international agencies such as the World Health Organization have latterly placed increasing emphasis upon community-based Primary Health Care; public health and sanitation; vaccination programmes etc., yet it cannot be denied that hospital medical care and diagnostic facilities must exist if only to provide a back-up to these ''grass-roots'' health systems.

Without blood transfusion, which underpins virtually all clinical services, modern hospital based care cannot be sustained.

Must these burgeoning services plod the same evolutionary path traversed by more advanced nations, and, in the time-worn phrase of first-year embryology, must ''Ontogeny recapitulate phylogeny''? Are there:
1. organization, or
2. technical short-cuts they can feasibly and cost-effectively adopt to accelerate their development?

The problems

There are, of course, myriad problems which beset the developing nations' health care planning and which inhibit the establishment of these infrastructural blood transfusion services.

Some of the most notable problems, perhaps are:
1. The enormous fragmentation and pluralism pervading blood transfusion practice. The lack of a national focal point for long term planning and organization; for establishment of standards and quality assurance programmes; creation of cadres and staff training; for problem-solving as a National Reference Centre and gathering of vital epidemiological and demographic data.

2. The failure of governments to integrate transfusion services into national health care plans and to commit adequate financial and human resources for the task. It may be that running costs alone (excluding the requisite capital expenditure and plasma fractionation) amount to over half a million US dollars per million population served.

3. Voluntary blood donor recruitment campaigns are poorly planned, unsystematic and unsufficiently funded. Unsustained, sporadic drives are carried out instead of professional, unified, long-term programmes. Little reliable information is available regarding commercialism in blood procurement, but the exploitation of sick, anaemic professional blood-donors by rapacious agents is still widespread and often uncontrolled. Where blood and funds are in short supply, the onus is often put upon the patient's relatives to supply the blood which is required. A number of countries have introduced compulsory blood donation for students, drivers license applicants and civil servants. Coercion may provide quick and relatively easy returns in the short term, but it will ensure public resentment and a permanent stable donor base may never develop.

4. Whatever the means of procurement may be, insufficient blood is available for the practice of modern medicine. In most of the Middle Eastern countries present needs are for up to five times more red cells, even when requirements for other blood components and plasma fractions are put aside.

5. Lack of trained manpower in transfusion services is a very acute problem. This, in turn, is due to the absence of career prospects for both doctors and technicians in this important branch of laboratory medicine. There are no formally constituted specialist training programmes in Blood Transfusion Science, and as a consequence, talented and ambitious young workers are not attracted to the field.

6. Finally, amongst the inhibitory factors, must be catalogued the many deficiencies of infrastructural services which all laboratories ultimately depend upon, such as equipment maintenance and repair; an efficient transport and communications network; adequate and above all stable power supplies; timely access to good quality laboratory reagents; access to the scientific and medical literature, and so forth.

Models of organization

Now there are a number of ways in which blood transfusion services may be organized and some of the advantages and drawbacks associated with each of these models of organization will be discussed. Needless to say, the demarcations between them are often blurred as they shade into each other, and indeed, several models co-exist in a number of countries.

Table 1. Models for blood provision.

---

1. The Hospital Blood Bank: buying or contracting for blood supply with an agent for professional donors.
2. The Hospital Blood Bank: collecting blood itself from relatives, volunteers or professional donors.
   Waste because of small turnover and limited use of components – a "hand to mouth" solution.
3. The Hospital Blood Bank: collecting as above, but also supplying a number of smaller, surrounding hospitals or clinics.
4. The Hospital Blood Bank: collecting as above, but subject to an Accreditation Programme, meeting certain government criteria and *accountable* to a central agency regulatory.
5. The Hospital Blood Bank: partially or wholly supplied with blood from an external *donor recruitment organization* (Red Crescent or Community based agency) which is responsible only for donor motivation and blood collection, but *no* testing, screening or processing of blood. Fragmentation in the continuum of blood provision and poor accountability to government, donor and recipient.

Hospital-based blood services (Table 1)

This, in itself, is a heterogenous group which ranges at one extreme, from the unregulated "free-for-all" of individual hospitals fending for themselves entirely, to a form of unity and regulation where the hospital blood bank is autonomous yet accountable to some central agency.

The latter model may be made to work successfully (as several Scandinavian countries have shown), but in general, small, scattered centres lead to mediocrity and poor standards, a high level of blood and plasma wastage and poor utilisation of financial resources. Duplication or even competition will inevitably develop in donor recruitment programmes, purchase of equipment and establishment of skilled personel. The essential weakness of this entire group is that no permanent mechanism is created which will undertake forward planning and long-term resolution of problems such as manpower development, teaching, quality assurance etc. These hospital based centres provide, at best, only a response to the transfusional needs of the day and represent therefore a "hand to mouth" solution.

Finally, within this category, are those hospital blood banks that are supplied by a non-profit community based or governmental organization (such as the Red Cross/Red Crescent) which undertakes only the recruitment and motivation of voluntary blood donors. These organizations are frequently not responsible for testing, screening and processing of blood for transfusion and this represents an undesirable fragmentation in the continuum of accountability which should ideally stretch from the criteria for selection and care of donors to the safe infusion of blood products to the patients.

Table 2. Models for blood provision.

---

1. A "confederation" of regional centres:
   Autonomously managing their own affairs.
   Loosely associated through a national committee to discuss:
   - Common problems
   - National standards and exchange of materials
   - Joint research projects
   - Industrial ventures of national interest:
     Plasma fractionation
     Reagent manufacture
     Blood bag manufacture, etc.
   - Training programmes and seminars.

Table 3. Models for blood provision.

---

2. A national reference centre: the *one-tier* approach:
   Functions as a problem-solvintg centre.
   Retains national rare donor file and cryopreserved rare blood units.
   Histocompatibility testing.
   Development of blood group serology and other laboratory agents.
   Does developmental and epidemiological research.
   Carries out teaching and training programmes and organizes seminars.
   Has delegated authority to accredit and inspect laboratories. Proficiency
     testing and quality control exercises, etc.
   (Plasma fractionation), etc.
   - Does *not* carry out:
     Donor recruitment, selection.
     Blood collection.
     Blood testing, screening and processing component preparation.
     Blood and blood product issue.
   - Blood for transfusion is provided from *pluralistic* sources.

Table 4. Models for blood provision.

---

3. A "two-tier" national service:

	National Blood Transfusion Centre	Tier 1

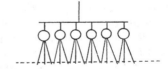

Few, large regional centres
of high standard, managed
and financed by national
service   Tier 2

Pluralistic Blood Transfusion Centres
(private, insurance, Red
Crescent, army, hospital
- based on free-standing)

The "confederation" of regional centres (Table 2)

Either for historical reasons or because of the sheer size and ethnic hetero-geneity of certain countries, the development of large, highly developed, autonomous regional centres may be the only practical solution. Here even though the centres manage their own affairs and are separately funded through their provincial authorities, yet they may be loosely associated through a national committee in order to discuss and agree upon certain common criteria, to co-ordinate their activities and to consider supra-regional, national requirements in the long term; exchange of sera; joint research projects etc.

The obvious dangers of this type of system lie in a lack of central leader-ship and a centrifugal state or loss of cohesion which makes it difficult to establish plasma fractionation, high quality reagent manufacture or to wield the kind of political "leverage" which is required to ensure adequate funding for future growth and development.

The "one-tier" approach – a national reference centre (Table 3)

This strategy comprises a responsibility limited to the scientific, industrial, monitoring and training activities, that will be alluded to later.

Where the reference centre actually shares in donor recruitment, blood processing and issue as well, acting, in this, as one participant amongst many, it may have a salutory exemplary role to fulfill.

In cases where tasks of recruitment and blood collection are delegated, one must have grave reservations about this approach, for the selection of donors; quality control of blood collection; adaptation to changing clinical needs and modes of cell harvesting are all divorced from blood processing; science and clinical medicine. Above all, the accountability to donors and patients is diluted and fragmented.

Certainly, it is better to have some national nexus, rather than none at all. However, the resulting pluralism in donor recruitment is undesirable and can only lead to conflicting messages being conveyed to the public; to destructive competition for donors and loss of good will and confusion amongst the potential donor population. As we have said before, it will also lead to a waste of blood components, as each blood centre seeks only to satis-fy its own, limited requirements. Finally, a national reference centre can all too easily become isolated, remote and bureaucratic if it is not intimately involved in the day to day business of providing a service.

The "two-tier" national service (Table 4)

A two-tiered system may be envisioned, where the national centre estab-lishes and directly manages, a very few major regional centres of high qual-ity, which undertake all but the most important or industrial tasks of the national centre such as plasma fractionation and reagent manufacture etc.

With the institution of a model such as this, all transfusion activity peripheral to the regional centre would be pluralistic (Red Crescent/Red Cross, private, insurance, armed forces, etc.), yet these disparate elements would all benefit from their association with the national service, and would, in turn, be subject to the quality assurance, proficiency-testing and other criteria established by the National Blood Transfusion Centre.

The multi-tiered, integral national service

Finally, the national service may provide an integral continuum, extending from donor recruitment, all the way to the delivery of service at the most peripheral district clinics. There are many advantages inherent in this approach: economies of scale, efficiency, pooling of scarce human resources, quality etc.

The functions of a national blood transfusion service

Essential national functions of the service

1. Organizational and administrative functions

a. Formation, establishment and implementation of appropriate legislation, code of practice and ethics governing all blood transfusion activity with government authorities.

b. Planning and implementing of a unified, persistent, voluntary donor recruitment campaign with common criteria for donor selection, blood collection and transport.
Exploiting and co-ordinating the resources of other agencies with community association such as the Red Crescent Society: Boy Scouts, religious and voluntary organizations, etc.

c. Formulating and applying national standards for blood and blood products, laboratory practice in both transfusion centres and hospital blood banks.
Monitoring and accrediting laboratories through authority delegated from the Ministry of Health by means of quality control and proficiency testing exercises, standard operating procedures, etc.

d. Long-range planning and budgetting for the entire service and negotiation of adequate financial support to ensure growth.

e. Long-term planning of overall manpower development and establishing specific attractive career prospects for transfusion personnel at a national level.

f. Negotiating close co-ordination with the armed forces: joint disaster planning, interchangeable equipment, standards and procedures, etc.

2. *Operational functions*

A. Provision of a problem-solving *"reference centre"* capability:
   a. Detection and identifying irregular red cell, platelet and white cell antibodies.
   Provision of laboratory standards and reference materials.
   b. Offering a tissue typing service.
   c. Selecting donors and reagents for histocompatibility testing, red cell serology, high titre plasma for specific immune-globulin, etc.
   d. Plasmapheresis of selected, well-documented donors to harvest these materials.
   e. Retaining national rare blood donor file and cryopreservation of rare blood units, lymphocytes, panel cells, etc.

B. Provision of teaching and training programmes:
   a. Introduction of transfusion technology into technician school curricula:
   – Training graduate technicians and offering specialized higher qualifications.
   – Making research opportunities, workshops, seminars available to technicians. Providing refresher courses to technicians employed in hospital blood banks.
   b. Introducing modern blood transfusion practice into nursing school curricula or upgrading existing programmes. On the job training of qualified nurses employed in hospitals.
   c. Strengthening the instruction of blood transfusion practice in medical school curricula. Holding seminars and refresher courses for practicing doctors in transfusion science.
   d. Offering specialized post-graduate training and research opportunities to doctors and science graduates in various fields: immuno-chemistry, virology, genetics, molecular biology, haemostasis, etc.

C. Research
   a. Carrying out developmental and basic research.
   b. Carrying out epidemiological and demographic research, liver disease, viral disease, population genetics, etc.
   Data processing and statistics.
   c. Organization of seminars, workshops, multicentre trials of therapeutic materials or test procedures, national and international scientific meetings, etc.

Regional functions of the national centre

1. Blood collection, utilizing a variety of modalities: mobile teams, collection at fixed sites, mobile trailers, plasmapheresis for specific donors, cytapheresis.
2. Blood processing, testing and screening.
3. Blood component production;
4. Issue and distribution of blood and blood products.
5. Carrying out an antenatal screening programme.

Industrial functions of the national service

1. Large scale production of ABH, Rh, HLA and other serological reagents, screening and panel cells, etc.
2. Diagnostic kits – hepatitis testing, haemostasis, etc.
3. Plasma fractionation or negotiation of advantageous terms for contract fractionation, organizing the collection and dispatch of crude plasma and the quality control and distribution of fractionated products.
4. Plastic bag manufacture for blood and intravenous fluids, dialysis fluids, wash solutions, etc.
5. Design and contracted or direct manufacture of materials and equipment used in transfusion centres: folding beds, trolleys, scales, packing and transport modules, racks, etc.

Functions in co-operation with others (Research Laboratories, Universities, etc.)

1. Library facilities, ensuring early and easy access to relevant scientific literature.
2. Repair and maintenance workshops with an adequate inventory of spares.
3. Laboratory animal breeding facilities providing access to specific breeds and to the necessary expertise.

The creation of an organization such as this requires the dedicated services of an individual with the necessary vision and drive, someone, above all, who is able to establish credibility amongst the public, the medical community, and governmental policy-makers.

No single model can be taken as universally valid, feasible or appropriate, although, in those countries where blood transfusion is embryonic, it is probable that *centrifugal* planning from a national service, offering strong leadership, is more likely to succeed than endeavours to establish dominion or control over a pre-existing, heterogenous system which has started at the periphery – the *centripetal* approach.

Thus, in the basic organizational matters at the core of the service, there are no easy short-cuts.

What can be done

Given the existence of a well-established, structured service, however, there *are* a number of technical procedures, devices and policies which can be implemented to good advantage in developing countries at relatively little cost.

Microplate technology [1 - 3]

It is often forgotten that the history of microplates goes back as far as 35 years and to Hungary, which has provided us with other innovations such as the Biro, the Rubick Cube and Kaposi's Sarcoma. In 1950, Takatsy described a 96-well plastic plate for use in microbiology. This became an inexpensive and efficient substitute for a rack of glass precipitin tubes. Microbiologists exploited these microplates long before transfusionists began to appreciate their value in the mid-sixties.

From these early efforts, microplate techniques have evolved rapidly into the sophisticated systems available today and which offer marked economies in reagent consumption, equipment costs and technician time, without loss of sensitivity in comparison with conventional techniques.

Originally developed simply as manual ABO/Rh typing systems, various additives were then employed to enhance agglutination reactions and reduce incubation times. Then automation for handling and dispensing antisera was introduced and, finally, automated microplate readers adapted from microbiology ELISA photometers were added. The full spectrum is now completed with the development of microcomputer software packages controlling sample handling, donor or patient identity, the functions of the reader, interpretation of results with direct data capture, processing and reporting.

These systems will be equally adept in handling the highly sensitive solid-phase immunoabsorbance techniques in the future and, given their compatibility with procedures in other related disciplines such as histocompatibility testing and virological screening, there is good reason to believe in their capacity for lateral applications. It may, for instance, be possible to replace the light source with a luminometer for chemi-luminescent enzyme immunoassays [4] or even with a time-resolved fluorometer [5] for a variety of highly sensitive immunoassays.

In summary, microplate technology is economical, compact, reliable and flexible in its applications.

1.   Kontron microgroupamatic

A semi-automated blood grouping and information management system which uses the standard 96-well microplate. It comprises a microplate photometer; DEC data processing unit driven by the GC5 programmer derived from the larger G 2000 software; a VDU and printer for hard-copy reporting. An option plate loader/stacker taking up to 10 plates is available and a light pen for entry of bar-coded plate numbers.

The system allows on-line editing which substantially reduces the rejection rate by visual interpretation.

This equipment bears a generic similarity to a number of other systems such as the Flow, Dynatech and Inverness machines. The latter, soon to be manufactured and marketed by MSE, probably has the most sophisticated scanning reader of them all.

2. Gamma STS – M system

This fully automated system will carry out 10 ABO/Rh determinations per hour. It brings the added security of a bar-coded positive sample identification capability in contrast to the previous group which rely upon a batch/plate identification.

Interpretation of the test reactions here depends upon the detection by photosensing device of streaming (negative) or the absence of streaming (positive) patterns of red cells in the microtear reaction wells after centrifugation.

3. Olympus PK 7100

A large machine, more suitable for a regional blood transfusion centre than the average hospital blood bank, which is essentially built around the non-standard 120 well Olympus microplate. The wells have an ingenious "stepped" configuration which provides a sharp discrimination between positive agglutination reactions and negatives. This 12-channel machine can handle 240 samples per hour.

4. Ortho immunoscan 100

This is an extremely sophisticated, ambitious machine making intensive use of microprocessors which offer great flexibility. It utilizes a refined image analysis system for reading reactions, scanning 256 imaging points and provides for individual bar-coded sample identification extending even to tiny 400 microlitre sample tubes.

Cell-washing and 37°C incubation can be carried out directly in the microwells, so that irregular antibody screening, identification, Coombs testing and compatibility testing can be performed.

Bar-coding [6,7]

Bar-coding has long been used by the larger supermarket and drugstore chains and it is only in the past decade that this and other automatic identification systems have been applied in transfusion services.

In this context, the provision of positive sample identification is of fundamental importance, irrevocably linking the donor, donation, samples, blood group laboratory and microbial screening results; blood component products and hospital issue data. Latterly, some hospitals have adopted light pens and computer terminals so that the integral chain between donor and recipient or recipients is completed. The integrity of the system can be further refined so that particular blood product issues can be linked to specific quality control data, reagent batches, etc.

This system clearly provides invaluable validation and confidence in countries where the concept of quality assurance is poorly established and accurate data capture without clerical transcription error is vital.

In Britain and the USA, the CODABAR system has found favour, whereas in Finland and Sweden, the OCR.B system is preferred. In the former case, the donation number is printed in both bar-coded and eye-readable forms. In the OCR.B system, the same number is readable by both eye and by automated equipment.

The bar-code consists of different lines and spaces (both thick and thin), arranged to represent different characters. The American Blood Commission (ABC) symbol is preferred. This is a linear bar code which consists of four bars and three spaces of varying width. Each set of seven wide and narrow bars and spaces represents one character. When an item of information is recorded, it must be preceded by a start code and ended by a stop code, although these are not part of the eye-readable information.

There is an extremely remote possibility (1 in 10^6) that a light pen may make an error by the substitution of one number for another. To prevent this from happening, a check digit is necessary, reducing the possibility of substitution error to 1 in 10^9.

Check digit

Calculation of check digit

The International Standard Organization (ISO) modulus 11-2 check digit is recommended. The method of calculation is as follows:

"Weighting" factors 765432

1. Multiply each digit of the donation number by the corresponding weighting numbers.
2. Sum the products from step 1.
3. Divide the sum by 11.
4. Subtract the remainder from 11.

Example:

Donation no.	=	2	2	8	9	5	7
Weighting factor	=	7	6	5	4	3	2
Products	=	14	12	40	36	15	14
Sum of products	=	131					
Divide by 11	=	11 remainder 10					
Subtract remainder from 11	=	1					
The check digit is therefore		1					

The full donation number for the Birmingham Centre would therefore be:

2 2 8 9 5 7 H 1

H is the code for Birmingham and 1 is the check digit

Microcomputers [8]

One of the most significant benefits to be gained from the use of computers in blood transfusion is the ability to retrieve data quickly.

With this facility for fast retrieval comes a reduction in the need for reliance upon legions of clerical staff. Furthermore, it increases the willingness and ability of staff to access and manipulate data which would be prohibitive using manual methods.

The coming-of-age of low-cost, high-performance, micro- and super-microcomputers, operating with standard communications protocols and having networking capabilities has provided, at reasonable cost, a suitable entry point for transfusion services into the field of information technology.

In addition, the development of fourth generation languages as "programme generators" and "report writers" allows non-computer specialists to develop applications in relatively short time scales.

Development of automatic identification systems, such as bar-coding, has added a high level of reliability and safety to the data capture process. Furthermore, it has taken data capture out of the data processing departments onto the bench, where staff, who understand the data they are handling, can record accurately the results of their work.

In countries where reliable documentation and good clerical support are difficult to obtain, the fast retrieval of data coupled with fast and accurate data capture methods have provided an attractive alternative to previous manual methods. They also ensure the error-free capability, so vital in the context of hepatitis and HTLV infection, of tracing donors of infectious blood components long after they have been issued.

The careful selection of the appropriate microcomputer systems can provide effective building blocks on which future corporate information strategies can be developed.

Although information technology is changing at an ever-increasing pace, providing the hardware is selected which has future growth potential, from a supplier with a good pedigree, then potential users should grasp the technologies now and gain the benefits today.

Monoclonal antibodies [9]

Many developing countries possess sufficient expertise, were it not scattered, to establish a high-technology "core" for the production of monoclonal antibodies. The obvious attraction of hybridoma technology in immunohaematology is the ability to produce continuously available, standardized reagents.

Monoclonal antibodies, whether mass-produced in large culture vessels or in peritoneal cavity of mice and rats have been shown to be stable on long-term storage on temperatures ranging from minus 79°C to 56°C and even after repeated freezing and thawing. Their reactivity and specificity are affected by changes in pH and temperature, however, and one must be careful (as with conventional immune sera) to provide assay conditions specified for each particular reagent.

Costs will undoubtedly come down as the problems of large scale production are resolved and the questionable ethics of hyper-immunizing donors will undoubtedly serve as a further spur to efforts in this direction.

In summary, these sera offer the advantages of unlimited supply of homogeneous material which can be used to obtain reproducible results and where specificity, affinity, class and subclass will not change from lot to lot.

Optimal additive solutions [10,11]

The use of whole blood has progressively given way to component therapy in developing countries as it did many years ago in Europe and the USA.

Unfortunately, the optimal storage requirements of the different constituents of blood conflict: oxygen is noxious to red cells, whereas platelets require it; red cells must be kept at 4°C, platelets at 22°C and plasma at − 40°C. Citrate is the present anticoagulant of choice, but it impairs factor VIII stability which is only partially mitigated by expensive refrigeration. Besides, not only are red cells deprived of a major part of their carefully tailored nutrients when red cell concentrates are produced, these concentrates become an unattractive viscous product on storage.

You are all familiar with Claes Högman's seminal concept of resuspending concentrated red cells in 100 ml of a nutrient medium made up of saline, adenine, glucose and mannitol (SAG.M). This flexible system responds to a variety of entirely different needs:
- good long-term red cell survival;
- good rheology;
- maximal plasma harvest;
- low citrate levels;
- the option of microaggregate removal, etc.

There are now many other variants of this system which have been spawned in the past ten years, and at least one permutation which offers ATP levels over 50% after 16 weeks storage, together with 70% to 80% 24-hour red cell survival and a haemolysis level of only 0.3% to 1%!

Reviewing the main elements of the red cell storage lesion, we have also been interested in devising a system, mainly catering for the needs of developing countries without access to plasma fractionation facilities and requiring long-dating of red cells to cover the prolonged dearth of donors for instance, during the month of Ramadan in Moslem countries.

Our experimental additive involves:
1. For the maintenance of glycolysis: fructose 1, 6 diphosphate and a Wellcome Foundation compound for shifting oxygen dissociation to the right [12].
2. To maintain a low calcium level: a minimal degree of citrate as a secondary anticoagulant, whilst maintaining polyphosphates to retain intracellular Ca^{++B} buffering and ATP to pump Ca^{++} out.
3. To deal with the free oxygen radicles such as H_2O_2, $O_2{\cdot}^-$, $HO_2{\cdot}$ and $OH{\cdot}$ which must be seen as major contributors to the storage lesion: removal of the buffy coat, but also, the addition of alpha-tocopherol,

a more potent oxygen radicle scavenger than mannitol or sorbitol, which intercalates with the lipid bilayer.

4. Since we know that factor VIII is a metallo-protein reliant for its integrity and stability upon a physiological level of the calcium ion, it is tempting to use heparin as a primary anticoagulant as Rock and Smit Sibinga have done, in order to foster the production of a stable, high yield cryoprecipitation [13,14].

Heparin is injurious to platelets, however, and we have been experimenting with low molecular weight heparin fragments as a primary anticoagulant [15], used in combination with an optimal additive solution containing a minimal level of citrate.

If this work proves to be feasible, a blood collection package will have been provided which would allow the most modest blood centre to deploy a full range of therapeutic materials without recourse to outside help.

Laboratory policies

1. Although, after A and B, the Rh antigen – due to its immunogeneicity – is the most important red cell antigen in populations with a relatively high frequence of D negative subjects, this is not the case everywhere. In some populations, Rh-typing is a "non-problem" due to the absence or low frequence of Rh negativity. (0 to 1% amongst Japanese, Chinese, Burmese, Maoris, American Indians, etc., etc.) Yet much effort and money is expended in D-typing and classifying donors and recipients with expensive anti-D reagents and techniques.

2. It is well known that C and E in the absence of D, are poorly immunogenic. Consequently, it is wasteful to type donors for these antigens as a routine, although this hallowed tradition is perpetuated in many countries.

There has been no good evidence suggesting that C and E typing are necessary to indicate Rh D status of either donors or recipients. Consequently, the term "positive donor/negative recipient" used in designate r' and r'' subjects in an obsolete concept leading to confusion and a waste of Rh-negative blood. If Rh-typing is restricted with anti-D, regardless of C and E status, the stocks of Rh-negative blood would be significantly increased.

3. The further "non problem" of D^u must also be mentioned. D^u is a quantative defect arising from a reduced number of D sites per red cell and leading to weakened expression of a normal antigen. D variants (such as category VI) on the other hand, are qualitatively defective red cells, with either missing, altered or replaced determinants of the D antigenic cluster or mosaic. Finally, D^u variant cases are those which share both quantitive and qualitative defects.

For many years, numerous blood centres have carried out elaborate tests to detect D^u samples without questioning the basis for applying these tests to donor samples until the poor immunogenicity of D^u was documented, showing that D^u testing of blood donors is not cost-effective.

In any case, not *all* the weak forms of D expression are detectable by indirect antiglobulin testing and many can only be discerned by elaborate fixation/elution techniques.

If we accept the relatively high risk of immunization to K, c, E by providing blood unmatched for these antigens, we can reasonably accept the risk of immunization of D^u and D variants with Rhesus positive blood. The knowledge of D^u status in routine work is unnecessary and segregation into D positive and D negative is probably quite sufficient [16].

4. Although it is important to critically examine many irrational and wasteful traditional laboratory policies, it is equally important not to err on the side of doing too little.

Much is made in some developing countries of the large numbers of emergency transfusions which are required, the urgency of which override the need for proper compatibility testing. Indeed, matching is often dispensed with entirely.

It may be true that deficient primary health care and poor communications frequently lead to delayed treatment and the admission of patients in extremes. Nevertheless, there is almost never any excuse for failing to ensure ABO compatibility and the absence of clinically significant allo-antibodies.

A number of polycationic potentiating systems which non-specifically and reversibly aggregate erythrocytes, are well known, which greatly speed up and facilitate detection of red cell antibodies (polylysine, protamine, polybrene)

The manual polybrene test developed by Lalezari [17] offers a simple, inexpensive, highly sensitive test system for routine antibody detection in the hospital blood bank. It is also an extremely rapid test, allowing specific agglutination reactions to be read within 3 to 5 minutes after antibody addition. The supplementary antiglobulin phase is necessary to make the manual polybrene test equivalent in sensitivity to standard techniques for detecting anti-K, so that the overall elapsed time is only 7 to 9 minutes.

A further advantage of this method is the selective failure to detect "nuisance" antibodies – most cold autoantibodies, M, N, P$_1$ and many Lewis. The reagents are cheap and easy to make up.

Conclusion

As transfusionists, we are living through an extremely fast moving, exciting era in the course of which many of our traditional roles will be profoundly altered. Most developing countries cannot wait for these glamorous advances and may never be able to afford them.

For these countries, one must emphasize that, although there are a number of technical means which will provide for economies and more rapid advance, yet there is no way of avoiding the sheer perseverance and dedication required to establish a well-organized framework for national transfusion services.

References

1. Wegmann TG, Smithies OA. A simple haemagglutination system requiring small amounts of red cells and antibodies. Transfusion 1966;6:67.
2. McCloskey RV, Zimjewski CM. A semi-micro technique for detection of human blood group haemagglutinins. Techni Bull ASCP 1967;37:184.
3. Sacchi R. Analysis of the economies realised with the adoption of micro methods for some immuno-haematology procedures. La Transf del Sangue 1982;27:35 – 8.
4. Nicless GG, Thorpe GHG, Kricka LJ, Whitehead TP, Wells LJ, Ala FA. A rapid chemiluminescent enzyme linked immunosorbent assay for cytomegalovirus IgG antibodies using instant photographic film. J Virol Methods 1982:12.
5. Siitari H, Hemmila I, Soini, Lovgren T. Detection of hepatitis B surface antigen using time-resolved fluoroimmunoassay. Nature 1983;301:258 – 60.
6. Committee for Commonality in Blood Bank Automation (CCBBA). Final report, Vol. 3, 1977.
7. Ibbotson RN, Jackson RE. Data capture by the use of bar-coding in a blood transfusion centre. Med Lab Sci 1980;37:237 – 42.
8. Clark IR, Parekh J, Peters M, Frew ID. A hospital blood bank laboratory data processing system. J Clin Path 1984;37:1157 – 66.
9. Voak D, Lennox E, Sacks S, Milstein C, Darnborough J. Monoclonal anti-A and anti-B: development as cost-effective reagents. Med Lab Sci 1982;39:109 – 22.
10. Högman CF, Akerblom O, Hedlund K, Rosen I, Wilund I. Red cell suspensions in SAG.M. medium. Vox Sang 1983;45:217 – 23.
11. Meryman HT, Hornblower M, Syring R. Prolonged storage of red cells a 4°C. Abstracts of the 18th Congress of the International Society of Blood Transfusion. Karger S Basel 1984.
12. Hyde RM, Patterson RA, Livingstone DJ, Batchelor JF, King WR. Modification of the haemoglobin oxygen dissociation curve in whole blood by a compound with dual action. Lancet 1984;i:15 – 6.
13. Rock GA, Cruikshank WH, Tackaberry ES, Palmer DS. Improved yields of factor VIII from heparinised plasma. Vox Sang 1979;36:294 – 300.
14. Smit Sibinga CTh, Das PC. Heparin and factor VIII. Scand J Haematol 1984;33(suppl.40):111 – 22.
15. Kakkar VV, Djazaeri B, Fox J, Fletcher M, Scully MF, Westwick J. Low molecular weight heparin and prevention of post-operative thrombosis. Brit Med J 1982;284:375 – 9.
16. Moore BPL. Does knowlegde of the D^u status serve a useful purpose? Vox Sang 1984;46(suppl.1):95 – 7.
17. Lalezari P, Jiang AF. The manual polybrene test. Transfusion 1980;20:206 – 11.

BAG DESIGNS, PLASTICS AND PRESERVATIVES

J.M. Anthony

When discussing bag designs, plastics and preservatives or, as we call them at Fenwal, plastics and juices, it is interesting to note that in fact Fenwal began as a manufacturer of glass containers back in the late 1930s and moved into the era of plastics in the late 1940s [1]. The first patent for a platic Blood-Pack® utilized an ion exchange column and almost immediately improvements and innovations took place such as attaching the needle to the Blood-Pack® and adding a liquid anticoagulant. Ultimately transfer packs were introduced and then in the late 1950s the multiple pack which has made our industry possible emerged.

When talking about product development we are really talking about one phase of marketing and marketing is something that all of us do to some degree in our everyday jobs. Whether it is marketing to a blood donor to give at a particular blood center or to a hospital to use a particular blood component or to take advantage of a distribution arrangement, we are all marketing products and services. Understanding the environment and the needs that evolve from that environment are the keys to successful marketing and while reviewing bag designs, plastics and preservatives, let us try to keep in mind the environment and the needs it generates. For Fenwal the environment is dictated by the donor, the collecting center, the clinician and ultimately the patient. Certainly our ability to research and develop in certain areas and to leverage existing resources also enters to equation as well as national programmes and reimbursement schemes. So considering all this as part of the environment this paper will discuss five topics: design, plastics, juices, innovation and the future.

Design

Almost everyday in every plant that manufactures Fenwal products within the Travenol organization there are subtle designs and changes being made so that the products continue to be made in a cost effective environment with the lates technologies. Some of these are evident to the ultimate consumer, many are not. In recent years we have introduced such design changes as packs with rounded corners, different designs to expedite buffy coat removal, new approaches to break-away cannulas and different methodologies of sampling the blood collected whether it be a specimen tube built into the line or a means to fill a separate specimen tube.

One of the more dramatic changes recently has been the new needle with "K-Koat" in a newly designed hub and cover. This innovation is becoming to standard for needle excellence. And when we think of changes to the product line we must not think exclusively of changes to the Blood-Pack® itself, but also the way it is presented. Certainly the Unitrack® method of packaging where each Blood-Pack® is individually packaged in its own plastic overwrap causing the pack to remain flat, dry and with reduced kinking in the tubing. We are also looking to different approaches as to the way we bulk-pack the Blood-Pack® as the demands from our customers change in terms of collection sites, labor and product mix changes.

Plastics

For Travenol Laboratories as a company, Fenwal fulfills a very special role in that the Division screens almost all plastic compounds for their usefulness with the Travenol medical devices area. One can think of no other process that is as important and vital to the company as the search for new and better plastics. Understanding, for instance, what has been demanded of PL-146® in terms of a plastic for Blood-Pack® applications underlines the rigorous requirements a plastic formulation must fulfill with Travenol. A plastic's physical properties, its ability to be used in a manufacturing process, certainly its toxicological properties and finally its suitability for blood storage and component preparation are all part of the Fenwal evaluation. In fact there is no other product line within Travenol that requires so much of a plastic material as the Fenwal pack line. Think for a moment what a Blood-Pack® goes through; not only in our manufacturing process where it is heated, sealed, etc., but also in the hands of the ultimate consumer where it is filled, spun, squeezed, cooled if not frozen and then transported all over the place. PL-146® has been and probably will be for the foreseeable future one of the gold standards in the plastic formulations area. But other formulas have emerged from Fenwal including PL-732® and PL-1240®. What separates these formulations from PL-146® is primarily the characteristic of higher gas permeability. Very clearly platelet concentrates need greater gaseous interaction with the environment in order to successfully survive longer storage periods and PL-1240® and to a much greater degree PL-732® present that permeability to platelet concentrates [2]. The PL-732® formulation has been key in the development of the CS-3000® closed system apheresis kit which permits 5 day storage of single donor platelet concentrates [3]. Another plastic formulation that has been utilized by Fenwal is the PL-325® which was designed into a special frozen plasma container, developed jointly by the Blood Transfusion Service at Elstree facility in the UK and Fenwal, which permits the freezing and rapid automatic removal of the plasma from the container in an optimal fashion. Will there be other plastics? Currently, we are looking at nearly a half dozen new plastic formulations as to their applicability for Fenwal applications if not other medical device applications but the process is not rapid and both the company's and the markets', requirements are tough.

Juices

The number of anticoagulant solutions and preservation solutions that Fenwal has introduced over the years are numerous indeed. In fact the list of ACD, CPD, CPDA-1, SAG, SAG-M and ADSOL is really a partial listing when one considers the specials we have also developed for individual customers [4,5]. The question then is what might the customer need that current anticoagulants/preservation solutions may not give them? That is, is there an ADSOL II? Is there a SAG-M II? The essence of the matter comes down mainly to the function of the red blood cell. In the past we have concentrated on maintaining ATP levels and extending storage time. Now there is renewed interest in the function of 2,3 DPG and the red cell's ability to function immediately upon transfusion. Work is going on in this direction, but it is sort of a good news, bad news situation. The ability to maintain ATP and 2,3 DPG at the same time is not an easy balancing act, one being sacrificed at the expense of the other. We are optimistic that a product can be developed that both gives high 2,3 DPG levels and maintains red blood cells over an extended period of time. The question then is what is this product's position in the marketplace? It is a more costly product to make and with studies concerning the clinical efficacy of higher 2,3 DPG levels seemingly impossible to design, what will be the market acceptance of this new preservation solution? We would probably all agree that this is better medicine but are we willing to make this formulation part of our everyday routine? Other areas of exploration for us in the juices area include additive solutions for platelet concentrates which might give us "better" platelets and certainly liberate additional plasma for the blood center and systems which will address the optimization of citrate content, the use of heparin and other system improvements.

Innovation

As has been eluded to in the discussion of improved preservation solutions many innovations are possible but the innovations must be of demonstratable market value. A good example of a product which was innovative but which did not achieve acceptability in the marketplace was Fenwal's product FRES™. Here was a rejuvenating solution for red cells that stimulated market interest but sold very poorly and ended up being discontinued. The challenge for people in marketing is to separate what is interesting from what is needed. One innovation we are currently developing and one for which we have received much encouragement is the sterile connector [6]. The sterile connector is comprised of two identical plastic parts connected to whatever containers or devices you wish to effect a sterile connection between (fig. 1). The parts are first mechanically locked together and then this connection is inserted into a piece of hardware which focuses a light beam on a part of the connection to effect a fusion and flow path between the two sides (fig. 2).

IDENTICAL PARTS ARE MECHANICALLY LOCKED

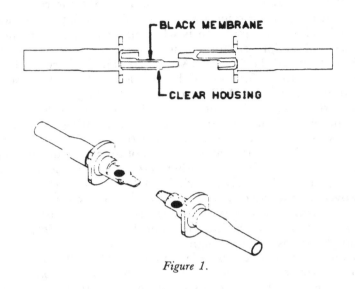

BLACK MEMBRANE

CLEAR HOUSING

Figure 1.

HARDWARE COMPONENT

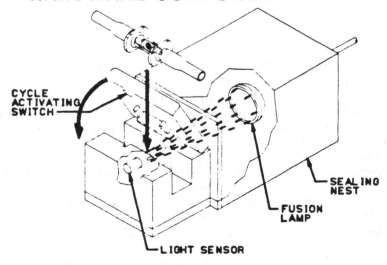

CYCLE ACTIVATING SWITCH

SEALING NEST

FUSION LAMP

LIGHT SENSOR

Figure 2.

That point of the connector is made out of a black plastic as opposed to the rest of the connector which is made out of clear plastic so that the heat is absorbed in the correct area. At 240°C the plastic melts fusing the connection and effecting sterility. The hardware device senses the hole formation and ends the fusing process when the hole is detected. Should a hole not be detected then the device signals a misconnection. Very briefly, a number of tests have been undertaken to ensure what we have here is in fact a sterile connection and Fenwal defines a sterile connection as a connection equal in sterility to that level we insist upon in our Blood-Pack® products, that is, having a log reduction sterility factor of 10^6. We have challenged sterile connections in various ways by smearing microbes on the black surfaces, by subjecting a completed connection to microbial ingress, by passing blood components through and comparing pre and post data, by placing connectors in the hands of non-laboratory types to understand functional integrity and reliability, and finally an entire battery of particulate matter and toxicology studies to ensure the safety of the device [7]. The Fenwal sterile connector system indeed looks promising. How might we use such a system? An Add-a-Pack or "build your own" system might be appropriate, certainly its use in pediatric applications will be considered, its use in cell separation systems is foreseen and certainly in other medical device applications where sterility is very important.

Future

As I see the future of blood banking and Fenwal, I look to see a blending of automation, which cell separators represent, and blood pack technology. If we examine the costs of running a blood collection center today, we see that only a small number of dollars go to material costs and a very large number of dollars go to salary and fringes as well as overhead. It is among these portions of the cost equation that Fenwal feels a blending of technologies may prove effective. In evaluating our experience with the CS-3000® Blood Cell Separator, we see automation as a means to leverage donor resources. For instance, in the United States where there are 12.3 million units of whole blood collected each year, if 8% of those collections could be performed on the CS-3000® with a closed system kit, virtually all the platelet needs of the United States could be filled. Imagine the effect of such a program on the logistics of mobile collections and the undoing of all the planning between collecting in doubles versus triples. Is this achievable? Of all donations 20% are collected in fixed sites now, so the donors are there. What is needed perhaps is some innovative thinking and adjusting of standard procedures to leverage what automation can bring to blood collection systems. If you do all the platelets at fixed sites, then automated systems to address red cell and plasma collections at mobile sites will be developed. But automation is not without risks. While it may reduce labor and leverage the donor base, it must be cost effective in today's environment. Additionally, automation requires capital so it is an investment not to be taken lightly.

And, as we approach the era of recombinant DNA blood components such as factor VIII and albumin, how much do we invest in automation to harvest human plasma? Undoubtedly, however, automation will enter blood banking more in the future not only from the perspective of the collection but also in terms of integrating collection, testing and information handling in one smooth system [8].

Other areas that Fenwal sees growing and will be participating in the coming years is bone marrow collection and tissue banking. We will leverage our experience with plastics and juices into better ways of collecting and processing bone marrow, bone, skin and other tissues which is essentially a glass or metal container business which is the anathema to anybody at Fenwal.

Finally, no matter what changes occur in our environment or markets, one principle remains constant – product quality must be superior and we at Fenwal define product quality as a feature of every product which is invisible to the user but permits him to accomplish his job in a repeatable fashion without interference. We are absolutely commited to this and it is perhaps the most important product we can bring to market.

Fenwal very much enjoys its relationship with people such as the blood-banking community and we look forward to a very bright future working together to provide the best in collection and processing products, services and systems. We encourage your input, suggestions and help as we go forward because you are very much the market that has the needs and together we can find answers to those needs.

References

1. Walter CW. Invention and development of the blood bag. Vox Sang 1984: 318 – 24.
2. Murphy S, Kahn RA, Holme S, Phillips GL, Sherwood W, Davisson W, Buchholz DH. Improved storage of platelets for transfusion in a new container. Blood 1982;60:194 – 200.
3. Buchholz DH, Porten JH, Grode G, Lin AT, Barber T, Brda J, Kozar I. Extended storage of single-donor platelet concentrate collected by a blood cell separator. Transfusion 1985;25:557 – 62.
4. Button LN, Kevy SV. The development and acceptance of the anticoagulant. CPD. Vox Sang 1985;48:122 – 5.
5. Heaton A, Miripol J, Aster R, Hartman P, Dettart D, Rzad L, Grapka B, Davisson W, Buchholz DH. Use of Adsol® preservation solution for prolonged storage of low viscosity AS-1 red blood cells. Br J Haematol 1984;57:467 – 78.
6. Smit Sibinga CTh. Sterile docking devices. International Congress ISH-ISBT, Budapest 1982:58 (abstract).
7. Bacehowski D, Brown R, Boggs D, Cerny D, Granzow D, Buchholz DH. Development of a docking device to permit the sterile transfer of fluids between two unconnected containers. Transfusion 1985;25:477 (abstract).
8. Wolf CFW, Salamon JL, Brown K, Brodheim E. Hospital blood bank automation: A bar code-based patient and blood product system. Transfusion 1985;25:495 (abstract).

IN VIVO KINETICS IN AUTOLOGOUS TRANSFUSION OF RED CELLS PRESERVED 42 AND 49 DAYS AT +4°C IN PAGGSS AND IN ADSOL-AS1

L. Noel*, O. Messian*, G. Fabre**, J. Saint-Blancard**, B. Saint-Paul*

Extending the storage period of red blood cells at +4°C will help to improve the supply in some countries and will simplify the development of autologous transfusion programmes. Transfused red blood cells (RBC) are expected to act as efficient substitutes; this implies the same capacity to bring oxygen to the tissues, and the same life span as normal red blood cells. The control of these properties is mandatory to the validation of new red cell preservation procedures. As the oxygen dissociation curve is a function of the 2,3 DPG level which will be regenerated if needed after 12 to 48 hours in the circulation [1], the RBC ability to actually deliver oxygen to the tissues depends on the red cells capacity to survive in the circulation. We studied the in-vivo kinetics of RBC stored at +4°C in ADSOL-AS1 (Fenwal Laboratories) and PAGGSS (Biotest Laboratories) for 42 and 49 days in autologous transfusion. PAGGSS and ADSOL-AS1 are two optional additive solutions according to the concept pioneered by Lovric and Högman [2,3]. ADSOL-AS1 is a variant of Högman's SAG-Mannitol [4] and PAGGSS contains phosphate adenine guanosine glucose saline and sorbitol according to Spielman and Seidl [5].

Measurement of the in vivo recirculation of preserved RBC has been a controversial subject over the last few years [6,7]. In order to give an accurate 24 hour recirculation percentage, the time zero amount of injected labelled cells in the circulation must be determined. If one relies on a log linear back-extrapolation at time zero from samples collected between 5 and 20 minutes after reinjection, assuming a simple log linear kinetics within this period, an immediate exaggerated destruction of stored RBC during the very first minutes might be overlooked (fig. 1). In order to take into account such a possibility we used a double isotope technique according to Mollison [8]: an aliquot of stored RBC labelled with 51Chromium (51Cr) was reinjected simultaneously with an aliquot of fresh autologous RBC labelled with 99mPertechnetate (99mTc). Thus an independant measure of the RBC volume could be obtained from the dilution of the 99mTc.

The ratio Rm, derived from the RBC volume as measured with stored cells over the RBC volume measured with fresh cells, is used to correct an eventually underestimated 51Cr time 0 activity.

* Centre de Transfusion et d'Hématologie de Versailles.
** Centre de Transfusion Sanguine des Armées, Jean Juiliard.

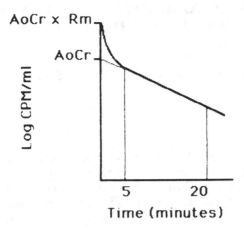

Figure 1. Diagram showing how an exaggerated destruction of transfused stored RBC within the first five minutes could be ignored if a single label is used. The Rm ratio is the ratio of the RBC volume as measured with the labelled stored cells (^{51}Cr) to an independent measure of the actual RBC volume (fresh cells, ^{99m}Tc).

Material and methods

450 ml of whole blood was collected in the primary bag of a closed triple bag system from 29 healthy male volunteers duly informed of the means and objectives of the study. The primary bag contained 63 ml of anticoagulant citrate phosphate dextrose solution, one of the satellite bags 100 ml of ADSOL-AS1 solution (n = 12) or PAGGSS solution (n = 17). Within 6 hours, RBC concentrates and platelet poor plasmas were prepared after centrifugation at 6000 g for 10 minutes at 20°C (RC-3B, Sorvall Instruments) and RBC concentrates resuspended in ADSOL-AS1 or in PAGGSS. Resuspended packed red cells with a mean hematocrit of 0.62 were immediately stored at + 4°C with a daily agitation, reproducing standard blood bank conditions for 42 or 49 days.

At the end of the storage period, just before labelling, preserved red cell concentrates were filtered through a standard 170 μ filter as we had previously noticed macroaggregates or small clots potentially harmful to the recipient [9]. Furthermore this filtration reproduces actual transfusion conditions. After thorough mixing, an aliquot of approximately 8 ml was labelled with 1295 KBq (35 μCi) of ^{51}Cr. The method used was according to the guidelines developed by the International Committee on Standardization in Hematology [10]. Meanwhile the volunteers were drawn 8 ml of blood on a trace of heparin and the fresh RBC were labelled with 925 kBq (25 μCi) of ^{99m}Tc according to Bardy [11], using a commercial stannous pyrophosphate kit (TCK 11 International-CIS, CEA). Both red cell suspensions were mixed together and injected with the same syringe. A single dilution of the mixtures was counted in order to limit errors.

Samples were collected from the opposite arm at 5, 10, 15 and 20 minutes post reinjection then at 24 hours, day 2, 4, 7, 14, 21, 28. Counting was realized on a single well 3 inches gamma counter (LKB or Intertechnique) with a precision in excess of 99%.

A correction was made for ^{51}Cr spill over in the Technetium channel. Activities were expressed in cpm/ml RBC according to the hematocrit. A_0Cr is the extrapolation at time zero of the logarithmic linear regression of ^{51}Cr activities at 5, 10, 15 and 20 minutes (least squares method). The RBC volume was calculated from the injected ^{51}Cr activity related to A_0Cr. The mean ^{99m}Tc activity of samples collected at 5, 10 and 15 minutes was used as the time zero ^{99m}Tc activity and the RBC volume as measured with fresh cells, similarly calculated. $A_0Cr \times Rm$ was used as the 100% time zero transfused cells activity in the circulation. The 24 hour sample activity related to this value, gave the 24 hour percentage of survival.

The T_{50} of the injected stored RBC was calculated as well as the T_{50} of the stored RBC fraction surviving after the first 24 hours (fig. 2).

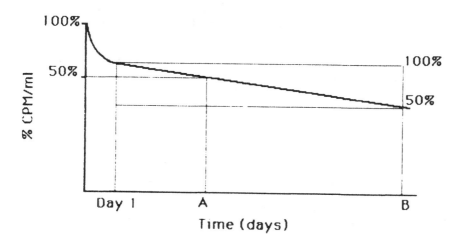

Figure 2. Diagram of a typical posttransfusion RBC kinetics study showing in a the T_{50} of the injected stored RBC and in B the T_{50} of stored RBC surviving beyond the first 24 hours.

Results

The 24 hour survival values for RBC stored for 42 and 49 days in PAGGSS and in ADSOL-AS1 are shown in figure 3. The 24 hour survival was $75 \pm 7\%$ (mean $\pm$ 1SD) for RBC preserved 42 days in ADSOL-AS1 (n = 5), $82.2 \pm 11.6\%$ after 42 days in PAGGSS (n = 7), $72 \pm 6.5\%$ after 49 days in ADSOL-AS1 (n = 5) and $78.2 \pm 8.5\%$ after 49 days in PAGGSS (n = 10).

The RBC volume measured with ^{99m}Tc is normally 1 to 3% larger than the RBC volume measured with ^{51}Cr when fresh red cells are used. This

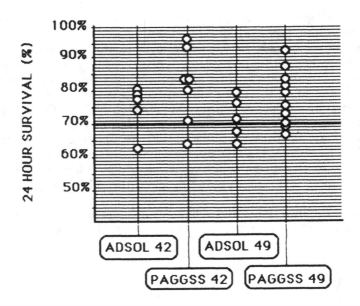

Figure 3. Twenty-four-hour survival levels of RBC stored in ADSOL-AS1 for 42 days (n = 5) and 49 days (n = 5), and in PAGGSS for 42 days (n = 7) and 49 days (n = 10).

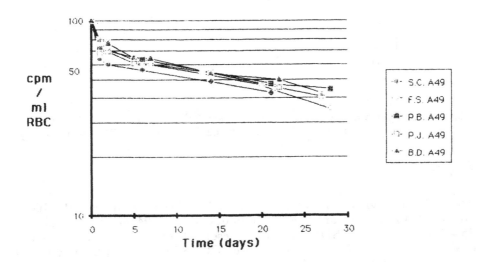

Figure 4. Autologous in vivo kinetics of RBC preserved for 49 days in ADSOL-AS1 and labelled with ^{51}Cr.

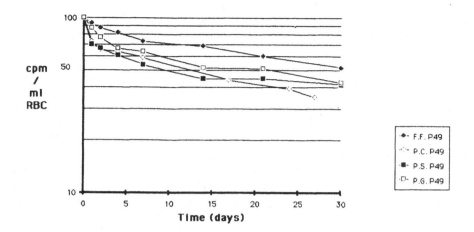

cpm / ml RBC

Time (days)

Legend:
- F.F. P49
- P.C. P49
- P.S. P49
- P.G. P49

Figure 5. Autologous in vivo kinetics of RBC preserved for 49 days in PAGGSS and labelled with [51]Cr.

has been observed by others and can be explained by an early elution of the label [12,13]. Rm ratios are 0.98 ± 0.02 with PAGGSS 42, 1×0.05 with ADSOL-AS1 42, 1.01 ± 0.03 with PAGGSS 49 and 1.05 ± 0.07 with ADSOL-AS1 49. After 49 days Rm ratios tend to increase.

The time in days for 50% of the ^{51}Cr activity at 24 hours to disappear from the circulation can be discribed as the half life of transfused RBC surviving after 24 hour assuming a mono exponential kinetics. In the four procedures studied this value was similar to fresh red cells half life when no correction for chromium elution is applied $(30 \pm 4 \text{ days})$. On a semilogarithmic graph of ^{51}Cr activities in the time, the survival curve after 24 hours is indeed usually linear (fig. 4). However we observed that in some cases with PAGGSS after 49 days the kinetics beyond the first 24 hours did not appear to be linear (fig. 5). A log/linear regression of ^{51}Cr activities of samples from day 2 to day 28, extrapolated to 24 hours ran clearly under the measured 24 hours percentage of survival.

The time in days at which 50% of th ^{51}Cr activity initially injected had disappeared was 20.2 ± 5.1 with PAGGSS 42 days, 19.1 ± 5.4 with ADSOL-AS1 42 days, 16.5 ± 3.4 with ADSOL-AS1 49 days, 18.6 ± 6.5 with PAGGSS after 49 days.

Discussion

We studied the in vivo kinetics of autologous RBC preserved 42 and 49 days in PAGGSS and in ADSOL-AS1 using a ^{51}Cr and ^{99m}Tc double label technique. Destruction of transfused cells in the first minutes after reinjection, as shown by a descrepancy between the two labels, was detected but in a lesser amount than described by Valeri with ADSOL-AS1 at 49 days, using a ^{51}Cr and ^{125}Iodine albumine double label technique [14]. We obtained with ADSOL-AS1 after 49 days on 5 individuals figures almost identical to those published by Beutler and West [15]. The 24 hour percentage of recirculation of RBC preserved in PAGGSS for 49 days confirms data obtained by Repucci with a single isotope technique [16] and comply with the recent FDA criterium requiring a minimum of a mean 75% 24 hour survival in 10 individuals. However the large standard deviation should be noted. Significant differences between donors in viability of red cells is a well known fact [17]. A stringent interpretation of the classical 70% criterium requiring the mean 24 hours recirculation minus two standard deviations to be above 70% is not met in these experiments.

Long term kinetics studies confirm that red cells surviving beyond the first 24 hours have a half life comparable to that of normal fresh cells. We noticed with PAGGSS after 49 days that in some individuals storage linked destruction seems to extend beyond the first 24 hours. This has not been observed with ADSOL-AS1 or with PAGGSS at 42 days. Is this storage linked phenomenon pure destruction or trapping and release? This needs confirmation and further studies. Half of the initially injected ^{51}Cr activity had disappeared after more than two weeks.

Conclusion

The ^{51}Cr and ^{99m}Tc double label technique appeared to be easy to use and did demonstrate some degree of early exaggerated posttransfusion destruction after 49 days of storage. Even if the use of a second label introduces a new source of errors in the result (variation in the ^{99m}Tc elution rate in healthy subjects) we believe that a double label technique should be prefered whenever investigating new procedures.

PAGGSS appeared to maintain the viability of stored red blood cells after 49 days at an acceptable level by present standards.

The large inter-donor variability requires a greater number of measures in the same conditions and there is no consensus today on a standardized methodologic technique. Paired studies in the same individual to compare an investigational product with a license recognized product is an elegant method though putting an extra strain on the volunteers. The possibility of intra-donor variations needs a careful study.

Finally, there appears to be a need for further studies of the posttransfusion kinetics of preserved RBC beyond the first 24 hours as well as correlation with morphological, biochemical, and rheological data.

References

1. Mollison PL. Blood transfusion in clinical medicine. 7th ed. Oxford. Blackwell Scientific Publications 1983.
2. Lovric VA, Prince B, Bryant J. Packed red cell transfusions improved survival quality and storage. Vox Sang 1977;33:346 – 50.
3. Högman CF, Hedlund K, Zetterstr8m MD. Clinical usefulness of red cells preserved in protein poor mediums. N Engl J Med 1978;299:1377 – 82.
4. Högman CF, Hedlund K, Salheström Y. Red cell preservation in protein-poor-media. III. Protection against in vitro hemolysis. Vox Sang 1981;41:274 – 81.
5. Spielmann M, Seidl S. Summary of clinical experiences in Germany with preservative anticoagulant solutions with newer additives. In: Greenwalt TJ, Jamieson GA eds. The human red cell in vitro. Grune & Staton, New York 1974:217 – 54.
6. Heaton A, Miropol J, Aster R, Hartman P, Dehart D, Rzad L. Use of adsol preservation solution for prolonged storage of low viscosity AS-1 red blood cells. Br J Haematol 1984;57:467 – 78.
7. Valeri CR. Measurement of viable ADSOL-preserved human red cells. N Engl J Med 1985;312:1392 – 3.
8. Mollison PL. Methods of determining the posttransfusion survival of stored red cells. Transfusion 1984;24:93 – 6.
9. Noël L, Messian O, Fabre G. Red cell survival techniques. Transfusion 1985;25:180(letter).
10. ICHS, International Committee for Standardization in Haematology. Recommended methods for radioisotope red cell survival studies. Blood 1971;38:378 – 86.
11. Bardy A, Fouye H, Gobin R. Technetium 99 labelling by means of stannous pyrophosphate application to bleomycin and red blood cells. J Nucl Med 1982;16:435 – 7.
12. Beutler E, West C. Measurement of the viability of stored red cells by the single-isotope technique using ^{51}Cr. Analysis of validity. Transfusion 1984;24:100 – 4.
13. Jones J, Mollison PL. A simple and efficient method of labelling cells with ^{99m}Tc for determination of red cell volume. Br J Haematol 1978;38:141 – 8.
14. Valeri CR. Measurement of viable ADSOL-preserved human red cells. N Engl J Med 1985;312:377 – 8.
15. Beutler E, West C. Measurement of viable ADSOL-preserved human red cells. N Engl J Med 1985;312:1392(letter).
16. Repucci AJ, Sondag-Thull D, Betz C, Andre A. Packed red blood cells stored in PAGGS sorbitol medium (Biotest): in vitro and in vivo survival studies. 18th Congr. International Society of Blood Transfusion, Karger Ag Basel 1984:174.
17. Dern RJ, Gwinn RP, Wiorkowski JJ. Studies on the preservation of human blood. Variability in erythrocyte storage characteristics among healthy donors. J Lab Clin Med 1966;67:955.

PLATELET FUNCTION DURING STORAGE IN PVC BAGS WITH INCREASED GAS PERMEABILITY

K. Koerner

Introduction

In the last few years new plastics have been formulated to increase the gas permeability properties of containers used in storing platelets. Various studies have shown that increased gas permeability has allowed the liquid preservation of platelets to be increased to 5 days [1 – 7]. An indicator of viability and function of platelets is the pH. Some studies have shown that a decrease of the pH-value below 6.0 is correlated to loss of viability of platelets. Maintaining pH at or near physiological levels, and decreasing glucose consumption with decreasing lactate production have increased platelet storage time and conserved platelet viability. Improved gas permeability has also been enhanced by increasing the surface area of the container [8].

We have studied platelet storage in a PVC container, the blood bag currently in use, which has a thinner foil of 20% than the standard bag. We compared our in-vitro results for those found using a container of standard thickness made of DEPH (di-2-ethyl-hexylphtalate) plasticized PVC and bags using TOTM (tri-2-ethyl-hexyl-trimellitate) plasticized PVC.

Methods

Preparation of platelet concentrate

Whole blood, 450 ml, was collected from normal healthy donors not taking drugs including salicylates. All units were drawn on CPDA-1 anticoagulants (Biotest Pharma, Frankfurt, FRG). Blood was centrifuged at 2400 xg for 4 minutes. Platelet rich plasma (PRP) was then pressed to the platelet satellite bag. Platelet concentrate (PC) was prepared by centrifugation of PRP at 1200 xg for 30 minutes. The platelet poor plasma was then removed into another bag leaving 70 ml of plasma with the platelet button. The button was allowed to stand undistrubed at room temperature for 60 – 90 minutes before carefully being resuspended by gentle manual agitation. The platelet concentration was adapted to $1.3 \times 10^{11}/l$ in all experiments.

Platelet bags*		
Nr.	Wall thickness	Material/plasticizer
F76	0.36	PVC/DEHP
F763	0.30	PVC/DEHP
F702	0.36	PVC/TOTM
F76/702	0.36	PVC/DEHP – PVC/TOTM label

DEHP : di-2-ethylhexylphtalat
TOTM : tri-2-ethylhexyl-trimellitat

* BIOTEST Pharma, Frankfurt, FRG

Figure 1. Composition of different bags used for platelet storage.

Storage of platelets

Platelet concentrates were stored at 20 – 22°C with agitation using a platelet mixer (Fisher model 348, Fisher Scientific, Munic, FRG) with 2.4 rpm circular rotation.

Types of bags used

Four different platelet bags were used (Biotest Pharma) (fig. 1):
1. F76-DEHP plasticized PVC, 0.36 mm thick.
2. F763-DEHP plasticized PVC, 20% thinner than the standard F76 bag.
3. F702 – TOTM plasticized PVC.
4. F76/F702 – the labelled side of DEHP plasticized PVC and the unlabelled side of TOTM plasticized PVC.

The dimensions and surface area of all four containers were the same. The volume was 300 ml.

The relative gas permeability is different for the standard bag to the three other bags [9]. If the gas permeability is assumed as 100% for the F763 bag, then the standard F76 bag is 80%, the F702 bag 95% and the F76/F702 bag 100%.

Platelet function tests

Samples of PC were drawn aseptically from the bags at daily intervals. Platelets were counted on a TOA counter (TOA-Medical Electronics, Japan). Platelet function tests were performed in duplicate. PC was diluted to $300 - 400 \times 10^9/l$ with autologous platelet poor plasma (PPP). The pH was measured using a micro pH electrode (EA147) fitted to a Metrohm E603 pH meter (Filderstadt, FRG).

Readings were done immediately after sampling at room temperature. Plasma glucose and plasma lactate concentrations were determined using the enzyme "test combination" of Boehringer (Mannheim, FRG). Platelet response to hypotonic shock measured as the rate of recovery, platelet aggregation induced by ADP or collagen and measurement of ^{14}C-serotonine uptake were done on PC as previously described [10].

In-vivo tests were carried out using the same blood bag materials and the same method for preparing PC by Repucci and Frere, University of Liège and Red Cross Blood Transfusion Center, Liège, Belgium [11]. Platelets were labelled with ^{51}Cr for estimating platelet in-vivo survival [12]. Platelet survival and platelet recovery of volunteers and the corrected count increment after transfusion into thrombocytopenic patients were determined after a storage time of 5 days.

Results and discussion

After 3 days storage platelet counts were similar in all bags tested. Platelet counts in the standard thickness F76 bag decreased by up to 20% after 5 days due to aggregates, where as there was only a slight 5 to 10% decrease in the platelet count in the other three containers over the 5 day period.

The pH values were at about the same average in the four containers at the beginning of the storage period (fig. 2). The pH fell below 7.0 on the first day of storage in the standard F76 container. Platelets stored in the other three bags had slightly increased pH values on the second and third days. The pH did not fall below 7.0 in any of the three containers over the 5 days period storage.

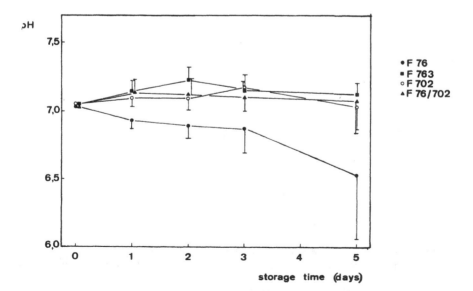

Figure 2.   pH values in plasma during platelet storage in 4 different bags ($\bar{x} \pm$ sd).

Table 1. Plasma glucose and lactate concentration during storage of platelets.

Day	F76	F763	F702	F76/702
Plasma glucose (mg(dl)				
(n = 6, × ± sd)				
3	233 ± 32	275 ± 33	275 ± 30	270 ± 25
5	110 ± 73	253 ± 23	226 ± 29	237 ± 60
Plasma lactate (mg/dl)				
3	156 ± 36	100 ± 10	117 ± 16	105 ± 3
5	269 ± 63	130 ± 63	148 ± 29	148 ± 29

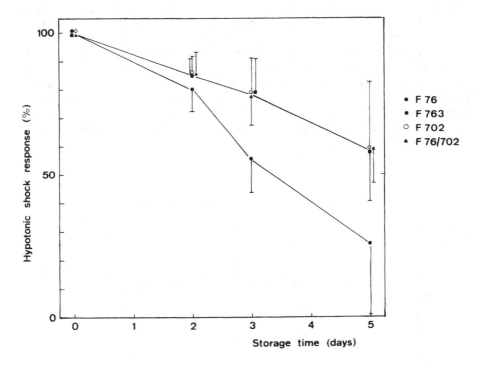

Figure 3. Hypotonic shock response of platelets during storage.

The glucose and lactate concentrations in plasma after 3 and 5 days of storage were shown in table 1. The glucose concentration of platelet concentrates stored in the standard thickness F76 plastic decreases more rapidly than that seen in the other 3 bags. On the other hand lactate levels increased at a greater rate in the F76 bag contrary to slower rates seen in the other bags tested.

The response to hypotonic shock solution decreased in all plastics over the observation period (fig. 3). A clear separation between the standard F76 container and the three other bags becomes apparent on the third day. After 5 days of storage the hypotonic shock responses of platelets stored in the thin-walled container is slightly better than that found on the third day in the standard thickness PVC container.

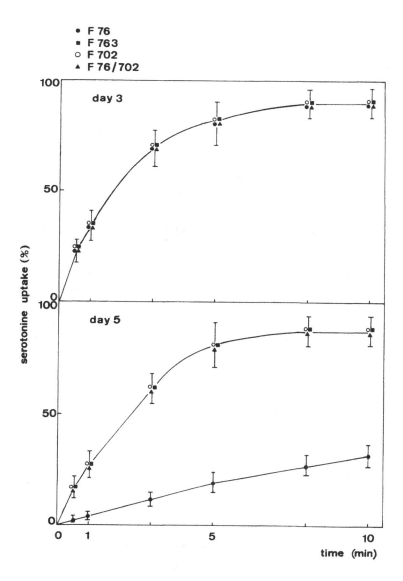

Figure 4. Kinetics of serotonine uptake during storage of platelet concentrates after 3 and 5 days.

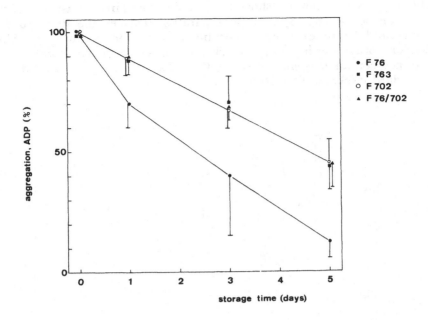

Figure 5. Aggregation induced with ADP during storage of platelets.

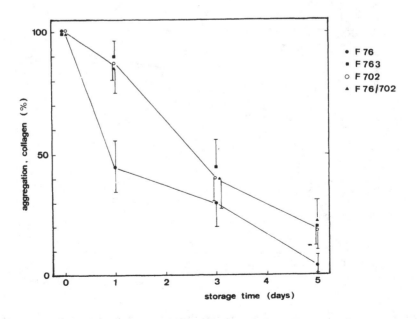

Figure 6. Aggregation induced with collagen during storage of platelets.

The kinetics of serotonine uptake of platelets after 3 days of storage were similar in all plastics studied (fig. 4). However, after 5 days storage there are great differences between the standard bag and the new bags. Platelet function in the F76 bag is significantly reduced whereas platelets stored in the three other containers maintained their serotonine uptake capacity through the 5th day.

The platelet aggregation response to ADP and collagen decreases during storage in all bags (figs 5,6). The aggregation response is better in the three new containers than in the standard material during storage.

Autologous transfusion of platelets labelled with ^{51}Cr in normal volunteers show that platelet viability is maintained during storage (table 2). The recovery was on the average about 50% for all three containers. The survival values of the thin-walled bag is slightly higher than for the other two bags. There are, however, no statistically significant differences between the values. These results are comparable to published data of platelet storage over a 5 day storage period [1 – 4].

Table 2. ^{51}Cr in vivo survival of platelets stored for 5 days (n = 6).

		In vivo recovery	Survival T½ (days)
Repucci et al.	1985		
F763		50 ± 11	3.8 ± 15
F76/F702		56 ± 9	3.6 ± 1.9
F702		49 ± 14	2.8 ± 0.2
Murphy et al.	1982	51	3.1
Simon et al.	1982	40	3.3
Archer et al.	1982	59	3.4 ± 1.5
Rock et al.	1984	58	5.1 ± 1.4

Table 3. In-vivo function of platelets in thrombocytopenic patients (n = 7).

	In-vivo recovery (%)	Corrected increment after 20 – 24 h × 10³/mm³
F763	32 ± 19	6.5 ± 4.9
F76/F702	35 ± 13	8.5 ± 3.3

Clinical results of transfusion of platelets stored 5 day in the thin-walled bag and the F76/F702 bag are shown in table 3. Platelets were transfused into thrombocytopenic patients with bone marrow failure or bone marrow suppresion induced by chemotherapy. Care was taken to select patients without sepsis, DIC, splenomegaly, fever, HLA antibodies or any combination of these.

The in-vivo recovery was at about 30% and the corrected increment measured after 20 hours was $6 - 8 \times 10^9/l$. This is not significantly different. These data are comparable with results already published for platelets stored 2 or 3 days in a standard blood bag or for platelets stored for 5 days in the new bags.

Summarizing we can say platelet concentrates can be stored at least over a 5 day period at room temperature in the thin-walled platelet PVC bag and still maintain viability.

References

1. Murphy S, Kahn RA, Holme S, Phillips GL, Sherwood W, Davisson W, Buchholz DH. Improved storage of platelets for transfusion in a new container. Blood 1982;60:194 – 200.
2. Simon TL, Nelson EJ, Carmen R, Murphy S. Extension of platelet concentrate storage. Transfusion 1983;23:207 – 12.
3. Archer GT, Grimsely PG, Jindra J, Robson JE, Jeribeiro A. Survival of transfused platelets collected into new formulation plastic packs. Vox Sang 1982;43: 223 – 30.
4. Rock G, Sherring VA, Tittley P. Five-day storage of platelet concentrates. Transfusion 1984;24:147 – 52.
5. Moroff G, Morse EE, Kakaiya RM. Platelet viability following storage for 5 days. Transfusion 1984;24:382 – 5.
6. Koerner K. Platelet function of room temperature platelet concentrates stored in a new plastic material with high gas permeability. Vox Sang 1984;47: 406 – 11.
7. Repucci AJ, Frere MC, Bevers EM et al. Platelet concentrate storage over five dags in the Biotest F76/F7092 bag in vitro, in vivo and clinical results. Proc. 18th congr. International Society of Blood Transfusion, Karger Ag, Basel 1984:126.
8. Kakaiya RM, Katz AJ. Platelet Preservation in large containers. Vox Sang 1984;46:111 – 8.
9. Walker WH, Netz M, Gänshirt KH. The gas permeability of various plastic sheetings intended for storage of platelet concentrates in bags. Proc. 18th congr. International Society of Blood Transfusion, Karger AG, Basel 1984:125.
10. Koerner K. Platelet function after shipment of room temperature platelet concentrates. Vox Sang 1983;44:37 – 41.
11. Repucci AJ, Koerner K, Frere M-C. Platelet storage over five days in a thin-walled DEHP plasticized PVC container. Transfusion: in press.
12. Aster RH, Jandel JH. Platelet sequestration in man. I. Methods. J Clin Invest 1969;43:843.

DEVELOPMENTS IN APHERESIS TECHNOLOGY

D.W. Huestis

Historical introduction

> "... to perform an act whereof what's past is prologue ..."
> (Shakespeare, The Tempest, II, i)

The earliest attempts at direct modification of the blood, or what we would now call hemapheresis, were carried out experimentally in France in the early years of this century [1], as indeed was the first recorded therapeutic intervention of this sort in a human [2]. The word "plasmapheresis" was coined soon after in the USA to designate the separation of plasma from whole blood with return of only the red cells to an animal subject [3]. The firest recorded clinical application of plasmapheresis was for the treatment of a patient with chronic renal disease, and was recorded as a success [2]. Later attempts on a variety of such patients were considered unsuccessful [4], and interest in this type of procedure seems to have waned after the mid-1920s [5] until the development of mechanical blood cell separators in the early 1950s. It is the biomechanical devices that are to be discussed today.

The first blood cell separator sprang from the conviction of Dr Edwin Cohn of Harvard University that all the various components and fractions of human blood could be stored better if they were first separated from the whole blood. He and his associates devised the Cohn fractionator for this purpose [6]. Some 16 fractionators were made and utilized in various blood research institutes [7]. This machine was designed to separate plasma from red blood cells, to wash red cells, or to collect platelets or white blood cells. The donor's blood was processed in batches, and the fractionator evolved and changed under Dr Cohn's associates and successors until it eventually gave birth to our familiar present-day Haemonetics intermittent flow blood cell separators, the first in 1971 to boast a fully disposable blood pathway and centrifuge bowl [8].

In the meantime, somewhat later, Judson and Freireich, with the IBM Corporation, developed the first continuous flow cell separator [9]. This was designed with a more specific aim in mind: The collection of granulocytes for transfusion to leukemic patients who became neutropenic and infected as a consequence of their chemotherapy. With the same purpose, Djerassi applied the principle of continuous blood flow through nylon fibers to entrap and subsequently elute granulocytes for transfusion, an ingenious noncentrifugal system [10].

In the late 1970s plasma filtration through porous membranes was devised as a means of separation of plasma from blood cells [11,12], and continuous flow systems of this sort are still under active development. The ultimate refinement is the perfusion of blood or plasma through filters or columns that selectively remove specific fractions by immunologic or physicochemical adsorption, thus enabling all other cells and plasma components to be returned to the donor or patient [13,14].

All of these biochemical systems have been devised in such ways that donor's or patient's blood is passed through the machine in an integral vein-to-vein, extracorporeal circuit that subjects the blood to a manipulative process, then returns the more or less modified blood to that person. General requirements for such devices are: Patient or donor safety, maintenance of sterility, ease of operation and maintenance, disposable blood pathway, reasonable economy, versatility, and portability.

Centrrifugal systems

Intermittent flow centrifugation (IFC)

The original IFC manufacturer (Haemonetics) produced and marketed worldwide a separator (its model 30) that offered a winning combination: mechanical simplicity, versatility, a disposable system, and reasonable cost [8], at a time when its competitors were comparatively complex, difficult to operate, expensive, and featured centrifuge bowls that had to be disassembled and sterilized with each use. A variant of the model 30 is still in production (the 30S), and many of the original ones are still in regular service. The heart of this device is the Latham disposable centrifuge bowl, which is a supremely efficient (if somewhat unselective) collector of buffy coats. Red cells and lymphocyte contamination may necessitate secondary centrifugation of the product obtained. As with other centrifugal systems, a macromolecular additive to donor blood is required for the collection of granulocytes. Dideco's IFC separator seems to be very similar, but few data have been published with respect to its efficiency. Plasma exchange with these systems tends to be a slow process because of the need for multiple operating cycles to remove adequate quantities of plasma.

Recent developments with this system have concentrated on microprocessor-controlled automation and technical modifications to improve the purity of platelet concentrates, these being now the blood component in major demand.

The principle technical improvement has been the development of a hydrodynamic step in the buffy coat collection, in effect an elutriative surge that boosts the platelets away from contaminating red cells and lymphocytes, providing a purer concentrate [15]. This is done by an additional pump that short-circuits a rapid surge of donor plasma into the centrifuge bowl just before the platelets are collected. Careful timing is essential, and computerized control is the best way to assure satisfactory operation of this surge system.

Automation of the IFC separator, the development of modified machines for plasma collection and for plasma exchange, and the addition of the surge procedure have brought these systems back to the forefront of cell separation technology, a position from which they had slipped a few years ago. Inevitably, the new machines are more complex and exacting from the service point of view than is the case with the older workhorse manual models.

It is likely that further refinements will take place and that IFC will remain a viable and useful procedure. Already we have seen the development of an all-purpose basic operating apparatus with selected microprocessor programmes and moduls for its disparate functions. One can envision its eventual use at a first stage for plasma perfusion filtration, or cryogelation procedures (see below). Simpler variants have been devised for the specific collection of plasma (with or without platelets), using a bowl of different geometry ("grenade" bowl). It is anticipated that these may become competitive with the manual methods of plasma collection that have persisted for economic reasons.

One of the inherent problems with all present IFC methods is their comparatively large extracorporeal blood volume. Perhaps computerized operation will allow the development of smaller, even miniaturized separation chambers that would overcome this significant limitation.

Continuous flow centrifutation (CFC)

The original NCI-IBM separator ("2990") was also manufactured essentially unchanged by Aminco as the "Celltrifuge", and some of both varieties are still in use [7]. Fenwal manufactured an improved Celltrifuge II, but this excellent machine has recently been discontinued. IBM then totally redesigned their CFC apparatus, with a different centrifugal geometry, as the model 2997 [16]. When IBM discontinued their biomedical division in 1984, the 2997 was taken over by Cobe Laboratories. Fenwal in the meantime produced their own automated, microprocessor-controlled CFC separator, the CS-3000.

In contrast to IFC separators, which are all based on the Latham bowl and its "grenade" variant, CFC systems offer striking geometric variety. The NCI-IBM, Celltrifuge I, and Celltrifuge II are clearly relatively minor variants of each other, the last-named having a disposable blood pathway, a seal-less rotary connection, and partial automation. But the others are markedly different.

The *Cobe/IBM 2997* has a rotating hoop-like or belt-like channel, including a component separation chamber that can be observed by the operator by means of a strobe light [16]. A very ingenious dual-stage variation of the regular channel is eccentrically shaped so that different centrifugal forces operate in the two halves of the channel, separating platelet-rich plasma from red cells in the first half, then extracting platelets from plasma in the second [17]. In its present form, this system is able to produce excellent platelet or granulocyte collections with the single-stage channel, and highly purified platelets with the dual-stage. In addition, the single-stage channel is probably the most reliable and fastest system for doing therapeutic plasma exchange. For cell component collection, this device has the disadvantage of requiring clos attention and constant minor adjustments by the operator, particularly with the dual-stage channel.

The *Fenwal CS-3000* is again totally different, with two chambers on opposite sides of the centrifuge bowl. Plasma containing platelets and/or granulocytes is separated from the red cells in the first container, then passes to the second, where the cells are extracted from the plasma. Connections between the two sides and with the fixed exterior are via an Adams-type sealless multilumen tube [18]. The controlling microprocessor is set for the alternative programmes, one for platelets, one for granulocytes. The default values can be overriden by the operator at the beginning of each procedure, permitting procedural alteration if desired.

This is undoubtedly the easiest cell separator to operate because of its degree of automation. It produces excellent granulocyte and platelet concentrates [19,20], the platelet programme giving platelet concentrates with a minimum of contaminating leukocytes or red cells. A disadvantage is that the operator cannot see the product as it collects inside the centrifuge, so that a malfunction occasionally produces surprising results. The original system was not well adapted to therapeutic cytapheresis or plasma exchange, but recent modifications promise to improve those functions.

Because existing systems work very well is no reason to suppose that improvements and new devices will not appear. The 2997 system calls out for microprocessor control, particularly for its dual-stage operation, and it would be surprising if that development were not forthcoming. As with IFC systems, although less urgently, a decrease in the overall size of equipment and extracorporeal volume would be welcomed. The Hemascience Company, which has already produced a miniature membrane-type plasma collector, is also developing a tiny continuous flow platelet collecting chamber with a volume of less than 10 ml.

Other centrifugal systems

Centrifugation combined with counterflow elutriation has had considerable application for the production of purified cell suspensions in research [21,22], and, as has already been pointed out, is the principle used in the IFC "surge" system for purifying platelet concentrates. This seems to be a technique with a great potential for the production of suspensions of one isolated cell type, which would be highly desirable for such purposes as adaptive immunotherapy with lymphocyte or monocyte lines, concentration of stem cells from peripheral blood, or removal of T lymphocytes from bone marrow collected for transplantation. The same principle has been applied to the purification of granulocyte concentrates for transfusion. Although commercial equipment has not yet been made available for this, the Beckman Company is currently working on its development.

Noncentrifugal systems

Membrane separation

Membrane technology has been used primarily in the field of hemodialysis, for the removal of non-protein-bound solutes from blood. More recently it has been increasingly applied to plasma exchange, primarily for removing protein-bound pathogenic substances. Obviously, to achieve this purpose, the membrane must be of such porosity as to permit the passage of plasma protein molecules while barring blood cellular elements. Many variables affect the operational efficiency of such systems (table 1).

Table 1. Efficiency factors in membrane plasma separation.

Geometry of flow pathway
Membrane structure and porosity
Blood flow rate
Pressure differential across the membrane
Area of blood-to-membrane exposure
Membrane composition: biocompatibility
Sterilizability
Cost

The membranes used are plastic structures of various thickness and porosity, sometimes with a thicker supporting membrane [12]. The configuration of devices using such membranes is either that of blood flowing between flat sheets of membrane (the ''sandwich'' type), or flowing through multiple capillary-like membranous tubules (hollow fiber type). With either type, the blood flow is parallel to the membrane surfaces with the flow of filtered plasma therefore at right angles or perpendicularly through the membrane. Sandwich-type, flat-sheet membranes require structural support to prevent dimensional changes as a result of hydrodynamic pressures, and may also require external compression or some other device to maintain uniform blood flow thickness and seal integrity. Hollow fibres have generally thicker walls and undergo minimal distortion at operational flow pressures.

The hydrodynamic force of blood flow results in a transmembrane filtration pressure leading to plasma flow through the membrane. This convective force towards the surface is countered by an opposing fluid shear force. These effects are complicated by a tendency for blood cells to pile up against the membrane, forming in effect a secondary membrane, the extent of which varies according to operating conditions [23]. Its importance is debatable. Mathematical formulas relating such variables have been derived, the practical value of which is still uncertain. A possible complicating factor is that of polarization concentration of protein molecules at the membrane surface, which may also affect the plasma flow through a membrane.

Membrane characteristics

In addition to permitting efficient plasma separation, membranes must be biocompatible. There should be no or minimal adverse effects on blood cells exposed to the membrane, no toxic effects, no harmful substances leached from the plastic, and minimal complement activation [24]. Various plastics and polymers are used.

The membrane should be porous enough to permit molecules as large as immune complexes to pass through, while retaining all blood cells. Permeability can be calculated as a "sieving coefficient", of which a figure of 1.0 defines total permeability, and zero indicates complete rejection. Maximum pore sizes of 0.2 to 0.6 microns are usually satisfactory. The sieving coefficient tends ot decrease as blood flow continues.

There is a greater variety of manufactured membrane separation devices than is the case with centrifugal blood cell separators. Of the hollow-fiber devices, there are about 11 manufacturers, five of them Japanese. There are three present manufacturers of flat plate type membrane separators (table 2). Most of these have a total extracorporeal volume of 115 to 285 ml.

Table 2. Manufacturers of membrane type plasma separators.

Hollow fiber type	Flat plate type
Dideco (Italy)	Cobe (USA)
Fenwal (USA)	Rhone-Poulenc (France)
Parker Beiomedical (USA)	Terumo (Japan)
Organon Teknika (USA)	
Fresenius (W. Germany)	Hemascience (USA)
Gambro (W. Germany)	(modified plate type)
Kuraray (Japan)	
Mitsubishi (Japan)	
Teijin (Japan)	
Asahi (Japan)	
Toray (Japan)	

One manufacturer (Hemascience, USA) has produced an ingenious modification of a flat plate device in which the very small membrane is of cylindrical configuration, inside a somewhat larger cylinder, and supported by an internal fluted cylinder to conduct away the filtered plasma [25]. Blood flows into the external chamber, while plasma filters through into the center. The unique feature of this device is that the membrane is constantly rotated by means of a magnet. This increases its filtration efficiency since the turbulence tends to prevent membrane clogging and cell buildup. This microprocessor-operated machine is designed for the collection of plasma, and can separate 500 ml of plasma very economically in about 30 minutes by an intermittent flow system [25]. A plasma exchange module has not yet been developed.

Filtration, adsorption, and precipitation systems

Obviously, the removal of whole plasma and its substitution or partial substitution by albumin or some similar product results in the depletion of many useful nonpathogenic proteins. In fact, the proportion may be about 100 g of useful protein removed with each gram of pathogenic material [14]. Furthermore, the replacement medium, usually albumin, is very expensive and its availability is dependent on commercial blood donation sources. More specific methods of extracting pathogenic substances from blood or plasma are highly desirable from the pathophysiologic as well as economic points of view. A great deal of work is indeed going on in this field, and represents an interesting marging and crossfertilization of hemapheresis and dialysis technologies.

A number of possibilities exists. For example, a simple off-line system can be employed for the removal of cryoglobulins and some immune complexes, whereby whole plasma is first removed from the patient by any process, substituting, for example, albumin. The plasma may then be subjected to a cryogelation or cryoprecipitating procedure, the cold insoluble material removed, and the modified plasma returned to the patient at the next plasmapheresis treatment [26]. The effectiveness of such a procedure is subject to many variables, e.g., the ability of the cryoglobulin to gel or precipitate at the selected temperature. Moreover, whatever the offline processing technique, these are cumbersome systems, requiring the capability to collect, treat, store, and separate large volumes of plasma.

Ultrafiltration

After the initial separation of plasma from red cells, the plasma is passed through a molecularly selective secondary membrane intended to allow passage of albumin but bar all large plasma protein molecules. This is also referred to as cascade filtration [27]. Presently available membranes can reject IgM proteins but usually allow passage of IgG, so their usefulness is limited to certain high molecular weight paraproteinemias or hypercholesterolemias. The need for exogenous albumin is obviated.

Problems with cascade filtration will probably be solved by the development of better membranes, i.e., those capable of barring passage of IgG molecules, and less prone to clogging by retained proteins. The possibility also exists of having several stages of progressively more selective membranes.

Cryogelation

In presently available systems (again, after initial plasma separation), aggregation and removal of certain plasma proteins is achieved by cooling at 4°C followed by micropore filtration at a pore size of about 0.1 micron [28]. Cryoglobulins and immune complexes can be removed by this technique. As with ultrafiltration, clogging of the micropore filter is a serious problem with this system. In addition, losses of noncryoglobulins (classical cryoprecipitate, fibrinogen complexes, entrapped gels) have continued to be a problem. Clinical application of the cryogelation technique has been reported predominantly in rheumatoid arthritis, but the studies have been neither controlled nor compared with conventional plasmapheresis.

Immunoadsorption

This technique has the possibility of exquisite specificity, i.e., of removing a pathogenic substance and nothing else [14]. The principle is of binding an antibody (usually covalently) to an inert solid matrix, then passing plasma through a column of such material while the bound antibody removes its corresponding antigen from the plasma. A wide variety of matrices can be used to hold sorbents of various sorts.

In addition to strictly immunologic sorbents, analogous biochemical and biophysical reactions can be employed in the same setting, sometimes with great efficacy. Much interest has attached to adsorption with Staphylococcal protein A, which has affinity for IgG classes 1, 2, and 4. There have been many experimental clinical applications of protein A immunosorption, not the least of which is in the area of cancer therapy: the attempt to bolster the immune defences against malignancy by releasing "blocked" tumoricidal antibodies [29]. The approach is controversial, but interesting and perhaps hopeful.

The whole field of immunoadsorption technology holds a great deal of promise, and is exciting much current research interest at both clinical and technological levels. It seems certain that a wide variety of sorbents will be developed for various clinical purposes. Table 3 lists some of the important current clinical applications.

Table 3. Some plasma immunoadsorption systems.

Sorbent	Matrix	Substance removed	Clinical disorder
Anti-LDL	Sepharose	LD lipoproteins (cholesterol)	Hypercholesterol-emia
Charcoal	Glass beads	Bile acids	Cholestatic pruritus
A and B substances	Silica	Anti-A, -B	Marrow trans-plant
DNA	Charcoalcollodion	ANA, immune complexes	Lupus
Protein A	Charcaolcollodion	Cancer "blocking agents", immune complexes	Cancer, Kaposi
Trytophane-PV alcohol resin		AChR antibody	Myasthenia gravis

Some important considerations with immunoadsorption are those of stability of columns, absorptive capacity, cost, possible elution of either matrix or sorbent into the patient's circulation, ability to recycle and re-sterilize (for re-use with the same patient), and selection of optimal flow geometry.

A special challenge is that of possible compatibility of immunoadsorbent materials with whole blood rather than plasma, which would have the enormous advantage that the preliminary separation of plasma from blood cells would become unnecessary. Some preliminary tests appear hopeful [30]. This would require some means of preventing the thrombocytopenia that is presently the result of many attempts at direct hemoperfusion.

Other systems
Various types of electrophoretic or electrodialytic techniques of plasma protein separation have been tried on a small scale [31] as have enzymatic systems. However, none of these seems to have reached a clinical stage and they remain as speculative possibilities for future development.

Conclusions

From a slow start over 30 years ago, cell separation technology has developed rapidly, and often in unforeseen ways. Intermittent flow systems originally intended to separate blood components for better storage were later seen as an optimal system for deglycerolizing frozen red cells, and are now primarily used to prepare platelets. A continuous flow machine originally designed for the collection of granulocytes evolved into the optimal centrifugal system for plasma exchange. Most newer cell separators are now microprocessor-controlled, thus reducing operator dependency. I am willing to predict a trend to miniaturization, to reduce extracorporeal blood volume. A merging of the efforts of nephrologists and hematologists has brought membrane plasma separation technology to a high level and still rising. Here too we can anticipate further geometric and membrane improvements, and probably miniaturization as well. Behind and supplementing both these cell and plasma separation technologies lie the exciting possibilities of more specific plasma modification by means of ultrafiltration, cryofiltration, and various immunoadsorption systems. Such manipulative technology amounts in essence to increasingly precise surgery on living blood.

References

1. Hédon E. Sur la transfusion, après les hémorragies, de globules rouges purs en suspension dans un sérum artificiel. Arch Med Exptl 1902;14:297 – 326.
2. Fleig C. L'auto-transfusion de globules lavés comme procédé de lavage du sang dans les toxhémies. Bull Mens Acad Sci Let. Montpellier 1909;1:4 – 9.
3. Abel JJ, Rowntree LG, Turner BB. Plasma removal with return of corpuscles (plasmaphaeresis). J Pharmacol Exp Therap 1914;5:625 – 41.
4. O'Hare JP, Brittingham HH, Drinker CK. Plasmaphaeresis in the treatment of chronic nephritis and uremia. Arch Int Med 1919;23:306 – 8.

5. Gilbert A, Tzanck A, Negroni. Emission sanguine avec restitution globulaire. Paris Med 1926;61:217 – 24.
6. Tullis JL, Surgenor DM, Tinch RJ et al. New principle of closed system centrifugation. Science 1956;124:792 – 7.
7. Huestis DW, Bove JR, Busch S. Practical blood transfusion (3rd ed), Boston: Little, Brown, 1981; Chapter 10.
8. Tullis JL, Tinch RJ, Baudanza P et al. Plateletpheresis in a disposable system. Transfusion 1971;11:368 – 77.
9. Freireich EJ, Judson G, Levin RH. Separation and collection of leukocytes. Cancer Res 1965;25:1516 – 20.
10. Djerassi I, Kim JS, Mitrakul C, Suvansri U, Ciesielka W. Filtration leukopheresis for separation and concentration of transfusable amounts of normal human granulocytes. J Med (Basel) 1970;1:358 – 64.
11. Solomon BA, Castino F, Lysaght MJ, Colton CK, Friedman LI. Continuous flow membrane filtration of plasma from whole blood. Trans Am Soc Artif Intern Organs 1978;24:21.
12. Stromberg RR, Hardwick RA, Friedman LI. Membrane filtration technology in plasma exchange. In: MacPherson JL, Kasprisin DO (eds). Therapeutic hemapheresis, Vol. I. Boca Raton FL, CRC Press, 1985:135 – 47.
13. Pineda AA (ed). Selective plasma component removal. Mount Kisco, NY: Futura, 1984.
14. Lysaght MJ, Samtleben W, Schmidt B, Gurland HJ. Closed-loop plasmapheresis. In: MacPherson JL, Kasprisin DO (eds). Therapeutic hemapheresis, Vol. I. Boca Raton FL, CRC Press, 1985:149 – 68.
15. Schoendorfer DW, Hansen LE, Kennedy DM. The surge technique: a method to increase purity of platelet concentrates obtained by centrifugal apheresis. Transfusion 1983;23:182 – 9.
16. Hester JP, Kellogg RM, Mulzet AP, Kruger VR, McCredie KP, Freireich EJ. Principles of blood separation and component extraction in a disposable continuous-flow single-stage channel. Blood 1979;54:254 – 68.
17. Reference 7, p. 329.
18. Stong CL. The amateur scientist. Scientific American 1975;233:120 – 4.
19. Loftus TJ, White RF, Huestis DW. Leukapheresis: increasing the granulocyte yield with the Fenwal CS-3000. J Clin Apheresis 1983;1:109 – 14.
20. Katz AJ, Genco PV, Blumberg N, Snyder EL, Camp B, Morse EE. Platelet collection and transfusion using the Fenwal CS-3000 cell separator. Transfusion 1981;21:560 – 3.
21. Lionetti FJ, Hunt SM, Lin PS, Kurtz SR, Valeri CR. Preservation of human granulocytes. II. Characteristics of granulocytes obtained by counterflow centrifugation. Transfusion 1977;17:465 – 72.
22. Contreras TJ, Jemionek JF, French JE, Shields LJ. Human granulocyte isolation by continuous flow centrifugation leukapheresis and counterflow centrifugation elutriation (DFCL/CCE). Transfusion 1979;19:695 – 703.
23. Chmiel H. The effects of pressure, flow conditions, and surface composition on the filtration properties of plasma separation modules. Plasma Ther Transfus Technol 1983;4:387 – 96.
24. Wegmüller E, Kazatchkine MD, Nydegger UE. Complement activation during extracorporeal blood bypass. Plasma Ther Transfus Technol 1983;4:361 – 71.
25. Rock G, Adams G, McCombie N, Tittley P. Plasmapheresis using the Hemascience Autopheresis-C plasmapheresis system. Proc. 18th congr. International Society of Blood Transfusion, Karger Ag, Basel 1984:130.

26. McLeod BC, Sassetti RJ. Plasmapheresis with return of cryoglobulin-depleted autologous plasma (cryoglobulinpheresis) in cryoglobulinemia. Blood 1980;55: 866 – 70.
27. Gregory MC, Shettigar UR, Kolff WJ. Theoretical value of cascade plasmapheresis. Plasma Ther Transfus Technol 1984;5:517 – 29.
28. Abe Y, Smith JW, Malchesky PS, Nosé Y. Cryofiltration: development and current status. Plasma Ther Transfus Technol 1983;4:405 – 14.
29. Terman DS. Immunoadsorbents in autoimmune and neoplastic disease. Plasma Ther Transfus Technol 1983;4:415 – 33.
30. Nilsson IM, Freiburghaus C, Sundquist SB, Sandberg H. Removal of specific antibodies from whole blood in a continuous extracorporeal system. Plasma Ther Transfus Technol 1984;5:127 – 34.
31. Bing DH. Chemical precipitation and removal of IgG and immune complexes. In: Pineda AA (ed). Selective plasma component removal. Mount Kisco, NY: Futura, 1984:139 – 68.

MANUFACTURING IN THE BLOOD BANK OF HIGH PURITY HEAT-TREATED FACTOR VIII CONCENTRATE FROM HEPARIN STABILIZED BLOOD AND ITS CONSEQUENCES FOR THE RED CELL AND SUPERNATE PLASMA COMPONENTS

K. Wallevik, J. Ingerslev, S. Stenbjerg Bernvil, S. Glavind Kristensen, J. Jórgensen, F. Kissmeyer-Nielsen

Introduction

The blood bank in Aarhus, Denmark, has since 1964 produced a freeze-dried cryoprecipitate in amounts of $1 - 2 \times 10^6$ IU factor VIII per year. The factor VIII depleted plasma has also been freeze-dried and used locally in conventional component therapy as an albumin substitute. Freeze-dried cryoprecipitate looses between 50 and 80% of its factor VIII activity by heating to 68°C for 24 h. Due to governmental regulations demanding for heat treatment of factor VIII preparations, we were obliged to discontinue production of cryoprecipitate and turn to the manufacturing of a high purity factor VIII concentrate.

For a year we have worked experimentally with the method originally developed in Groningen by Smit Sibinga and co-workers [1] using heparinized blood as the starting material, and we have succeeded in producing on the blood bank level a high purity factor VIII concentrate withstanding heat-treatment. Collecting blood in heparin, instead of in citrate has of course great implications on the organization of the blood bank. Before such changes are introduced it is necessary to demonstrate that the side products (red cell concentrate and factor VIII depleted plasma) are useful components.

Manufacturing of factor VIII

Figure 1, part A, summarizes the principal steps in the Groningen method. Crude plasma contains around 5 IU of heparin per ml plasma. The first precipitation is a conventional cryoprecipitation. After removal of the supernatant plasma, the cryoprecipitate is dissolved in residual plasma plus a small amount of saline.

The pooled cryoprecipitate is subjected to a second precipitation at 0°C for two hours. After centrifugation the supernatant is easily separated from the heavy precipitation and discarded. The second precipitate is dissolved at 37°C in a redissolving buffer, filtrated and freeze-dried in appropriate aliquots. Table 1 shows that we were able to reproduce the results of Smit Sibinga with respect to yield and specific activity. However, after dissolving of the second precipitation at 37°C, we were often hampered by a very heavy precipitation which rendered the final filtration difficult.

Heparin in plasma ($\sim$ 5 IU/ml)

A

1st precipitation = cryoprecipitation

Dissolving of cryoprecipitate in residual plasms
+ *"2nd precipitation solution"*

2nd precipitation at 0°C for 2 hours

Dissolving of precipitate (CIG) in *"redissolving buffer"*

3rd precipitation at 10°C for ½ hour

Filtration of supernatant, optional: addition of
protectives, freeze drying

Heat treatment (68°C, 24 – 72 hours)

B

Figure 1. The precipitation steps involved in the manufacturing of factor VIII according to the method of Smit Sibinga et al. (part A) and Danativ® , Aarhus (part B).

Table 1. Factor VIII preparation manufactured in Aarhus according to the method of:

	Smit Sibinga et al. [1]	Danativ®
Yield (%)	64 ± 3	52 ± 6
Specific activity (factor VIII IU/mg)	0.9 ± 0.3	2.4 ± 0.6
Fibrinogen (g/l)	14 ± 4	2.1 ± 0.4
Protein (g/l)	26 ± 9	11.2 ± 3.3

	Factor VIII IU/ml	Total protein g/l	Specific activity IU/mg
Redissolved CIG (37°C)	23.2	25	0.9
Supernatant after ½ hour precipitation at 10°C	23.6	14	1.7
Freeze-dried, reconstituted	23.6	14	1.7

Figure 2. Effect of a third precipitation of the redissolved CIG at 10°C on factor VIII activity and specific activity in the supernate. The CIG was dissolved in the buffer solution used by Smit Sibinga et al. with citrate omitted and Ca^{++} ions added to a molarity of 2 mM.

2nd Precipitation	a. ionic strength	
	b. pH value	
3rd Precipitation	a. ionic strength	
	b. $CaCl_2$ concentration	
	c. pH value	
	d. glycin concentration	
	e. glucose concentration	

Figure 3. Parameters checked systematically in experiments designed to constitute the conditions for optimal purification of factor VIII.

	Smit Sibinga et al. [1]	Danativ®
2nd Precipitation solution		
NaCl (g/l)	9	25
Heparin (IU/ml)	9	1
"Redissolving solution"		
Glycine (g/l)	10	15
NaCl (g/l)	3.4	0
Trisodium citrate (g/l)	6.6	0
Dextrose (g/l)	13	0
Phosphate (M)	0	0.015
$CaCl_2$ (M)	0	0.002*
Heparin (IU/ml)	1	0
pH value	6.5	6.4
Protectives		
Amino acids Amodex® (Pharmacia)] (ml/ml)	0	0.05

* $CaCl_2$ is added separately to avoid calciumphosphate precipitation.

Figure 4. Solutions applied in manufacturing of factor VIII concentrate according to the methods.

We recognized that the amount of this precipitate had no influence on the factor VIII activity which suggested that a third precipitation step should be introduced for further purification. Figure 2 shows an experiment in which the second "0°C-precipitate" (CIG) after dissolution is kept at 10°C for half an hour.

During this incubation a dense precipitate is formed. After freeze-drying of the supernatant the reconstituted concentrate has the same factor VIII

Table 2. Characterization of Danativ® factor VIII concentrate. Three batches of ~ 15,000 IU heat treated 24 hours at 68°C.

Factor VIII related parameters (IU/ml)	
Factor VIII (Chromogenic assay) CoA	25.2 ± 1.2
C	26.7 ± 4.2
v. W. factor (Risto cofactor)	20.8 ± 3.9
Proteins (g/l)	
Total protein	11.2 ± 3.3
Fibrinogen	2.1 ± 0.4
Fibronectin	4.1 ± 0.4
IgG	1.7 ± 0.2
Albumin	3.3 ± 0.3
Prothrombin	0.0023 ± 0.0007
Specific activity (factor VIII Coa) IU/mg	2.4 ± 0.6
Yield (factor VIII Coa) (%)	52 ± 6
Miscellaneous	
Reconstitution time (min)	4 ± 2
Appearance	dissolved; turbid
Appearance after 6 hours, 21°C	fine flocculation
pH	7.14 ± 0.05
Iso-agglutinins (titer)	
Anti-A 37°C saline	0
Anti-A 37°C + i.c.	4 – 8
Anti-B 37°C saline	0
Anti-B 37°C + i.c.	2 – 4
Heparin (IU/ml)	1.06 ± 0.05
Inorganic salts (μM/l)	
NA^{++}	61 ± 5.
K$^+$	1.9 ± 0.3
Ca^{++}	1.26 ± 0.02
Al^{+++}	1.8

activity per ml as the dissolved second precipitate, but the specific activity (factor VIII IU/mg protein) is doubled.

Figure 1 (B) illustrates the diversion from the Groningen method introducing the third precipitation step.

By varying the physico-chemical parameters of the solutions indicated in figure 3 we were able to select conditions during the second and third precipitation steps to give optimal purification of factor VIII. Figure 4 shows the buffers and conditions we have selected for preparing three batches of each 15,000 IU factor VIII produced for clinical trial of our heat treated factor VIII concentrate Danativ® .

There are substantial changes in the composition of the solutions of the Groningen method compared to our principle. Most important, Ca^{++} has

Table 3. Yields of factor VIII in three batches of Danate-H, each processed from 120 blood donations.

Batch	Plasma		Danate-H factor VIII concentrate			
	Amount ml × 10⁻³	Total factor VIII Coa IU × 10⁻³	Amount ml	Factor VIII Coa IU/ml	Total factor VIII Cao IU × 10⁻³	Yields* %
850924	32.3	29.0	558	24.7	13.8	47 (43)
850930	31.4	30.0	663	26.6	17.6	58 (55)
851001	32.7	29.9	649	24.2	15.7	52 (48)
				x̄ 25.2 ± 1.2		52 ± 6 (48 ± 6)

* The yield is calculated on basis of the factor VIII activity in citrated plasma collected in 10 ml pilot tubes just after draining of the blood portion. The average of factor VIII activity in the pooled starting plasma should according to the unit definition of factor VIII be one, but is measured to 0.92. The yields calculated on basis of the theoretical factor VIII content in plasma are indicated in the brackets.

been added to the redissolving solution as it protects factor VIII activity [2], and glucose was omitted as it turned out to caramelize during the heating procedure. Finally, a mixture of amino acids was added to the factor VIII concentrate before freeze-drying for protection of factor VIII during the heat treatment and for better solubility of the freeze-dried heat treated preparation [3].

Characterization of the factor VIII concentrate

Table 2 summarizes the characteristics of the three batches mentioned.

Factor VIII related parameters were comparable in the three batches. The concentrations of fibrinogen was low while the concentration of fibronectin was high compared to other high purity factor VIII preparations. The iso-agglutinin-titres were low and the solubility properties of the preparation were acceptable in spite of a small non soluble residue retained in the filter needle. The calculation of yield is shown in table 3.

The impact of heparinized blood on the blood bank routine

Because of the high yield and the high specific activity obtained in the heat treated factor VIII concentrate, we have decided to initiate a production based on the method described.

We designed a routine in which 3 – 4 technicians are able to process 96 blood donations per day for 4 days a week. The fifth day is used for the final pooling and preparing of a week batch of some 50,000 units of factor VIII.

Table 4. Heparin in freeze dried plasma products after reconstitution in H_2O.

	IU/ml
Plasma (300 ml)	3.8 ± 0.4
Factor VIII concentrate (25 ml)	2.8 ± 0.4
Factor VIII concentrate 68°C 24 hours (25 ml)	2.2 ± 0.2

The heparin content measured in the derived blood components is shown in table 4. The heat treated factor VIII concentrate contains a total of 40 – 70 IU of heparin in the reconstituted 500 IU solution. This is equal to the quantity found in many commercial high purity preparations and will be of no clinical importance.

We decided to combine the SAGMAN storing conditions with the heparin stabilized blood as shown in figure 5. The main bag contains 1,500 units of heparin in 300 ml phosphate buffered saline (as used in the Groningen method). The "SAGMAN bag" further contains 10% of the "main bag" CPD of the original "SAGMAN four bag system". Plasma is collected in one of the dry bags, buffy coat in the other. One hundred ml SAGMAN-COD is drained into the erythrocyte concentrate to make an erythrocyte suspension which apart from the heparin and phosphate, is close to the original SAGMAN-suspension. Smit Sibinga et al. [4] have studied the consequences of the small amounts of heparin in erytrocyte concentrate and they found no change in the in vitro storage properties or the in vivo survival of the erythrocytes.

The differences in conditions for the erythrocytes of the two storing systems are small; however, investigations on the in vitro and in vivo characteristics of the erythrocytes in the SAGMAN-CPD system are in progress in our laboratory.

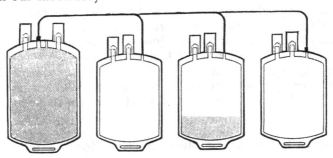

Heparin 1500 IU
in phosphate buffered saline 30 ml

SAGMAN + CPD
(10% of original formula) → 100 ml

Figure 5.

Freeze-dried plasma

The plasma bag and the empty SAGMAN bag are frozen and stored at $-40°C$ for later production of cryoprecipitate. The cryodepleted plasma is collected in the empty SAGMAN bag and later transferred to 500 ml glass bottles to be spin-frozen and freeze-dried. After reconstitution with 300 ml of water the cryodepleted plasma will be used in the clinic as an ordinary plasma substitute. Since 1965 our hospital has used around 10,000 units per year of freeze-dried cryodepleted citrated plasma as a spin off of our traditional cryoprecipitate production and only very few clinical complications have been observed. The heparin stabilized freeze-dried plasma dissolves as easily as the citrate stabilized plasma. Storage for one year does not change the dissolving properties nor the heparin content.

Freeze-dried heparin plasma reconstitutes well after heat treatment at $68°C$ for 24 hours. Electrophoretic or clinical investigations on the heat treated preparations are in progress.

According to table 4 1000 – 1200 IU of heparin will be infused per unit plasma. When this amount of heparin is diluted into a plasma volume of 3500 ml the maximum in vivo plasma concentration will be 0.3 IU/ml. In practice it will be considerably smaller because of binding of heparin after infusion and due to the short half life of heparin in vivo (90 min). Our clinicians have concluded that infusion of 1 – 2 units of reconstituted freeze-dried heparinized plasma will represent no bleeding risk for the patient. If larger amounts are given, neutralization of heparin with protamin chloride may be considered.

To confirm these statements clinical investigations on the influence of infusion of heparinized plasma on the coagulation parameters of the patient are in progress.

References

1. Smit Sibinga CTh, Welbergen H, Das PC, Griffin B. High-yield method for production of freeze-dried purified factor VIII by blood banks. Lancet 1981;ii: 449 – 50.
2. Rock GA, Cruickshank WH, Tackaberry ES, Ganz PR, Palmer DS. Stability of VIII:C in plasma: the dependence on protease activity and calcium. Thromb Res 1983;29:521 – 35.
3. Margolis J, Eisen M. Stabilising effect of aminoacids on factor VIII in lyophilised cryoprecipitate. Lancet 1984;ii:1345.
4. Smit Sibinga CTh, Das PC. Heparin and factor VIII. Scand J Haematol 1984; 33:111 – 22.

HEATING OF DOUBLE COLDPRECIPITATED FACTOR VIII CONCENTRATE FROM HEPARINIZED PLASMA

C.Th. Smit Sibinga, J. Notebomer, P.C. Das

Factor VIII (FVIII) concentrates have been produced from heparinized plasma by double coldprecipitation. In clinical trials these FVIII concentrates have showed normal FVIII recovery and half-life in stable hemophiliac patients, and good hemostatic effect during acute surgical procedures in hemophiliac patients. It is a high-yielding (50%) freeze-dried product with specific activity of 0.5 to 0.8. Most of its protein content is due to fibrinogen and fibronectin [1]. Repeated exposure to FVIII concentrate carries the potential risk of virus infections such as hepatitis. Despite the fact that our product is derived from small pools [2] the recent publicity on HTLV III and AIDS has necessitated the introduction of a virus inactivation procedure on this material [3]. Heating was chosen since it is easily adaptable to our system. HTLV III seems to be exquisitely sensitive to heating at 56°C in the liquid stage [4]. Dry heating is also effective but requires a longer time and higher temperature, for instance 68°C for 24-48 hours [5,6], although 60°C for 10-30 hours may also be effective for dried FVIII concentrates [7,8].

Most of the published reports, however, concentrate on spiking experiments where virus is added to the final material and heating results are presented as log inactivation of virus loss [4 – 6]. Very little information is available about the loss of biological activity of FVIII during heating and how to prevent such. Most commercial FVIII concentrates are now heat-treated [8,9], and understandably industries protect their recipes.

The production of FVIII concentrate from heparinized plasma has been described previously [1]. The frozen plasma is first cryoprecipitated; the precipitates from 12 donations are then pooled and allowed to form a second precipitate by keeping the pool at 0°C for 2 hours. Following centrifugation the pool-precipitate is collected and a routine freeze-drying buffer (citrate, glycine, glucose, pH 6.5) is added. The liquid final product is disposed in glass vials, snapfrozen and subsequently freeze-dried.

Our first attempt was to heat the final product in a liquid state at 56°C. The result was a disaster. In half an hour the solution precipitated into an insoluble gel like mass. This is not surprising since in liquid state fibrinogen, which is a major component of the product, is highly precipitable at about this temperature [10].

For heating in the dry state two batches were chosen, one with a higher FVIII content than the other. They were freeze-dried in routine buffer containing glucose, glycine and citrate, pH 6.5 (table 1). Heating at 64°C over 24 hours led to significant loss of FVIII activity; more loss occurred for the

104

Table 1.   Composition of routine freeze-drying buffer.

NaCl	0.34%
Trisodium citrate 2H$_2$O	0.66%
Glycine	1.00%
Dextrose	1.3 %
pH 6.5	

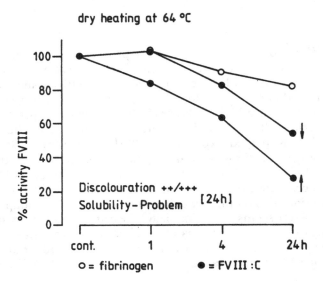

Figure 1.   Dry-heating at 64°C of FVIII concentrate derived from heparinized plasma, freeze-dried in routine buffer. Two concentrates were heated; FVIII content was higher (↑) in one, and lower (↓) in the other. Non-heated controls were run parallel which were kept at room temperature. Material was discoloured at 24 hours heating.

material with the higher FVIII content. This material also showed caramelization and solubility problems (fig. 1). When heated at 68°C almost all FVIII activity and fibrinogen disappeared with an insoluble chocolate colour material left (fig. 2). So, the routine glycine and glucose buffer is not protective to FVIII, when heat is applied. Sorbitol is thought to be protective to FVIII moieties [11,12]. A batch was produced where in the routine freeze-drying buffer glucose was replaced by sorbitol (table 2). Heating at 68°C for 24 hours suggested that sorbitol did indeed provide significant protection to both FVIII and fibrinogen, but discolouration did appear and the material is still difficult to reconstitute (fig. 3). These encouraging results stimulated the development of two major lines of action:
a. to optimalize the stability of FVIII by changing the freeze-drying buffer;
b. to improve the purity of our preparation by reducing protein content.

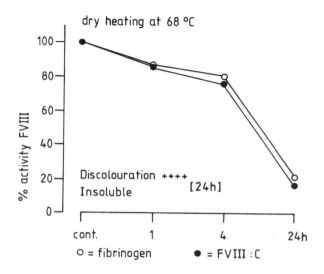

Figure 2. Dry-heating at 68°C for 24 hours. Other conditions: see fig. 1.

Table 2. Composition of freeze-drying buffer with added sorbitol as a stabiliser.

NaCl	0.34%
Trinatriumcitrate 2H$_2$O	0.66%
Glycine	1.00%
Sorbitol	1.2 %
pH 6.5	

Various combinations of buffers for freeze-drying were tried (table 3). Figure 4 shows an experiment with a 2% sucrose buffer and heated at 68°C for 24 – 48 hours. This indeed provided significant protection of FVIII with a loss of about 10 – 15% activity. The same heated product was kept at 4°C for 3 weeks and appears to remain reasonably stable (fig. 4a). The heated product easily dissolves with 10 – 15 minutes. Immunoelectrophoresis showed no changes in fibrinogen, immunoglobulin and albumin between the heated and non-heated product.

An independent second line of thought we persued is to produce a next generation product by further purification of the present material. In a two-level factorial design, one could experiment with all possible combinations of determining factors like pH, temperature, time of precipitation and heparin concentration [13]. A series of experiments suggested that an additional reprecipitation step would result in further purification by removal of significant amounts of fibrinogen and fibronectin; the end product is a clear solution that can be sterile filtered. A very preliminary experiment suggests

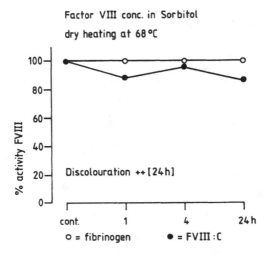

Figure 3. As a stabiliser sorbitol was added in the freeze-dried buffer. The freeze-dried powder was heated at 68°C for 24 hours. Controls were samples without heating kept at room temperature in parallel. Heated samples were discoloured at 24 hours.

Table 3. Composition of freeze-drying buffer with added sucrose as a stabiliser.

NaCl	0.34%
Citric acid 1H₂O	0.55%
Na phosphate 12H₂O	4.607%
Sucrose	2.00%
pH 6.5	

that it could also sustain wet-heating at 56°C (fig. 5). There may be some advantage in wet-heating since there is a claim that wet-heating may be more effective against non-a non-B hepatitis [14], which may not be completely eliminated by dry-heating [15].

Conclusion

For heating of FVIII a stabiliser is needed. Under conditions of vacuum in the freeze-dried state glucose easily caramelizes where sorbitol has a more promising protective effect. However, related to time some discolouration occurs resulting in loss of FVIII activity. Sucrose seems to protect effectively FVIII stability at 68°C over a 48 hours heat exposure in the freeze-dried state.

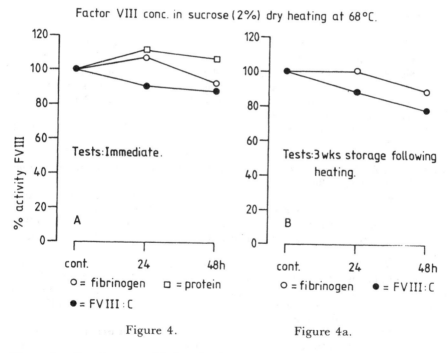

Figure 4.   Figure 4a.

Figure 4.   Sucrose was added to the freeze-drying buffer. Following freeze-drying the FVIII concentrates were heated at 68°C for 48 hours. Controls were run in parallel without heating but kept at room temperature over 48 hours. Tests were done immediately after heating (fig. 4); the heated samples and controls were stored at 4°C for 3 weeks and retested (fig. 4a).

108

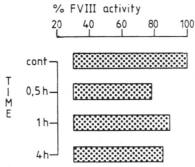

% FVIII activity

"Wet heating" of further purified factor VIII
conc. (↓) prepared at the SRBG-D

Figure 5. Routine FVIII concentrate derived from heparinized plasma was further purified by precipitation of fibrinogen and fibronectin. An experimental material in liquid state was heated at 56°C for 4 hours. The same non-heated material was used as controls.

References

1. Smit Sibinga CTh, Das PC. Heparin and Factor VIII. Scand J Haematol 1984;33(suppl 40):111 – 22.
2. Smit Sibinga CTh, Das PC. Small pool versus large pool in plasma fractionation: Reevaluation of a concept. In: Smit Sibinga CTh, Das PC, Seidl S (eds). Plasma fractionation and blood transfusion. Martinus Nijhoff Publ. Boston/Dordrecht/Lancaster 1985:43 – 6.
3. Anonymous. Blood transfusion, haemophilia and AIDS (editorial). Lancet 1984;ii:1433 – 5.
4. Spire B, Dormont D, Barré-Sinoussi F, Montagnier K, Chermann JC. Inactivation of lymphadenopathy associated virus by heat, gamma rays and ultraviolet light. Lancet 1985;i:188 – 9.
5. Levy JA, Mitra G, Mozen MM. Recovery and inactivation of infectious retrovirus added to Factor VIII concentrate. Lancet 1984;ii:722 – 3.
6. Levy JA, Mitra G, Mozen MM. Inactivation of wet and dry heat for AIDS associated retroviruses during purification from plasma. Lancet 1985;i: 1456 – 7.
7. Petriciani JC, McDougal JC, Evat BL. Case for concluding that theat treated licensed anti haemophiliac Factor is safe from HTLV III. Lancet 1985;ii:890 – 1.
8. Fielding P, Nilsson IM, Hansson BG, Biberfeld G. Absence of antibodies to LAV/HTLV III in haemophiliacs treated with heat treated Factor VIII concentrate of American origin. Lancet 1985;ii:832 – 3.
9. Mozen MM, Louic RE, Mitra GA. Heat inactivation of viruses in anti haemophiliac factor concentrate. Presentation XVI international congress of the World Federation of Haemophilia, Rio de Janeiro, August 24 – 28, 1984.
10. Ellis BC, Stranski A. A quick and accurate method for the determination of fibrinogen in plasma. J Lab Clin Med 1961;58:477 – 8.
11. McLeod AJ, Dickson IH, Foster PR. Pasteurisation of coagulation factor concentrates. Thromb Haemost 1983;50:432.

12. McLeod AJ, Cuthbertson B, Foster PR. Pasteurisation of Factor VIII and IX concentrates. Abstr. 18th congr. ISBT Munich. Karger Basel 1984:34.
13. Uithof J. Optimalisation of Factor VIII preparation from heparinized plasma. Red Cross Blood Bank Groningen-Drenthe, 1985.
14. Kernoff PB, Miller EJ, Savidge GF, Machin SF, Dewar MS, Preston FE. Wet heating for safer Factor VIII concentrate. Lancet 1985;ii:721.
15. Colombo M, Mannucci PM, Carnelli V, Savidge GF, Gazengel C, Schimf K. Transmission of non A non B hepatitis by heat treated Factor VIII concentrates. Lancet 1985;ii:1 – 4.

PRACTICAL ASPECTS OF ICE-FREE CRYOPRESERVATION*

G.M. Fahy, T. Takahashi, H.T. Meryman

Low temperatures are used by biologists primarily because they slow or prevent unwanted physical and chemical events. Unfortunately, the utility of low temperatures is usually compromised by the inconvenient fact that cooling also leads to the crystallization of water and thereby creates new and unwanted physical and even chemical events which may injure the system the biologist wishes to preserve. Although the penalties imposed by freezing are in many cases acceptable, ice formation renders biological preservation generally imperfect and sometimes inconvenient.

Here we will consider an alternative to this situation. It is now possible, after suitable pretreatment, to prevent ice formation in biological systems during cooling to liquid nitrogen temperature in such a way that when these systems are warmed rapidly, little or no injury is observed. Instead of forming ice, these systems become glassy rather than crystalline, an event known as vitrification.

Vitrification

Figure 1 illustrates how the viscosity of highly concentrated solutions of cryoprotective agents rise dramatically during cooling. The elevated viscosity corresponds to decreased molecular mobility which makes the rearrangement of water into a crystalline form more and more difficult as the temperature is lowered. Evenutally, at around 10^{13} poise [1], molecular mobility becomes essentially nil. At that point the liquid is considered to have become a glassy solid and is said to have vitrified or undergone a glass transition [1]. Unlike freezing, vitrification involves no biologically significant changes in solution structure or composition. At temperatures of the order of $10 - 20°C$ below the glass transition temperature, biological systems should be stable indefinitely.

* This work is contribution No. 688 from the American Red Cross Blood Services Laboratories and was supported in part by NIH Grants BSRG 2 S07 RR05737 and GM 17959.

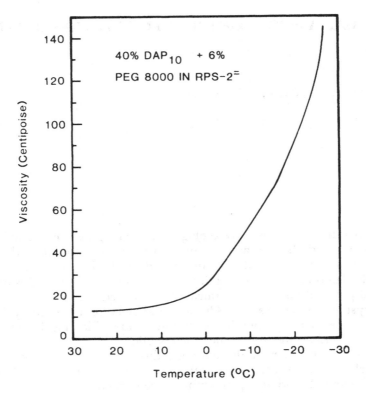

Figure 1. Viscosity of the vitrifiable solution VS2 as a function of temperature. VS2 = 15.5% w/v acetamide + 20.5% w/v dimethyl sulfoxide + 10% w/v propylene glycol + 6% poly (ethylene glycol) (MW = 8000) with RPS-2 as the cellular support base solution. RPS-2 contains 3.2% w/v glucose, which adds to the vitrifiability of the solution. Viscosity was determined using a Dip-N-Read viscosimeter (National Instrument Company, Baltimore, Maryland).

Advantages of vitrification

The advantages of vitrification are considerable. Since no ice forms, an empirical search for optimal cooling and warming rates is unnecessary. Vitrification and warming can generally be accomplished by immersing the specimen directly into baths of the appropriate temperature, in contrast to the sometimes lengthy processes of freezing and thawing. There is no need to purchase expensive controlled rate freezing machines and to tolerate the serious deficiencies that these machines generally possess. The results of vitrification and warming should in general be more predictable than the results of freezing and thawing, since fewer events and therefore fewer potential complications occur during vitrification and warming. Finally, since ice does not form, vitrification offers a unique advantage for systems which are subject to mechanical injury from ice crystals.

Disadvantages of vitrification

There are however several disadvantages to vitrification. One is the need to use very high concentrates of cryoprotective agent [2]. The required levels (~ 5 – 9 molar) may well prove to be too toxic for many systems. Furthermore, at these high concentrations, the cryoprotectants must be added and removed with much greater caution than is required for the comparatively low concentrations needed for conventional cryoprotection, possibly necessitating a cold room to minimize toxicity during addition and removal of the cryoprotectant [3]. It should be noted, however, that the degree to which it is necessary to use cryoprotectants to erect kinetic barriers to the thermodynamically favored processes of ice crystal nucleation and growth depends on the time avaible for these processes to occur. Hence, for small samples, rapid cooling and warming can be used in place of some of the cryoprotectant, thereby potentially avoiding toxicity.

Another disadvantage is the requirement during warming for a heating rate of 300 – 3000°C/min in order to avoid crystallization (divitrification) of the sample during recovery from the vitreous state [2 – 5, unpublished observations]. At present this means that the sample must be either very small or very thin. A variety of techniques are now being explored to heat large vitrified objects such as human kidneys at the required rates, but this technology is not yet in hand.

A further disadvantage for macroscopic samples may be the need for storage temperatures in the vicinity of – 130 to – 160°C. Direct exposure of most vitrified samples to liquid nitrogen temperature results in fracturing. Unfortunately, commercial equipment designed to maintain steady temperatures between – 135°C and – 160°C is not available, and practical experience with this temperature range is limited. But this problem probably applies only to generally organized tissues, since cells in suspension will generally be unaffected by fracturing of the suspending medium.

A final disadvantage for many systems may be the need to use high pressure equipment to facilitate vitrification, as will be described below.

Vitrification solutions

As noted above, very high concentrations of cryoprotectant are necessary for vitrification. Examples of several solutions which are sufficiently concentrated to support essentially complete vitrification at ambient pressures are shown in table 1. It can be seen that the concentration needed for vitrification (CNV) varies from one agent to another, and that the CNVs for the relatively non-toxic polyols glycerol and ethylene glycol are particularly high.

Figure 2 shows how the CNV of mixtures of cryoprotectants varies as a function of the composition of the solution. Composition is expressed here in terms of the mole percentages of the components other than water. In general, the CNV of a mixture varies in direct proportion to the composition of the mixture and may be considered to be a weighted average of the CNVs of the individual component solutions. Hence, the CNV of a mixture

114

Table 1. Concentrations needed for vitrification (CNV)*

	Molality	Molarity	Percentage w/v
Acetamide	23	10.3	61
Ethylene glycol	18	8.9	55
Glycerol	15	7.1	65
DAP$_{10}$	15	7.4	52
Dimethyl sulfoxide	12	6.3	49
Propylene glycol	10	5.7	44

* CNV determined in RPS-2 or R-delta solution (formulas given in [6]), at atmospheric pressure. DAP$_{10}$ = 10% w/v propylene glycol + 18.1% acetamide + 23.9% dimethyl sulfoxide.

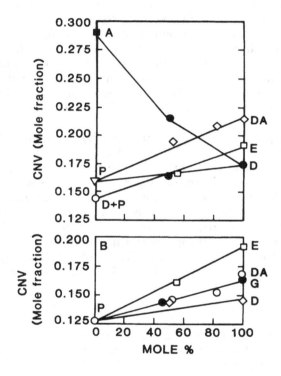

Figure 2. CNV as a function of the proportion of cryoprotectants in a mixture. The CNV for individual aqueous components (including components such as DA, which can be treated as a single substance when mixed with another cryoprotectant) are given in the mole % = 0 and mole % = 100 lines. G = glycerol; P = propylene glycol; E = ethylene glycol; D = dimethyl sulfoxide; A = acetamide; DA = equimolar mixture of A and D; D + P = equal weights of D and P. Upper panel = 1 atm except for the mixtures of E with D + P, which are for 1000 ATM and in the presence of 6% PVP. Lower panel = 1000 atm and in the presence of 6% w/v PVP. All CNVs obtained in the presence of RPS-2 or R-delta carrier solutions. Data from [2] and from unpublished studies.

is fairly predictable given the CNVs of the component solutions. This is true both at 1 atmosphere (upper panel) and at 1000 atmosphere (lower panel).

Experience at formulating mixtures of cryoprotectants which are not only vitrifiable but are also non-toxic is still limited, but the following generalizations appear to apply.

First, it seems generally advantageous to use mixtures of cryoprotectants rather than single cryoprotectants for vitrification because individual agent has disadvantages at high concentrations which can generally be minimized in an appropriate mixture. For example, propylene glycol is a good glass-forming agent but it is too toxic to use by itself [7,8]. In a mixture, however, it can enhance glass-forming ability without having toxic effects [2].

Second, it appears that certain additives are able to partially neutralize each other's toxicity. The best documented examples are dimethyl sulfoxide-amide mixtures, which have been discussed in detail elsewhere [2,7,9 – 11]. For example, an 8 molal solution of dimethyl sulfoxide is roughly three times more toxic to kidney tissue than a 9.1 molal solution composed of equimolar amounts of dimethyl sulfoxide and acetamide [7]. Another example of specific toxicity reduction is prevention of irreversible binding of dimethyl sulfoxide to proteins by dextrose [12].

Third, it appears generally advantageous to use nonpenetrating additive as part of the mixture [2]. Figure 3 shows that polyvinyl pyrrolidone can significantly lower the CNVs of selected penetrating cryoprotectant solutions. Normal intracellular proteins similarly lower the amount of intracellular penetrating cryoprotectant required for intracellular vitrification. By using polymer extracellularly the concentration of extracellular penetrating cryoprotectant can be reduced to the minimum value consistent with intracellular vitrification, thereby minimizing the intracellular concentration of additive.

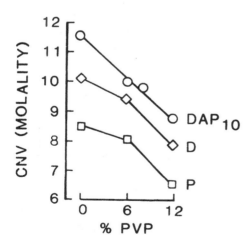

Figure 3. Effect of polyvinyl pyrrolidone (PVP K30) concentration on the apparent CNV of various solutions. Data from [2] and from unpublished studies. DAP_{10} = 10% w/v propylene glycol + DA; other abbreviations as in figure 2.

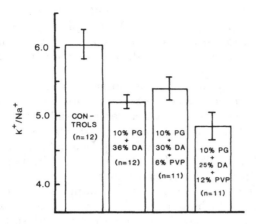

Figure 4. Effect of CNV reduction by polymer on the toxicity of vitrification solutions. The K^+/Na^+ ratio is a viability index for kidney slices. The improvement in recovery seen with 6% PVP was unusually small in this particular experiment but is visible. 12% PVP, however, was not beneficial. Cryoprotectant introduction schedule = 10% penetrating agent (pa) for 30 min at 0°C; 20% pa for 60 min at 0°C; vitrification solution (vs) for 40 min at 0°C. Washout schedule = 20% pa + 300 mM mannitol (20% +) for 20 min at 0°C; 15 +, 10 +, 5 +, and 0 + for 20 min each at 0°C; 0% pa (RPS-2), 0°C. Polymer was present during loading and unloading in proportion to the pa. For example, in the 12% PVP group, the polymer concentration during loading was $(10/35) \times 12$, $(20/35) \times 12$, and 12% w/v in the 10%, 20%, and 35% solitions, respectively. PG in the loading and unloading steps varied in proportion to the total pa concentration. For example, PG level was $(10/35) \times 10$ in the 10% step for the 35% group, but $(10/47) \times 10$ in the 10% step for the 46% group. Unpublished results.

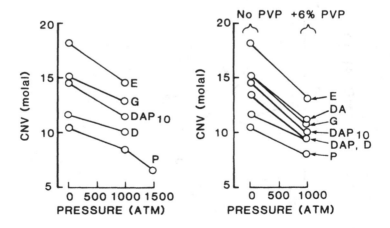

Figure 5. Left side: Effect of high pressure on the CNV of various solutions. Data from [2]. CNV of PG at 1500 atm estimated. Abbreviations as in previous figures. Right side: Effect of pressure + polymer on CNV. Data from [2].

The practical limit to the concentration of nonprenetrating agent appears to be in the vicinity of 6% w/v. Higher polymer concentrations are associated more with a reduction in the size of ice crystal nuclei than with a reduction of the number of nuclei. At the apparent CNV, the solution is therefore in all probability heavily nucleated by ice particles too small to be seen with the naked eye. When such nucleated glass is warmed, rapid devitrification (freezing) is likely. In addition, polymer concentrations above 6% seem to convey no advantage in terms of improved viability (fig. 4).

The role of high pressures

Hydrostatic pressure, like cryoprotectants, inhibits the freezing of water and can lower CNV [2,13,14], providing a potentially essential alternative when a system is subject to serious toxicity from cryoprotectants at their CNVs and, particularly, when the system is too large to allow CNV to be relaxed by the use of very high cooling and warming rates. High pressures also inhibit devitrification, which may prove to be of equal importance. Although high pressures may of themselves be damaging, we have found that high concentrations of cryoprotectants can prevent injurious effects of high pressure, at least in kidney slices [2,13].

Figure 5 (left side) shows the effect of pressure on the CNVs of several vitrification solutions. On the average, 1000 atm reduces CNV by about 17% in our hands [2], which could represent a decisive advantage for many systems in view of the intense concentration dependence of cryoprotectant toxicity [2]. This effect is superimposable on the effects of polymers and propylene glycol (fig. 5, right side). The vitrification of suspensions of sensitive cell types utilizing a combination of cryoprotectants and high pressures would certainly be technically feasible and inexpensive.

Specific examples

1. Monocytes, granulocytes, and erythrocytes

Recently, Takahashi et al [4] have studied the vitrification of human monocytes at atmospheric pressure. Although monocytes may have useful clinical applications in view of their many functions [15,16], we offer the following results primarily to illustrate the feasibility of vitrification using a cell type familiar to blood bankers. The fact that monocytes are relatively freezing tolerant [17 – 19] suggested that they would be good candidates for vitrification.

In the studies of Takahashi et al., monocytes were purified (>95% pure) by a combination of Ficoll-Paque separation and counterflow centrifugal elutriation using a J2-21 centrifuge (Beckman Instruments, Palo Alto, Calif.) equipped with a JE-6 elutriator rotor. The vitrification solution was VS1 [3,4], and consisted of 20.5% dimethyl sulfoxide (the primary cryoprotectant), 15.5% acetamide (the "toxicity neutralizer"), 10% propylene

Table 2. Viability of monocytes before and after vitrification*

Test	Controls	Treatment VS1	Vitrified	Vit/con × 100%
Cell #	93.9 ± 3.0	92.0 ± 2.	91.8 ± 2.5	*97.8*
FDA/EB	97.8 ± 1.5	95.2 ± 1.9	94.5 ± 1.7	*96.6*
Phagocytosis	96.5 ± 1.8	92.3 ± 2.1	92.2 ± 2.9	*95.5*
Chemotaxis	99.7 ± 4.7	93.5 ± 4.5	95.8 ± 6.8	*96.1*

* Data from [4].
Cell # = cell number recovery (%); FDA/EB = % of cells surviving based on fluorescein diacetate/ethidium bromide staining assay; phagocytosis = % of cells phagocytosing more than 5 *E. coli*; chemotaxis = number of cells migrating through polycarbonate filters in response N-formyl-methionyl-leucyl-phenyl-alanine (as % of control). Values given are mean ± SD (n).
Cells cooled to 0°C, stirred two hours, and centrifuged similarly to VS1 and vitrified groups. Cell number recovery was normalized to controls which were simply chilled to 0°C for 2 hours (taken as 100%).
VS1 added and removed at 0°C, cells not vitrified.
Vitrified by cooling at 600°C/min and warmed at 560°C/min in an ice bath (storage time at − 196°C: 30 days).
Recovery of vitrified/warmed monocytes as a percentage of the controls. Note lack of difference between VS1 and vitrified groups.

glycol (the vitrification enhancer) and 6% w/v PEG 8000 (the nonpenetrating agent), in Hanks' balanced salt solution carrier. VS1 was added dropwise to the monocytes at 0°C over the course of 10 minutes, yielding a final suspension equal to 94% of VS1. The monocytes were cooled by immersion of the 0.8 ml suspension in a 12 cm length of 3/16″ OD silastic tubing into liquid nitrogen (cooling rate, ∼600°C/min). After warming by immersion in an ice bath (∼560°C/min), the cryoprotectants were diluted out gradually at 0°C and functional recovery assessed.

The results are shown in table 2. Simple addition and removal of this 13 molal cryoprotectant solution at 0°C caused minimal loss of cells, of membrane integrity (as assessed by the FDA/EB assay), of phagocytosis, and of chemotaxis. When the cells were also cooled to − 196°C and warmed, no further damage was induced. No effect of storage time in liquid nitrogen was observed.

Granulocytes might also be susceptible to preservation by vitrification. In contrast to monocytes, these cells are quite sensitive to freezing [20,21], since they are subject to chilling injury, thermal shock, and dilution shock, and are particularly sensitive to hyperosmotic stress, rendering successful freezing extremely difficult if not impossible [21]. However, granulocytes do tolerate high concentrations of cryoprotectant [22], which is the only prerequisite cryopreservation by vitrification. It remains to be seen whether cryopreserved granulocytes would be of sufficient clinical value to warrant their use.

Vitrification of human eryti.rocytes was reported in 1968 by Rapatz and Luyet [23]. These authors exposed red cells to 8.6 M glycerol at room temperature and at ambient pressure and plunged them in capillary tubes into a – 150°C freon bath. No ice was observed in cells or in the suspending medium using freeze-fracture techniques, and they had previously found (unpublished observations) that cells treated in this way survived in high proportions.

2. Embryos, ova, and sperm

Mouse embryos have also been vitrified successfully at ambient pressure [3]. VS1 was introduced in steps: quarter-strength VS1 at room temperature for 15 min followed by half strength VS1 at 4°C for 10 min followed by VS1 itself at 4°C for 10 min. The embryos were then cooled at 20, 500, or 2500°C/min to – 196°C. VS1 was removed by reversing the VS1 introduction protocal. At all cooling rates studied, survival as judged by growth to expanded blastocysts in cultures was the same after vitrification and warming as it was before cooling to – 196°C (81 – 88%). Subsequent studies showed that previously vitrified embryos could develop into normal live young after transfer to foster mothers [24].

Various laboratories around the world are now attempting to apply vitrification to sperm and ova and to embryos of other species including man. Results of these studies are not yet available.

3. Tissues

Kidney slices exposed to a solution (40% DAP_{10} + 6% PEG 8000) which will vitrify at 1000 atm show an $80 \pm 10\%$ recovery based on their ability to re-establish a normal K^+/Na^+ ratio. In unpublished studies conducted circa 1972 in the laboratory of B.C. Elford and M.J. Taylor in the UK, taenia coli intestinal smooth muscle strips recovered full contractile strength after having been vitrified and warmed in the presence of 60% w/v dimethyl sulfoxide at ambient pressure. Attempts to vitrify pancreatic islets using VS1 have recently been undertaken but have not as yet been successful [25]. Attempts to vitrify human skin using VS1 are also now in progress.

4. Organs

As yet, no solid mammalian organs have been subjected to vitrification and successfully recovered in a viable condition. Both guinea pig uteri [26] and frog hearts [27] can tolerate concentrations of cryoprotectant which are high enough for vitrification even at atmospheric pressure. Other organs, however, are not likely to be able to withstand the concentrations of cryoprotectant required for vitrification at one atmosphere and will in all likelihood require the use of high hydrostatic pressures for both cooling and rewarming. Even if toxicity were not a limiting factor for achieving vitrification for organs such as the kidney, heart, and liver, it is quite possible that the use of high pressure would still be required in order to minimize the rate of devitrification during warming from the vitreous state.

Pitfalls to avoid

Although vitrification can be simple, quick, and effective, success will generally require strict adherence to the following basic rules.

(1) Vitrification solutions are nontoxic *only* when used at low temperatures and for a limited time. Therefore, the following points should be kept in mind.

a. Adding room temperature vitrification solution (VS) to chilled cells may allow the cells to warm to a damaging temperature in the process. The use of chilled VS, preferrably in a cold room, is safer. Adding warm cells in ¼ or ½ strength VS to chilled VS suffers from the same potential problem. It is better to cool the cells before mixing them with chilled VS. Pipetting cells using warm pipets can also be lethal.

b. Do not allow any cells to remain in contact with the VS for longer than necessary at 0°C. Some cells are killed in 20 min at 0°C [3].

c. Cells should not be in the vicinity of the portion of the container to be heat sealed or otherwise allowed to warm above 0°C before vitrification.

d. Cells in straws or test tubes should not be handled with bare hands since this may warm them.

e. Samples should *not* be warmed in a 37°C bath or even in a 25°C bath. Only a 0 – 10°C bath (preferrably composed of half-strength VS) should be used to avoid overheating the sample.

f. After warming to 0°C, cells should be diluted at 0°C to ½ or ¼ strength VS before the tempeature is allowed to rise further.

(2) Vitrification solutions contract greatly upon cooling. This contraction will tend to draw liquid nitrogen into the sample if the sample is inadequately sealed. Upon warming, the nitrogen will suddenly vaporize with the potential to explode the sample. Insemination straws, for example, must be heat sealed, not sealed with powder plugs.

(3) Devitrification (crystallization) of formerly vitrified cells during warming is lethal [3,4]. Warming rates of at least 300°C/min and possibly of 3000°C/min may be needed to prevent devitrification. Therefore:

a. Samples must have as large a surface/volume ratio as possible to maximize warming rate.

b. The container should be thin-walled and thermally condicutive.

c. The warming bath should vigorously stirred during sample rewarming if possible. The sample itself should also be vigorously agitated in the warming bath.

(4) Death associated with devitrification may be caused by an inadequate concentration of cryoprotectant prior to vitrification. The CNV found in reference tables such as table 1 is the *minimum* concentration needed for essentially complete vitrification. Lower concentrations may allow survival after cooling and rapid warming [3,4] and will appear optically transparent upon quenching but will be heavily nucleated and will devitrify at an accelerated rate during rewarming. If VS at its CNV is added to a cell suspension or tissue, the resulting mixture of VS and cells will have a concentration below its CNV and may therefore be subject to problems from devitrification. To avoid this, the VS added must have a concentration greater than its CNV or it must be added to cells in great excess, or the supernatant must be removed and fresh VS added a second time.

(5) Vitrification solutions can cause osmotic damage if added and/or removed too rapidly. Control experiments on cryoprotectant permeation into the cells of interest should be carried out before vitrification is attempted, and cryoprotectant loading and unloading protocols should be designed that take permeation rates into account. If problems persist, optimum holding times at each concentration step should be determined.

Conclusion

Vitrification has become a successful method for cryopreserving human monocytes and erythrocytes, murine embryos, and guinea pig smooth muscle and is likely to be useful for other cell types and tissues relevant to blood banking. It can be a simple, quick, inexpensive, and reliable process when carried out properly, but it must be executed carefully. Only the future will decide the limits of applicability of this relatively new approach to cryopreservation.

References

1. Kauzmann W. The nature of the glassy state and the behavior of liquids at low temperatures. Chem Rev 1984;38:653 – 6.
2. Fahy GM, MacFarlane DR, Angell CA, Meryman HT. Vitrification as an approach to cryopreservation. Cryobiology 1984;21:407 – 26.
3. Rall WF, Fahy GM. Ice-free cryopreservation of mouse embryos at – 196°C by vitrification. Nature 1985;313:573 – 5.
4. Takahashi T, Hirsh A, Erbe EF, Bross JB, Steere RL, Williams RJ. Vitrification of human monocytes. Cryobiology 1986;23.
5. Boutron P. Stability of the amorphous state in the system water-1, 2-propanediol. Cryobiology 1979;16:557 – 68.
6. Fahy GM. Cryoprotectant toxicity: biochemical or osmotic? Cryo-Letters 1984;5:79 – 90.
7. Fahy GM. Prevention of toxicity from high concentrations of cryoprotective agents. In: Pegg DE, Jacobsen IA, Halasz NA (eds). Organ preservation, basic and applied aspects. Lancaster: MTP Press, 1982:367 – 9.

8. Pegg DE, Jacobsen IA, Diaper MP, Foreman J, Hunt CJ. Some observations on rabbit kidneys exposed to solutions containing propane-1, 2-diol. Cryobiology 1985;22:608.

9. Baxter SJ, Lathe GH. Biochemical effects on kidney of exposure to high concentrations of dimethyl sulfoxide. Biochem Pharmacol 1971;30:1079 – 91.

10. Fahy GM. Cryoprotectant toxicity neutralizers reduce freezing damage. Cryo-Letters 1983;4:309 – 14.

11. Fahy GM. Cryoprotectant toxicity reduction: specific or nonspecific? Cryo-Letters 1984;5:287 – 94.

12. Clark P, Fahy GM, Karow AM Jr. Factors influencing renal cryopreservation. II. Toxic effects of three cryoprotectants in combination with three vehicle solutions in non-frozen rabbit cortical slices. Cryobiology 1984;21:260 – 73.

13. Fahy GM, Hirsh A. Prospects for organ preservation by vitrification. In: Pegg DE, Jacobsen IA, Halasz NA (eds). Organ preservation, basic and applied aspects. Lancaster: MTP Press 1982:399 – 403.

14. MacFarlane DR, Angell CA, Fahy GM. Homogeneous nucleation and glass formation in cryoprotective system at high pressures. Cryo-Letters 1981;2: 353 – 8.

15. van Furth R (ed). Mononuclear phagocytes in immunity: infection and immunity. London: Blackwell Scientific Publ. 1975.

16. Carr I, Deams WT (eds). The reticuloendothelial system: A comprehensive treatise. Vol. 1. Morphology. New York: Plenum Press 1980.

17. van der Meulen FW, Reiss M, Stricker EAM, Elven EV, von dem Borne AEGKr. Cryopreservation of human monocytes. Cryobiology 1981;18: 337 – 43.

18. Hunt SM, Lionetti FJ, Valeri CR, Callahan AB. Cryogenic preservation of monocytes from human blood and platelet pheresis cellular residues. Blood 1981;57:592 – 8.

19. Takahashi T, Hammett MF, Cho MS, Williams RJ, Meryman HT. Cryopreservation of monocytes. Cryobiology 1982;19:676.

20. Takahashi T, Inada S, Pommer CG, O'Shea JJ, Brown EJ. Osmotic stress and the freeze-thaw cycle cause shedding of Fc and C3b receptors by human polymorphonuclear leukocytes. J Immunol 1985;134:4062 – 8.

21. Takahashi T, Hammett MF, Cho MS. Multifaceted freezing injury in human polymorphonuclear cells at high subfreezing temperatures. Cryobiology 1985;22:215 – 36.

22. Takahashi T, Bross JB, Shaber RE, Williams RJ. Effect of cryoprotectants on the viability and function of unfrozen human polymorphonuclear cells. Cryobiology 1985;22:336 – 50.

23. Rapatz G, Luyet B. Electron microscope study of erythrocytes in rapidly cooled suspensions containing various concentrations of glycerol. Biodynamica 1968;10:193 – 210.

24. Rall WF, Wood MJ, Kirby C. In vivo development of mouse embryos cryopreserved by vitrification. Cryobiology 1985;22:603 – 4.

25. Rajotte RV, DeGroot TJ, Ellis DK, Rall WF. Preliminary experiments on vitrification of isolated rat islets of Langerhans. Cryobiology 1985;22:602 – 3.

26. Farrant J. Mechanism of cell damage during freezing and thawing and its prevention. Nature 1965;205:1284 – 7.

27. Rapatz G, Keener R. Effect of concentration of ethylene glycol on the recovery of frog hearts after freezing to low temperatures. Cryobiology 1974;11:571 – 2.

PROPERTIES OF HEMOGLOBIN INTERDIMERICALLY CROSS-LINKED WITH NFPLP*

J.C. Bakker, W.K. Bleeker, H. van der Plas

Introduction**

Stroma-free hemoglobin (Hb) solutions may be used as an oxygen-carrying plasma expander. The efficacy to transport and release oxygen is governed by the affinity of Hb for oxygen and the persistence of Hb in the circulation.

Free Hb leaks out of the circulation mainly via the kidneys. Bunn et al. [1] have shown that this occurs in the dimeric form of Hb, and that the leakage can be decreased by cross-linking the dimers with bis-(N-maleimidomethyl) ether. This modification, however, resulted in a increased oxygen affinity, as shown by a P50 value of 3 mm Hg. Thus, the oxygenated form of this compound will not release its oxygen to the tissues.

Coupling of the β chains by an organic phosphate compound with two aldehyde groups, i.e. 2-nor-2-formyl-pyridoxal 5'-phosphate (NFPLP) [2], might solve both the problem of Hb leakage and oxygen affinity.

From laboratory data measured at 20°C [2] it might be expected that the oxygen affinity of HbNFPLP will be close to normal under physiological conditions. We have tested the hypothesis that binding of NFPLP to Hb will decrease the oxygen affinity of free Hb and thus improve tissue oxygenation and increase the vascular retention time of Hb.

Methods

Preparation of hemoglobin solutions and coupling to NFPLP

Packed erythrocytes made leukocyte-free by filtration via cellulose-acetate columns [3], were washed three times with a physiological saline solution to remove traces of plasma proteins and platelets. The erythrocytes were lysed by addition of two volumes of cold distilled water. Membrane fragments were removed by tangential flow filtration (0.45 μm) and subsequent filtration through sterile 0.22 μm membrane filters. The resulting solution was dialysed against either 0.1 M Tris-HCl (pH 7.0) or against a perfusion

* This study was supported in part by the Foundation for Medical Research FUNGO, which is subsidized by the Netherlands Organization for the Advancement of Pure Research

** Abbreviations used in this paper: Hb = hemoglobin; NFPLP = 2-nor-2-formyl-pyridoxal 5'-phosphate; HbNFPLP = hemoglobin cross-linked with NFPLP.

medium (see below), and stored at 4°C as solutions of 7 g% stroma-free Hb.

The coupling of NFPLP to Hb is esseitally the same as that of pyridoxal 5'-phosphate to Hb as described by Benesch et al. [4]. A 7 g% stroma-free Hb solution in 0.1 M Tris-HCl (pH 7) was deoxygenated in a rotating flask under a stream of nitrogen. NFPLP was added in a molar ratio of 1:1 to Hb. After 3 hours of rotating under nitrogen, a 40-fold excess of sodium borohydride in 1 mM KOH was added, and incubated for another 30 min. Thereafter, the solution was oxygenated by a stream of air during 15 min. After filtration through 0.22 μm membrane filters and dialysis against the perfusion medium, the solution was stored at 4°C.

NFPLP was synthesized in a five-step procedure, starting from pyridoxal hydrochloride, as described [5,6], with some modifications for synthesis on a gram scale (van der Plas et al, in preparation).

Analytical methods

P50 values were calculated from the oxyHb dissociation curves recorded with the Dissociation Curve Analyser (type I, Radiometer, Copenhagen, Denmark) in diluted Hb samples [7,8] at standard conditions of pH 7.4, PCO_2 40 mm Hg and 37°C. The degree of coupling of Hb with NFPLP was determined on a mono Q-HR 5/5 high-resolution anion-exchanger (FPLC system, Pharmacia, Uppsala, Sweden). Samples of 750 μg in 0.01 M Tris-HCl (pH 8.3) were applicated, and eluted by a salt gradient. The percentage coupling was defined as the ratio of the surface area of the HbNFPLP peak divided by the total surface area of the two main peaks, times 100%.

Liver perfusions

To evaluate the oxygen transport and release capacities of Hb and NFPLP, rat livers were perfused with these solutions under conditions of normoxia and stagnant hypoxia (hypoxia induced by a decrease of the perfusion flow rate). The following oxygen-dependent parameters were tested:
– venous PO_2;
– oxygen consumption;
– bile flow rate;
– lactate/pyruvate ratio, as a reflection of the redox level in the cytoplasm;
– β-hydroxybutyrate/acetoacetate ratio, as a reflection of the redox level in the mitochondria.

Exchange transfusions

To determine the vascular retention of free Hb and HbNFPLP, exchange perfusions were performed in rats. The animals were anesthetized with pentobarbital. The arterial blood pressure and heart rate was monitored continuously. Nine ml of blood was exchanged with 9 ml of coupling mixture, in which the ratio of Hb to HbNFPLP had been adjusted to about 1. During 5 hours, blood samples were taken for the determination of hematocrit, erythrocyte number, and the concentration of free Hb and HbNFPLP in the plasma. Urine was collected via a catheter for the measurement of the volume and Hb concentration.

Results

Oxygen affinity and liver perfusions

The described coupling method of Hb and HbNFPLP resulted in a mixture of 65% HbNFPLP and 35% Hb, as derived from the FPLC analysis. The P50 values of the non-modified and the cross-linked solutions were 15 and 40 mm Hg, respectively (at pH 7.4, 37°C and PCO_2 = 40 mm). The latter P50 is close to the normal P50 of erythrocytes, which is 27 mm Hg. The Hill factor n was 2.0 for the HbNFPLP coupling mixture, 2.3 for Hb and 2.7 for erythrocytes. The main results of the two series of liver perfusions with the Hb and the Hb/HbNFPLP solutions were as follows.

1. The NFPLP-induced decrease in oxygen affinity was reflected in a higher venous PO_2 during normoxia and during stagnant hypoxia: the PO_2 in the hepatic vein at time 70 min were 22.0 ± 2.2 and 14.4 ± 1.5 mm Hg for the livers perfused Hb/HbNFPLP and unmodified Hb solutions, respectively. The O_2 consumption of both groups did not differ significantly: 0.81 ± 0.11 and 0.76 ± 0.06 ml O_2/min liver.
2. All O_2-dependent parameters were decreased during stagnant hypoxia. Table 1 shows the response of venous PO_2 and of O_2 consumption.
3. The coupling of NFPLP to Hb did not result in a change in rheological properties of the Hb solutions, since no differences in perfusion flow rate and pressure were found between the two series.

Exchange transfusions

The vascular retention of Hb HbNFPLP after exchange transfusion of 9 ml of rat blood with 9 ml of coupling mixture is shown in figure 1. The upper part shows the time course of the decrease of the Hb and HbNFPLP concentration in the rat plasma. The concentration of Hb and HbNFPLP was decreased to 50% after 100 and 300 min, respectively. However, for the proper estimation of the vascular retention time, the change of plasma volume should also be taken into account. From the corrected data, shown in the lower part of the figure, half-disappearance times of 65 and 190 min were calculated for Hb and HbNFPLP, respectively. In the urine samples only very small amounts of HbNFPLP were detected when compared with Hb: less than 5% of the transfused mainly coupled product after 5 hours.

Table 1. Parameters of isolated perfused rat livers at different flow rates.

Perfusion time	70 min	100 min	130 min
Series	A/B	A/B	A/B
PO_2 of inflowing perfusate (mm Hg)	96.8 ± 1.5 97.7 ± 1.6	103.9 ± 3.2 95.2 ± 2.0	96.9 ± 5.0 99.2 ± 2.1
Perfusion flow rate (ml/min)	18.0 ± 0.2 18.2 ± 0.3	9.0 ± 0. 9.1 ± 0.	6.0 ± 0 6.0 ± 0.
O_2 supply (ml O_2/min)	1.41 ± 0.03 1.24 ± 0.04	0.71 ± 0.01 0.60 ± 0.02	0.46 ± 0.01 0.41 ± 0.01
Venous PO_2 (mm Hg)	14.4 ± 0.5 22.0 ± 0.8	10.2 ± 0.6 11.6 ± 0.9	8.1 ± 0.6 9.3 ± 1.5
O_2 consumption (ml O_2/min)	0.81 ± 0.24 0.76 ± 0.02	0.56 ± 0.01 0.51 ± 0.02	0.39 ± 0.01 0.36 ± 0.01

Values are means ± SEM of 8 separate perfusion experiments with non-modified Hb solutions (columns A) and 8 experiments with modified Hb solutions, containing 65% HbNFPLP and 35% Hb (columns B). In each experiment, the flow rate was decreased to 9 ml/min at t = 75 min until t = 105, and then a flow rate of 6 ml/min was maintained for another 30 min.

Discussion and conclusions

The hypothesis that coupling of NFPLP to Hb might decrease the oxygen affinity and improve tissue oxygenation, as well as improve the vascular retention time appears to be correct.

The cross-linking of Hb with NFPLP induced a substantial decrease in oxygen affinity. In-vivo, this change was reflected in a higher venous PO_2, an indicator for tissue oxygenation. No difference in O_2 consumption was observed. Although it has a high oxygen affinity, unmodified Hb released almost 90% of its oxygen in this model. When compared with erythrocyte perfusions during stagnant hypoxia [9], it can be concluded that Hb solutions allow better tissues perfusion and oxygenation. This is probably due to the lower viscosity of the Hb solutions, which is especially important during low-flow perfusions.

Benesch et al. [10] observed a higher O_2 extraction in heart perfusions when they compared a diluted HbNFPLP solution (1 g/100 ml) with a diluted Hb solution. These investigators observed less than 50% O_2 extraction with the latter solution, and values up to 80% with the cross-linked solution. Apparently, oxygen affinity is a limiting factor in this model. In our liver model, perfused with isooncotic Hb solutions of 7 g/100 ml, oxygen affinity is not a limiting factor for O_2 release to the tissue. Theoretically a low oxygen affinity is of advantage for O_2 release to tissue. Our experiments show that it is not always a critical factor. It is difficult to predict

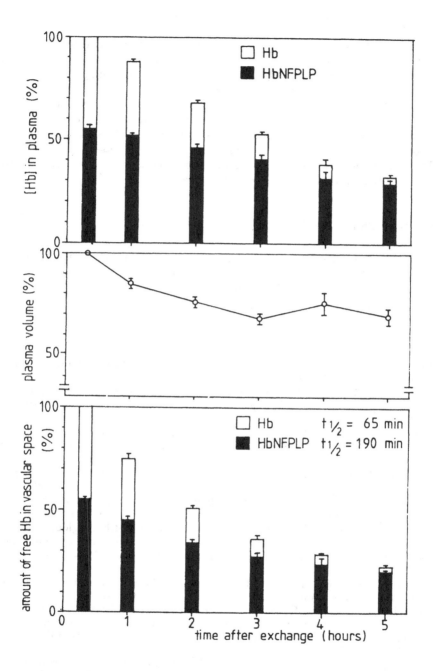

Figure 1. Vascular retention (means ± SEM, n = 5) of free Hb and HbNFPLP after exchange transfusion of 9 ml blood with 9 ml of coupling containing about 50% Hb and 50% HbNFPLP. Hb and HbNFPLP were determined by FPLC analysis. The plasma volume was calculated from the hematocrit.

under which clinical circumstances oxygen affinity will play a crucial role in O_2 transport.

The second part of our hypothesis has been confirmed most strikingly. The vascular retention time of HbNFPLP is three times as long as that of Hb. This is most probably due to the prevention of leakage of the cross-linked Hb molecules through the kidney. It is clear, however, that the cross-linked Hb molecule still disappears from the circulation, albeit at a reduced speed. The question remains which mechanisms are responsible for its disappearance: for instance, diffusion to the interstitial space, uptake by macrophages or uptake by liver cells. Since the infusion of large amounts of Hb may overload certain clearance mechanisms, this question requires an answer before clinical trials can be started.

Acknowledgements

The authors thank mr J. Ageterberg, mr A. van Hamersveld, mrs G. Rigter and mrs A. de Vries-van Rossen for skilfull technical assistance and dr D. Roos for critically reading the manuscript.

References

1. Bunn HF, Esham WT, Bull RW. The renal handling of hemoglobin. I. Glomerular filtration. J Exp Med 1969;129:909 – 24.
2. Benesch R, Benesch RE, Yung S, Edalji R. Hemoglobin covalently bridged across the polyphosphate binding site. Biochem Biophys Res Commun 1975;63: 1123 – 9.
3. Diepenhorst P, Sprokholt R, Prins HK. Removal of leucocytes from whole blood and erythrocyte suspension by filtration through cotton wool. Vox Sang 1972;23:308 – 20.
4. Benesch RE, Benesch R, Renthal RD, Maeda N. Affinity labelling of the polyphosphate binding site of hemoglobin. Biochemistry 1972;11:3576 – 82.
5. Pocker A. Synthesis of 2-nor-2-formylpyridoxal 5'-phosphate, a bifunctional reagens specific for the cofactor site in proteins. J Organ Chem 1973;38:4295 – 9.
6. Benesch R, Benesch RE. Preparation and properties of hemoglobin modified with derivatives of pyridoxal. In: Antonini E, Rossi-Bernardi L, Chiancone E (eds). Methods in enzymology. Vol. 76. Academic Press, New York 1981:147 – 59.
7. Duvelleroy MA, Buckles RG, Rosenkaimer S, Tung S, Laver MB. An oxyhemoglobin dissociation analyzer. J Appl Physiol 1970;28:227 – 33.
8. Teisseire B, Lousance D, Soulard C, Herigault R, Teisseire L, Laurant D. A method of continuous recording on micro-samples of the Hb-O_2 association curve. I. Technique and direct registration of standard results. Bull Eur Physiopathol Resp 1975;11:837 – 51.
9. Bakker JC, Gortmaker GC, Offerijns FGJ. The influence of the position of the oxygen dissociation curve on oxygen-dependent functions of the isolated perfused rat liver. II. Studies at different levels of hypoxia induced by decrease of blood flow rate. Pflügers Arch 1976;366:45 – 52.

10. Benesch R, Triner L, Benesch RE, Kwong S, Verosky M. Enhanced oxygen unloading by an interdimerically cross-linked hemoglobin in an isolated perfused rabbit heart. Proc Natl Acad Sci USA 1984;81:2941 – 3.

PRODUCTION OF HEMATOPOIETIC CELLS IN CULTURE*

E.D. Zanjani, J.C. Schulman, L.C. Lasky

Despite many advances in blood banking technology, our ability to support patients with blood products remains severely limited because they can only be obtained by harvesting mature cells from the peripheral blood of individual donors. The supply of all cell lines is threatened by occasional shortages and the unavailability of unusual antigen types. White blood cell transfusions have the added problems of inadequate yields, despite advances in leukapheresis, and poor granulocyte function after manipulation, so that white cell transfusions remain of marginal clinical utility [1]. Availability is further limited by the lack of storage techniques for platelets and white cells. Disease transmission remains a problem with conventional techniques [2]. The recent adoption of HTLV-III antibody screening should lessen the transmission of AIDS, but non-A non-B hepatitis remains a frequent complication of transfusion, as is CMV in the immunosuppressed [3] and malaria in Third World countries

The needs of some patients, moreover, are best served by the provision of hematopoietic progenitors. Those rendered aplastic by disease or chemotherapy can be treated with bone marrow transplantation, but this technique is limited by unavailability of suitable donors, graft-versus-host disease, occasional failure of engraftment, and our inability to support patients through a period of prolonged, profound leukopenia with mucosal defenses damaged by conditioning regimens of chemotherapy and radiation [3,5]. Long-term bone marrow cultures (LTC) hold the potential for changing this situation by providing a continuous supply of fresh, functional and disease-free mature blood cells, as well as hematopoietic progenitors capable of reconstituting the hematopoietic system in the recipient. If malignant progenitors can be separated from normal cells in culture, as has been demonstrated in cases of acute and chronic myelogenous leukemias in man [6,8], LTC-derived autologous transplant or blood product support would make increasingly aggressive chemotherapy possible.

The LTC has been well established for the murine system [9]. These cultures produce abundant numbers of committed myeloid (CFU-GM) and erythroid progenitors (BFU-E) and large numbers of multipotent stem cells (CFU-S) capable of reconstituting lethally irradiated mice [10]. In addition, under appropriate conditions, fully functional mature granulocytes, macro-

* Supported by Veterans Administration, and grants AM24027 and CA23021 from the national Institutes of Healths. LCL is supported by Clinical Investigator Award 5K08-HL01054 from the National Heart, Lung and Blood Institute.

phages and erythrocytes can be formed in LTC for long periods [11 – 18]. Megakaryocyte precursors (CFU-MK) are also amplified several-fold in LTC [17]. The system also generates mature T and B lymphocytes as well as their progenitors [18 – 20]. Overall, significant net production of hematopoietic progenitors and mature blood cells can be documented in murine LTC for periods of several months.

By contrast, while net production of hematopoietic progenitors and mature blood cells occurs in human LTC [11,21 – 25] and the granulocytes produced appear to be functionally normal [26], the overall production of these elements is significantly less than seen in murine LTC, and the cultures begin to decline after 4 – 6 weeks and rarely persist for more than 20 weeks.

In the murine system the longevity and productivity of the cultures are critically dependent upon the development and maintenance of a functional adherent stromal layer [27 – 29]. The stromal layer, which is composed of, among others, fibroblastoid, endothelial, macrophagic, and fat cells, appears to mimic events that normally function to insure the survival and orderly proliferation and differentiation of hematopoietic progenitors in vivo. In the absence of an adherent stromal layer, adequate hematopoiesis can not be maintained to any significant degree. The importance of the adherent stromal layer in human LTC is also well established. However, the stromal layer of human LTC has been noted to be sparser and less developed than that of the murine culture. It is possible that the relative short-term nature of human LTC results from the difficulty in establishing a well-developed adherent stromal layer.

Although the mechanism(s) by which the stroma effects hematopoiesis is poorly understood, it is clear that the cellular elements of the stroma can exert profound influence on the proliferative activity of blood progenitors. In this regard, the stromal layer in murine LTC has been shown to produce/secrete factors that facilitate CFU-S survival [30]. Similarly, the endothelial cells present in this layer are well known producers of a variety of growth factors that regulate the hematopoietic progenitor activity at several levels [31]. Thus, in addition to providing the matrix upon which hematopoiesis occurs, the stromal layer appears to be involved in several aspects of the finely tuned regulatory processes necessary for blood cell production.

It is likely that as our knowledge of the regulatory events controlling hematopoiesis expands, improved procedures for developing a well-formed stromal layer and a more productive human LTC will become possible.

The production of adequate numbers of blood cells requires the orderly proliferation and differentiation of the pluripotent and committed hematopoietic stem cells. The regulatory signals that control these events are both of the well defined humoral types (e.g., erythropoietin, Ep) [32], and involve cellular interactions [33,34]. The role of cell-cell interactions in the regulation of hematopoiesis, originally suggested by the in vivo observations of Trenton [33], has been firmly established as the result of studies utilizing the in vitro clonal assays for hematopoietic progenitors [34 – 37]. The development of these clonal assays has refined and expanded our concepts of the regulation of hematopoiesis and provided a powerful tool for the study of the role of cellular interactions in blood cell production. Studies using these techniques have shown that cell-mediated events affect the proliferation and/or differentiation of a number of hematopoietic progenitors; the clonal growth of the human multipotential stem cell (CFU-GEMM/MIX) in vitro can be achieved only in the presence of media conditioned by mitogen-stimulated mononuclear cells (PHA-LCM) [38,39)]. Similarly, the clonal growth of CFU-GM is dependent upon a family of glycoproteins generally known as colony-stimulating activity (CSA) which is produced by a variety of cell types [40 – 42].

Cell-mediated factors also modulate erythropoiesis [31,34 – 37,43,44]. There is considerable evidence to indicate that the growth of the more mature progenitor CFU-E is critically dependent on Ep [45,46]. By contrast, the proliferative activity of the more primitive BFU-E appears to be regulated by accessory cell populations [31,34 – 37,43,44]. Thus, T lymphocytes [35,36], monocytes-macrophages (MO) [34,37,47], vascular endothelial cells (EC) [31], and other stromal cells [48], all normal components of marrow micro-environment, have been shown to modulate the proliferative activity of BFU-E through the production of a factor(s) commonly designated as the burst promoting activity (BPA). The mechanism of BPA production by these cells is not known. The amount of BPA produced by normal immuno-competent cells is significantly increased when they are activated to undergo rapid proliferation by mitogenic factors such as PHA.

Activated T lymphocytes and monocytes can also exert significant inhibitory effects on hematopoiesis [49,50]. Immuno-mediated suppression of erythropoiesis and granulopoiesis mediated by T lymphocytes have been demonstrated in aplastic anemia [50], in red cell aplasia associated with T cell CLL [51], and in some leukopenic patients [52]. Monocyte-mediated suppression of erythropoiesis has been reported in patients with disseminated histoplasmosis (fig. 1) [44]. In these studies, patients' T cells and/or MO were found to suppress the development of BFU-E and/or CFU-E derived colonies by patients and normal human bone marrow in vitro.

The delineation of the role of normal T cells and MO in hematopoiesis in general and erythropoiesis in particular has been hampered by the absence of pure populations of precursor cells, as well as defined culture conditions. As a result some controversy exists as to the type of effect these cells exert on hematopoietic progenitors. For example, Nathan et al. [35] showed that human blood BFU-E lack membrane characteristics of B or T lymphocytes, are isolated with the null cell fraction, but would not grow in the absence of T cells. We confirmed the null cell characteristics of blood BFU-E but were unable to demonstrate an obligatory role of T cells for their growth in vitro [53]. Similarly Zuckerman [37] reported that T cells were not required for the optimal growth of BFU-E in vitro. By contrast, Magnan et al. [54] and Haq et al. [55] presented evidence supporting the T cell need for optimal BFU-E development in vitro. In our initial studies we employed two procedures for removing T lymphocytes, SRBC rosetting and OKT3 anti-T cell antibody. However, in the former case significant numbers of T cells, recognized by different monoclonal antibodies, are present in the depleted fraction, which may have accounted for our inability to demonstrate

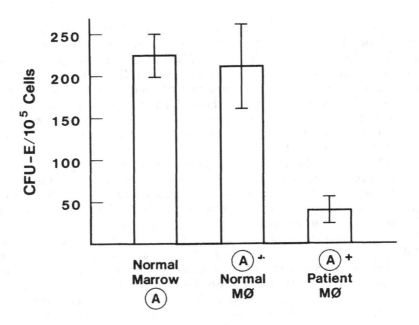

Figure 1. Suppression of normal human bone marrow erythropoiesis by mono-cyte/macrophages (MO) from patients with histoplasmosis. Isolated marrow MO were co-cultured with normal human bone marrow (A) at concentrations ranging from 2 – 8% of total nucleated cells in culture. Cells were cultured in plasma clot in the presence of 0.5 IU erythropoietin.

a significant effect of T cells in blood BFU-E development [53]. The use of OKT3 proved to be more effective in removing a greater percentage of T cells, and in this case we were unable to detect significant BFU-E growth in the T cells depleted fraction. However, the addition of autologous T cells to these cultures did not result in the stimulation of BFU-E growth. We found that this inability of T cells to promote BFU-E growth was related to the mitogenic influence of OKT3. When isolated T cells pretreated with OKT3 were co-cultured with autologous bone marrow or blood mono-nuclear cells, significant inhibition of erythroid colony formation occurred (fig. 2). This suppressive activity, which was directly dependent on the number of OKT3-treated T cells added to the culture, was similar to effects produced by PHA-stimulated autologous T cells [49] (fig. 2). More recent-ly, we employed a mixture of three monoclonal anti-T cell antibodies (TA1, UCHT1, T101) conjugated to the toxin ricin [56] to achieve near total T cell depletion and were able to demonstrate a significant role of T cells in the optimal growth of blood BFU-E in vitro (fig. 3); these antibodies either singly or in combination did not exhibit significant T cell mitogenic effect. The use of ricin-bound antibodies also permits the delineation of the role of endogenously produced T cells in BFU-E growth. We have found that when T-depleted bone marrow cells are cultured in the presence of

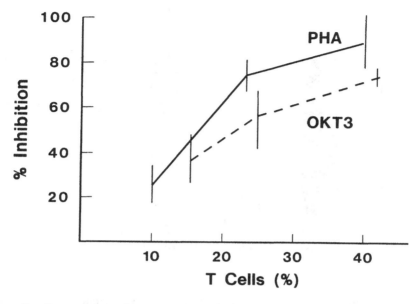

Figure 2. Suppression of normal human bone marrow erythropoiesis by PHA- or OKT3-activated autologous T-lymphocytes. T cells were exposed to PHA or OKT3 for 1 hour at 37°C, washed 2 × and co-cultured with autologous marrow in the presence of 0.5 IU erythropoietin in plasma clot.

PHA-LCM, significant numbers of T cells are produced by day seven of culture. Whether the continued production of T cells by marrow cells may explain the reported difference for T cell requirements of blood and marrow BFU-E [57] is not known. Thus the inadequacies of the depletion procedures and changes in the functional characteristics of T cells should be considered in the interpretation of the results obtained in such studies.

These studies and those reported by others, bring out an important feature of the role of accessory cell populations in the modulation of hematopoiesis; the same biologic event that causes these cells to produce/release factors (BPA, CSA, PHA-LCM) that promote the growth of hematopoietic progenitors may render the cells inhibitory to the hematopoietic process. Thus while normal T cells can augment the growth of hematopoietic progenitors under certain experimental and clinical conditions these cells can be made to be highly inhibitory to the hematopoietic process. For example, as mentioned above, activation of normal T cells by exposure to mitogens such as PHA, PWM, Con A or certain of the monoclonal anti-T cells antibodies (e.g. OKT3) can render these cells inhibitory to hematopoietic progenitors in vitro [49]. Suppressor activity resulting in the inhibition of erythropoiesis is also generated by allo-sensitized immuno-reactive cells in both a genetically restricted and unrestricted manner [58]. Both helper

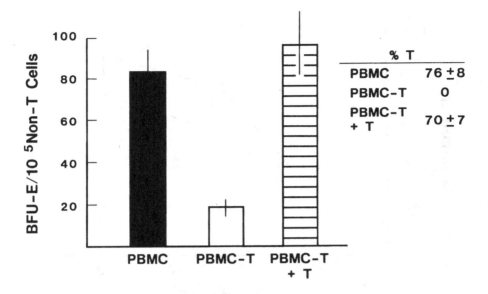

Figure 3. Stimulation of BFU-E derived erythroid colony formation by T cells depleted normal human peripheral blood mononuclear cells by autologous T lymphocytes. Whole peripheral blood mononuclear cells (PBMC) were depleted of T cells by sheep red cell rosetting and the use of ricin-conjugated anti-T cell monoclonal antibodies, and of monocytes by adherence. T cells used in co-culture studies were obtained from the SRBC-rosetting step. Autologous monocytes were added back to all cultures at concentrations similar to that present in whole mononuclear cell preparations.

(OKT4) and suppressor (OKT8) T lymphocytes are equally effective in producing inhibitory activity when exposed to plant lectins.

The mechanism(s) by which "activated" accessory cells affect hematopoiesis is not known. Clearly their "helper" effect can be mediated via the production factors such as CSA and BPA. It is possible that the "suppressor" effect is also humorally mediated; media conditioned by MO from patients with histoplasmosis were found to inhibit erythropoiesis to the same degree as when intact MO were added to the culture [44]. Activated monocytes and T cells produce a variety of bioactive agents including interleukin 1, endogenous pyrogen, and interferon, among others. Experimental evidence suggest that the detrimental influence of these accessory cells may be, at least in part, mediated via one or more of these agents.

Several lines of evidence indicate that γ-IFN may play a significant role in the mediation of the inhibitory effects of activated normal and abnormal T cells. Hoffman et al. [50] reported that lymphocytes from patiens with aplastic anemia suppressed erythropoiesis by normal human bone marrow in vitro, suggesting that at least in some cases, aplastic anemia was the end result of an immune-mediated pathogenic process. Recently, Zoumbos et al. [59,60] provided data to support the notion that γ-IFN may be involved in the inhibitory process. Interferon was detected in the circulation of some patients with aplastic anemia but not in control subjects, Moreover, higher than normal levels of IFN were present in bone marrow of these patients. That γ-IFN may be a mediator of hematopoietic suppression in these patients was demonstrated by the fact that the addition of anti-γ-IFN antibody patients' bone marrow resulted in the augmentation of hematopoietic colony formation [59,60].

Further evidence in support of a role for γ-IFN in the pathogenesis of aplastic anemia has been provided by the studies of Herrman et al. [61]. This group isolated an interleukin 2 dependent T cells line (SMAA) from a patient with aplastic anemia which inhibits the formation of hematopoietic colonies by human bone marrow in vitro. It was found that:
1. the addition of 10^4 neutralizing units of anti-γ-IFN antibody completely blocked the inhibitory properties of these cells; and
2. the suppressive effecst of SMAA cells on hematopoiesis in vitro could be duplicated by the addition of 10^4 U/ml of a preparation of recombinant DNA-derived human γ-IFN to the cultures.

In this regard, a possible direct association between IFN administration and bone marrow suppression in vivo was decribed by Mangan et al. [62]. The administration of IFN to a patient with well-differentiated lymphocytic lymphoma resulted in severe pancytopenia characterized by reduced marrow CFU-E activity and increased numbers of marrow suppressor T cells (OKT8). Immunosuppressive therapy caused marked improvement in peripheral blood count, an increase in marrow CFU-E and a decrease in marrow OKT8 cells. Whether IFN therapy was directly responsible for these finding remains unclear. However, depression of peripheral blood counts is frequently seen in patients undergoing IFN therapy [63].

Interferons are biologically active molecules that are produced by nucleated cells in response to viral infections, as well as a number of other stimuli [64]. As a class of molecules, IFN are capable of a diverse range of functtions both in vivo and in vitro. It has become increasingly obvious that, although initially recognized and defined by their anti-viral properties, this group of glyoproteins may play a significant role in cellular proliferation and differentiation, including those of the hematopoietic progenitors [64 – 66]. In this regard, IFN have been shown to inhibit the proliferation/ differentiation of normal human bone marrow multipotent (CFU-GEMM), as well as committed (CFU-GM, BFU-E, CFU-E) hematopoietic progenitors in vitro [65,66].

To examine the mechanism(s) underlying the inhibitory effect of IFN on hematopoiesis, we studied the influence of different doses (5 – 10,000 U/ml) of a highly purified preparation of recombinant-DNA produced human γ-IFN (Biogen, Inc., Cambridge, MA) on erythroid colony formation by normal human bone marrow BFU-E and CFU-E in the presence and absence of monocytes and/or T cells in vitro [66]. The addition of γ-IFN to whole marrow caused the suppression of BFU-E (6 – 63%) and CFU-E

(31 – 79%) in a dose-dependent fashion. This inhibition occurred both with the direct addition of and pre-exposure of marrow cells to γ-IFN followed by washing of the cells; at the highest concentration of IFN used (10,000 U/ml), near maximal inhibition of colony formation occurred with as little as 15 minutes of incubation. The removal of monocytes and/or T lymphocytes prior to the addition of γ-IFN resulted in a significant decrease in the inhibitory effects of this lymphokine on both BFU-E and CFU-E activity. Our findings suggested that the inhibitory effect of γ-IFN on erythropoiesis was mediated, at least in part, through monocytes and/or T cells. A direct demonstration of the role of these accessory cells in the mediation of γ-IFN effect on erythropoiesis was achieved by the use of co-culture studies. Co-culture of purified autologous monocytes or T cells, preexposed to γ-IFN, with either whole marrow or marrow depleted of monocytes and T cells resulted in highly significant suppression of erythroid colony formation. This was the case even when these γ-IFN treated cells comprised <1% of the total nucleated cells in culture. These results, once again, reveal the profound influence these accessory cells can exert on the hematopoietic process.

It is well documented in the murine LTC that the removal of the non-adherent cells (mainly mature cells) combined with the replacement of the "old" culture medium with fresh medium stimulates CFU-S mitosis [67 – 69]; an inhibitor of CFU-S proliferation has been detected in the "old" medium [68,69]. Although it is not known what cell(s) produces this inhibitory factor(s), it is possible that the production of these types of factors is a reflection of the negative feedback control on the hematopoietic process normally exercised by the mature blood cells.

Normal in vivo hematopoiesis is associated with the constant migration of mature blood cells from the bone marrow into the systemic circulation. Dead and senescent cells are promptly removed along with any toxic by-products of these cells. In the restricted milieu of the LTC, however, prolonged exposure of the hematopoietic progenitors to mature cells and their by-product occurs. Improved productivity of the LTC, unless accompanied by procedures to insure near constant removal (harvesting) of the mature cells, may exacerbate the stituation leading ultimately to the death of the system. The harvesting system should also allow for the needed removal of mature cell by-products. Considerable evidence exists which implicates neutrophils and their secretory products in the suppression of hematopoiesis. In short-term cultures neutrophils have been shown to inhibit myelopoiesis through the production/release of lactoferrin and acidic isoferritin [70,71].

The possibility also exists that the effect of "activated" accesory cells, including neutrophils, on hematopoietic progenitors may be mediated through the production of reactive oxygen metabolites. It is known that phagocytic leukocytes, including cells, of monocytic series, can produce potent oxidizing molecules capable of destroying normal and neoplastic cells [72,73]. The generation of oxygen intermediates, low in resting potential, increases during phagocytosis or after specific stimulation of the phagocytic membrane and is accompanied by a burst of oxygen consumption. The primary species generated are the univalent or divalent products of oxygen, superoxide and hydrogen peroxide [73]. These metabolites play an important role in the generation of other radicals and halide oxidation products [73]. The cytotoxic acity of these oxygen intermediates on eukaryotic cell and the findings that γ-IFN mediated activation of monocytes results not only in increased tumoricidal activity and suppression of normal hematopoietic precursors, but also enhanced secretion of H_2O_2 [74] suggest that the reactive oxygen metabolites should be evaluated as possible effectors of activated accessory cells. These molecules cause oxidant damage by reacting with DNA, unsaturated and thiol-containing aminoacids, carbohydrates in cell surface receptors, and lipids [73]. It has been previously shown that in vitro growth of erythroid progenitors is increased in a low-oxygen atmosphere [74,75], revealing the possible susceptibility of hematopoietic progenitors to oxidant damage.

We found that the addition of H_2O_2 to normal human bone marrow cells in vitro caused marked inhibition of erythroid colony growth. This inhibition was partially reversed by catalase or the iron chelator deferoxamine; iron catalyzes the Haber-Weiss reaction whereby the extremely toxic hydroxyl radical is generated. In other system, deferoxamine has also been noted to ameliorate oxidant-induced cellular damage [76]. We also found that when normal human marrow was exposed to a source of superoxide radical, xanthine oxidase and hypoxanthine, CFU-E and BFU-E growth was significantly inhibited; this was reversed by a variety of oxygen radical scavengers. Similarly, the addition of autologous neutrophils (PMN) activated with N-formyl methionyl leucyl phenylalanine (FMLP) to normal

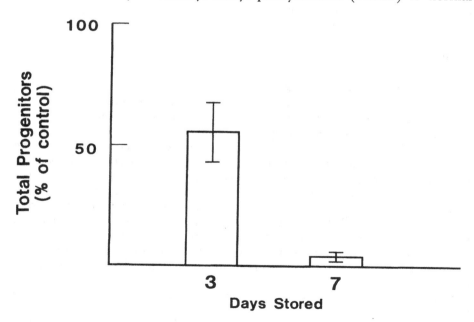

Figure 4. Loss of hematopoietic progenitors following storage of normal human bone marrow cells at 37°C, 5% CO_2 in humidified air.

human bone marrow in vitro significantly decreased growth of erythroid progenitors. In order to determine whether this inhibitory effect of activated PMN is mediated through the elaboration of $H_2O_2$and/or other oxygen radical species, we pretreated these cultures with either catalase, peroxidase or radical scavengers such as deferoxamine, mannitol, superoxide dismutase, or autologous red blood cells; in all cases near normal erythroid growth was restored. Although the in vivo importance of oxygen radical-mediated inhibition of hematopoiesis remains to be established, it is tempting to speculate that it may play a role, along with the other products of activated accessory cells, in the relatively poor hematopoietic progenitor profile of human LTC. Neutrophils and macrophages, well known producers/secretors of these reactive oxygen metabolites, are the more readily formed cells in human LTC. The production/release of these metabolites may lead to toxicity directed towards innocent neighbouring by-standers, including hematopoietic stem cells and other surrounding, but otherwise helpful, accessory cells.

We have found that the significant loss of hematopoietic progenitors that occurs when normal human bone marrow is stored under conditions not too dissimilar to LTC (fig. 4) is caused, at least in part, by the presence of toxic oxygen metabolites. When normal human bone marrow was stored ($37°C$, 5% CO_2 in air) in the presence of deferoxamine, a significant improvement in the recovery of hematopoietic progenitors was noted. Because, in these studies bone marrow cells were routinely processed, it is evident that similar release of these bioreactive agents can readily occur in the milieu of human LTC with similar negative influences.

Summary

The development of in vitro clonal assays for hematopoietic progenitors has refined our concepts of the regulation of blood cells production by permitting the operational identification and quantitation of different classes of progenitors, and of the regulatory signals that control their proliferation and differentiation. In addition,these techniques have opened the way for the evaluation of production/expansion of the hematopoietic stem cell pool and their mature progenies in more enduring culture systems. Although the long term culture of human hematopoietic cells is in its infancy, there are reasons to believe that the system may prove useful in providing expanded numbers of blood cells for use in clinical settings. Murine long term culture systems are capable of producing committed progenitors and mature granulocytes for long periods. When properly stimulated with erythropoietin and/or anemic serum formation of red cells can also be observed in this system.

While the optimum culture parameters for human cells remain to be worked out, some success is already apparent. Mature, functional granulocytes have been produced in such cultures which have been maintained in excess of six weeks with net production of hematopoietic progenitors. It is possible that the rate of production of blood cells and the longevity of the culture and of the progenitors may be dramatically improved by enabling the system to counteract the toxic secretory products of the produced cells. Interactions of progenitors with other cells, both normal and activated, and with various humoral factors may be important in establishing hematopoiesis in vitro. Past studies of such interactions are applicable and more studies are indicated. As the system improves, it may provide not only mature cells for traditional clinical transfusion purposes, but also sufficient numbers of progenitors cells for achieving hematopoietic reconstitution in man. In such an improved proliferative culture system it may also become possible to modify, by genetic and/or biochemical manipulations, the antigenic profile(s) of the blood cells produced in vitro.

References

1. Young LS. Prophylactic granulocytes in the neutropenic host. Ann Int Med 1982;96:240 – 2.
2. Kahn RA, Allen RW, Badassare J. Alternate sources and substitutes for therapeutic blood components. Blood 1985;66:1 – 12.
3. Hersman J, Meyers JD, Thomas ED, Buckner CD, Clift R. The effect of granulocyte transfusions on the incidence of cytomegalovirus infection after allogenic marrow transplantation. Ann Int Med 1982;96:149 – 52.
4. Storb R, Thomas ED. Allogeneic bone marrow transplantation. Immunol Rev 1983;71:77 – 102.
5. O'Reilly RJ. Allogeneic bone marrow transplantation: current status and future directions. Blood 1983;62:941 – 64.
6. Coulombel L, Eaves C, Gupta C, Kalousch D, Eaves A. Long-term marrow culture of cells from patients with acute myelogenous leukemia. J Clin Invest 1985;75:961 – 9.
7. Colombel L, Kalousek DK, Eaves CJ, Gupta CM, Eaves A. Long-term marrow culture reveals chromosomally normal hematopoietic progenitors cells in patients with Philadelphia-positive chronic myelogenous leukemia. New Engl J Med 1983;308:1493 – 8.
8. Dube ID, Kalousek DK, Coulombel L, Gupta CM, Eaves CJ, Eaves A. Cytogenetic studies of early myeloid progenitor compartments in Ph' positive chronic myelogenous leukemia. II. Long-term culture reveals the persistence of Ph' negative progenitors in treated as well as newly diagnosed patients. Blood 1984;63:1172 – 7.
9. Wright DG, Greenberger JS (eds). Long term bone marrow culture. New York: Alan R. Liss, Inc. 1984.
10. Spooncer E, Dexter TM. Transplantation of long term cultured bone marrow cells. Transplantation 1983;35:624 – 7.
11. Greenberger JS, Sakakeeny M, Parker LM. In vitro proliferation of hemopoietic stem cells in long term marrow cultures: principles in mouse applied to man. Exp Hematol 1979;7:135 – 48.
12. Mauch P, Greenberger JS, Botnick L, Hannon E, Hellman S. Evidence for structured variation in self-renewal capacity within long term bone marrow culture. Proc Nat Acad Sci (USA) 1980;77:2927 – 30.
13. Williams N, Jackson H, Rabellino EM. Proliferation and differentiation of normal granulopoietic cells in continuous bone marrow cultures. J Cell Physiol 1977;93:435 – 40.

14. Dexter TM, Testa NG, Allen TD, Rutherford T, Scolnick E. Molecular and cell biologic aspects of erythropoiesis in long term bone marrow culture. Blood 1981;58:699 – 707.

15. Eliason JF, Dexter TM, Testa NG. The regulation of hemopoiesis in long term bone marrow culture. III. The role of burst forming activity. Exp Hematol 1982;10:444 – 50.

16. Eliason JF, Testa NG, Dexter TM. Erythropoeietin-stimulated erythropoiesis in long term bone marrow culture. Nature 1979;281:382 – 4.

17. Williams N, Jackson H, Sheridan APC, Murphy MJ, Elste A, Moore MAS. Regulation of megakaryopoiesis in long term murine bone marrow cultures. Blood 1978;51:245 – 55.

18. Schrader JW, Schrader S. In vitro studies on lymphocyte differentiation. I. Long term in vitro culture of cells giving rise to functional lymphocytes in irradiated mice. J Exp Med 1978;148:823 – 8.

18a. Jones-Villeneuve E, Phillips RA. Potentials for lymphoid differentiation by cells from long term cultures of bone marrow Exp Hematol 1980;8:65 – 76.

19. Dorshkind K, Phillips RA. Maturational state of lymphoid cells in long term bone marrow cultures. J Immunol 1982;129:2444 – 50.

20. Whitloch CA, Robertson D, Witte ON. Murine B cell lymphopoiesis in long term culture. J Immunol Methds 1984;67:353 – 69.

21. Hocking WG, Golde DW. Long term human bone marrow cultures. Blood 1980;56:118 – 24.

22. Coulombel L, Eaves Ac, Eaves CJ. Enzymatic treatment of long term human marrow cultures reveals the preferential location of primitive hemopoietic progenitors in the adherent layer. Blood 1983;62:291 – 7.

23. Gartner S, Kaplan HS. Long term culture of human bone marrow cells. Proc Natl Aced Sci (USA) 1980;77:4756 – 9.

24. Toogood IRG, Dexter TM, Allen TD, Suda T, Lajtha LG. The development of a liquid culture system for the growth of human bone marrow. Leuk Res 1980;4:449 – 61.

25. Moore MAS, Sheridan AP. Pluripotential stem cell replication in continuous human, prosimian, and murine bone marrow culture. Blood Cells 1979;5:297 – 311.

26. Greenberg HM, Newburger PE, Parker LM, Novak T, Greenberger JS. Human granulocytes generated in continuous bone marrow culture are physiologically normal. Blood 1981;58:724 – 32.

27. Bentley SA, Foidart JM. Some properties of marrow derived adherent cells in tissue culture. Blood 1980;56:1006 – 12.

28. Zuckerman KS, Wicha MS. Extracellular matrix production by the adherent cells of long term murine bone marrow cultures. Blood 1983;61:540 – 7.

29. Song ZX, Quesenberry PJ. Radioresistant murine marrow stromal cells. a morphological and functional characterization. Exp Hematol 1984;12:523 – 33.

30. Blackburn MJ, Patt HM. Influence of a marrow stromal factor on survival of hemopoietic stem cells in vitro. Exp Hematol 1980;8:77 – 82.

31. Ascensao JL, Vercelloti GM, Jacob HS, Zanjani ED. Role of endothelial cells in human hematopoiesis: modulation of mixed colony growth in vitro. Blood 1984;63:553 – 8.

32. Krantz SB, Jacobson LO. Erythropoietin and the regulation of erythropoiesis. Chicago: Univerity of Chicago Press, 1970.

33. Trentin JJ. Influence of hematopoietic organ stroma (hematopoietic inductive microenvironments) on stem cell differenatiation. In: Gordon AS (ed). Regulation of hematopoiesis. New York: Appleton-Century-Crofts, 1970:159 – 84.

34. Gordon LI, Miller WJ, Branda RF, Zanjani ED, Jacob HS. Regulation of erythroid colony formation by bone marrow macrophages. Blood 1980;55: 1047 – 50.
35. Nathan DG, Chess L, Hillman DG, Clarke B, Beard J, Merler E, Housman D. Human erythroid burst-forming unit: T-cell requirement for proliferation in vitro. J Exp Med 1978;147:324 – 37.
36. Golde DW, Bersch N, Quan SG, Lusis AJ. Production of erythroid potentiating activity by a human T-lymphoblast cell line. Proc Nat Acad Sci (USA) 1980;77:593 – 6.
37. Zuckerman KS. Human erythroid burst-forming units. Growth in vitro is dependent upon monocytes but not T-lymphocytes. J Clin Invest 1981;67: 702 – 9.
38. Fuaser AA, Messner HA. Granulo-erythropoietic colonies in human bone marrow, peripheral blood, and cord blood. Blood 1979;53:1243 – 8.
39. Ash RC, Detrick RA, Zanjani ED. Studies of human pluripotential hemopoietic stem cells (CFU-GEMM) in vitro. Blood 1981;58:309 – 16.
40. Burgess AS, Metcalf D. The nature and action of granulocyte-macrophage colony stimulating factors. Blood 1980;56:947 – 58.
41. Quesenberry PJ, Gimbrone MA. Vascular endothelium as a source of granulopoiesis: production of colony-stimulating activity by cultured human endothelial cells. Blood 1980;56:1060 – 7.
42. Bagby GC, McCall E, Bergstrom KA, Burger D. A monokine regulates colony-stimulating activity production by vascular endothelial cells. Blood 1983;62:663 – 8.
43. Kurland JI, Meyers PA, Moore MAS. Synthesis and release of erythroid colony- and burst-potentiating activities by purified populations of murine peritoneal macrophages. J Exp Med 1980;151:839 – 51.
44. Zanjani ED, McGlave PB, Davies SF, Banisadre M, Kaplan ME, Sarosi GA. In vitro suppression of erythropoiesis by bone marrow adherent cells from some patients with fungal infection. Brit J Haematol 1982;50:479 – 90.
45. Hara H, Ogawa M. Erythropoietic precursors in mice under erythropoietic stimulation and suppression. Exp Hematol 1977;5:141 – 8.
46. Iscove NN. The role of erythropoietin in the regulation of population size and cell cycling of early and late erythroid precursors in mouse bone marrow. Cell Tissue Kinet 1977;10:323-34.
47. Reid CDL, Baptista LC, Chanarin I. Erythroid colony growth in vitro from human peripheral blood null cells: evidence for regulation by T-lymphocytes and monocytes. Brit J Haematol 1981;48:155 – 63.
48. Porter P, Ogawa M, Leary A. Enhancement of the growth of human early erythroid progenitors by bone marrow conditioned media. Exp Hematol 1978;8:83 – 8.
49. Banisadre M, Ash RC, Ascensao JL, Kay NE, Zanjani ED. Suppression of erythropoiesis by mitogen-activated T lymphocytes in vitro. In: Baum SJ, Ledney GD, Khan A (eds). Experimental hematology today. New York: S. Karger 1981:151 – 9.
50. Hoffman R, Zanjani ED, Lutton JD, Zalusky R, Wasserman LR. Suppression of erythroid colony formation by lymphocytes from patients with aplastic anemia. New Engl J Med 1977;296:10 – 3.
51. Hoffman R, Kopel S, Hsu SD, Dainiak N, Zanjani ED. T-cell chronic lymphocytic leukemia: presence in bone marrow and peripheral blood of cells that suppress erythropoiesis in vitro. Blood 1978;52:255 – 60.
52. Bagby GC, Gabourel JD. Neutropenia in three patients with rheumatic disorders. J Clin Invest 1979;64:72 – 82.

53. Nomdedieu B, Gormus BJ, Banisadre M, Rinehart JJ, Kaplan ME, Zanjani ED. Human peripheral blood erytrhoid burst-forming unit (BFU-E): evidence against T lymphocyte requirement for proliferation in vitro. Exp Hematol 1980;8:845 – 52.
54. Mangan KF, DesForges JF. The role of T lymphocytes and monocytes in the regulation of human erythropoietic peripheral blood burst forming units. Exp Hematol 1980;8:717 – 27.
55. Haq AU, Rinehart JJ, Balcerzak SP. T-cell subset modulation of blood erythroid burst-forming unit proliferation. J Lab Clin Med 1983;101:53 – 7.
56. Vallera DA, Ash RC, Zanjani ED, Kersey JH, LeBien TW, Beverely PCL, Neville DM, Yule RJ. Anti-T cell reagents for human bone marrow transplantation: ricin linked to three monoclonal antibodies. Science 1983;222: 512 – 5.
57. Lipton JM, Reinherz EL, Kudisch M, Jackson PL, Schlossman SF, Nathan DG. Mature bone marrow erythroid burst-forming units do not require T cell for induction of erythropoietin-dependent differentiation. J Exp Med 1980;152:350 – 8.
58. Torok-Storb B. T-cell effects on in vitro erythropoiesis: immune regulation and immune reactivity. In: Young NS, Levine AS, Humphries RK (eds). Aplastic anemia: stem cell biology and advance in treatment. New York: Alan R. Liss, Inc. 1984:163 – 72.
59. Zoumbos NC, Djeu JY, Young NS. Interferon is the suppressor of hematopoiesis generated by stimulated lymphocytes in vitro. J Immunol 1984;133: 769 – 74.
60. Zoumbos N, Gascon P, Djeu P, Young NS. Interferon is a mediator of hematopoietic suppression in apalstic anemia in vitro and possibly in vivo. Proc Nat Acad Sci (USA) 1985;82:188 – 92.
61. Herrmann F, Meuer S, Griffin JD. Establishment of an interleukin-2 dependent cell line from a patient with aplastic anemia which inhibits hematopoiesis. Blood 1984;64:105a.
62. Mangan KF, Zindar B, Ziegler Z, Winkelstein A, Shadduck RK. Interferon-induced aplasia: role of suppressor T cells and recovery after treatment with horse anti-human thymocyte globulin (ATG). Clin Res 1984;32:414a.
63. Kirkwood JM, Ernstoff MS. Interferons in the treatment of human cancer. J Clin Oncol 1984;2:336 – 52.
64. Preble OT, Friedman RM. Biology of disease: interferion-induced alterations in cells. Relevance to viral and non-viral diseases. Lab Invest 1983;49:4 – 18.
65. Broxmeyer HE, Lu L, Platzer E, Feit C, Juliano L, Rubin BY. Comparative analysis of the influences of human gamma, alpha and beta interferons on human multipotential (CFU-GEMM), erythroid (BFU-E) and granulocyte-macrophage (CFU-GM) progenitor cells. J Immunol 1983;131:1300 – 5.
66. Namus SW, Beck-Schroeder S, Zanjani ED. Suppression of normal human erythropoiesis by gamma interferon in vitro. Role of monocytes and T lymphocytes. J Clin Invest 1985;75:1496 – 1503.
67. Dexter TM, Wright EG, Krizsa F, Lajtha LG. Regulation of haemopoietic stem cell proliferation in long-term bone marrow cultures. Biomed 1977;27:344 – 9.
68. Wright EG, Lord BI, Dexter TM, Lajtha LG. Mechanisms of haemopoietic stem cell proliferation control. Blood Cells 1979;5:247 – 58.
69. Tokosoz D, Dexter TM, Lord BI, Wright EG, Lajtha LG. The regulation of hematopoiesis in long-term bone marrow cultures. II. Stimulation and inhibition of stem cell proliferation. Blood 1980;55:931 – 6.

70. Broxmeyer HE, Moore MAS, Ralph P. Cell-free granulocyte colony inhibiting activity derived from human polymorphonuclear neutrophils. Exp Hematol 1976;5:87 – 92.

71. Broxmeyer HE, Smithyman A, Eyer RR, Meyers PA, deSousa M. Identification of lactoferrin as the granulocyte-derived inhibitor of colony-stimulating activity production. J Exp Med 1978;148:1052 – 67.

72. Freeman BA, Crapo JD. Biology of disease: free radicals and tissue injury. Lab Invest 1982;47:412 – 26.

73. Weiss SJ, LoBuglio AF. Biology of disease: phagocyte-generated oxygen metabolites and cellular injury. Lab Invest 1982;47:5 – 18.

74. Nathan C, Horowitz C, de la Harpe J, Vadhan-Raj S, Sherwin S, Krown S. Administration of recombinant-"G" interferon enhances the ability of cancer patients' monocytes to secrete H_2O_2. Clin Res 1985;33:559a.

74a. Rich IN, Kubanek B. The effect of reduced oxygen tension on colony formation of erythropoietic cells in vitro. Brit J Haematol 1982;52:579 – 88.

75. Bradley TR, Hodgson GS, Rosenthal M. The effect of oxygen tension on haemopoietic and fibroblast cell proliferation in vitro. J Cell Physiol 1978;97: 517 – 22.

76. van Asbeck BS, Marx JJM, Struyvenberg A, van Kats JH, Verhoef J. Deferoxamine enhances phagocytic function of human polymorphonuclear leucocytes. Blood 1984;63:714 – 20.

DISCUSSION

Moderators: C.F. Högman and P.C. Das

J.A. van der Does (The Hague): In the Red Cross Blood Bank at the Hague, we have started a hollow fiber filtration plasmapheresis project. From this plasma, we produce a normal wet cryoprecipitate. We pool the cryoprecipitates of three plasmas. Our yield then is 53% in the routine. We have also tried to go to heat-treatment. We have lyophilized our cryoprecipitate and heated it for 24 hours at 68°C with the buffers described by Dr. Das from Groningen. So, starting from a wet cryoprecipitate with a recovery of 53%, freeze-dried cryoprecipitate has a recovery of 50%, and after heat-treatment we end up with a yield of 42%.

C. Th. Smit Sibinga (Groningen): Mr. Anthony, what do you think is the future of the pack design, now that you have described your sterile connection device as basically a single pack with a pigtail?

J.M. Anthony (Deerfield): I really think that depends on a market-by-market analysis. In the United States, 88% of the blood is spun at least once into plasma and red cells, so for this marketplace a double pack might well be the base pack. In various regions of Europe, perhaps the single pack is the best one to begin with. It is very flexible; we can make the design practically any way we want. The key here is that you want to make it so it is most economical for a particular operation.

C. Th. Smit Sibinga: How do you see the connection of your device to a plastic of another manufacturer?

J.M. Anthony: I do not see that.

C. Th. Smit Sibinga: Dr. Bakker, I was very much intrigued by your presentation and would like to congratulate you. However, one thing I missed from the presentation: What is your expectation of the oxygen release capacity of this hemoglobin analogue?

J.C. Bakker (Amsterdam): That is difficult to explain. From the in vitro data, you see a shift of the oxygen hemoglobin dissociation curve to the right. Of the mixture, the position of the curve – at least the p50 – is very close to the p50 of normal erythrocytes. That is an important improvement. When you compare this to non-modified hemoglobin, it has a p50 of around 12 to 15. This is an in vitro observation.

But, the oxygen hemoglobin dissociation curve in our case was a little bit flatter. That means that at the arterial po2 of 100, not 100% of the hemoglobin is saturated. Normally, that is not a disadvatage; it is only a disadvantage in case the loading of oxygen is the problem. So, in cases of arterial hypoxemia it is disadvantageous when the curve has shifted too much to the right.

C. Th. Smit Sibinga: So there is a perspective for the release of oxygen when using this material.

J. C. Bakker: Yes. One can imagine under certain circumstances, for example during extracorporeal circulation, when the blood is cooled, it is of great advantage that the curve is shifted to the right, because temperature decrease will shift it to the left. Then one perhaps will end up at 28°C at normal p50.

C. F. Högman (Uppsala): Do you have any comment on any kidney problem, or dosage problem? What if you try to transfer the animal data to possible use in humans?

J. C. Bakker: The few clinical data derived from humans, show some kidney problems, although in those studies there was very minor contamination of stroma. The problem is that you have to remove all the stroma contaminants. The probable explanation is that it is still a little toxic and will cause damage to kidneys. I reported on the liver, but we also have to solve the toxicity issue as far as the kidney is concerned. The problem is: How do you determine the stroma contamination? We tried several markers, for instance a hemagglutination inhibition test, which is used in quality control of albumin products to see how much membrane fragments are still present. The sensitivity of that test was not sufficient to detect low levels of contamination. We used cholesterol as a marker of membrane lipid, and we ended up with less than 0.5% of membrane lipids still present in our solution. But, we still do know whether or not that is sufficient.

T. J. Greenwalt (Cincinnati): Dr. Fahy, about 18 or 20 years ago, I visited Dr. Perry Blackshear at the University of Minnesota. He was freezing human red cells – in very small quantities, of course – under high pressure. He claimed that once he had frozen them, he could reduce the normal atmospheric pressure and they would still store. This sounded very encouraging to me. What has happened to these observations?

G. M. Fahy (Bethesda): I do not think that that work was followed up. The general experience with using high pressures to facilitate freezing is not very positive. Generally speaking, the results are equal to what you get without the pressures or worse. I am not that familiar with Blackshear's work, but if he did have some positive results, it probably is true that you could release the pressure and still store, provided that the temperature was down below the glass transition temperature of water when you did that. That is also true with the vitrification approach: If one uses high pressures to vitrify, one can release the pressures for storage, but you have to be below the glass transition temperature to allow that.

P. C. Das (Groningen): Dr. Wallevik, after you have heat-treated the factor VIII, did you study stability on storage, let us say for six months.

K. Wallevik (Århus): We have not studied the solubility after six months' storage in the freeze-dried heat-treated state, because we have not yet heat-treated for six months. I do not think that will change the product.

C. Th. Smit Sibinga: Dr. Lasky, this technique might come in place of our donor population, to a certain extent. What do you see as a major source of the pluripotent stem cells, and what do you see as the technique for yielding enough cells to really meet the needs for transfusion purposes?

L. C. Lasky (Minneapolis): That is really far in the future, I think. It could be a combination of two things. One is that, currently, people are starting to put together HLA-typed stored collections of cadaver bone marrow. You can get cadaver bone marrow in vast quantities from individuals who are brain dead, or are donating their kidneys or livers. That would be a great source of hematopoietic progenitors and down-the-line blood cells. One of the neat things about the blood system is that from one progenitor cell, you can get lots and lots of mature granulocytes or red cells – in theory – if we get the system working. The other one is with genetic engineering techniques.

III. Labortory aspects

MACHINE-READABLE SYMBOLS IN BLOOD TRANSFUSION

H.K. Prins

Objective and prerequisites of blood transfusion practice

The objectives of the transfusion of a blood component are
- effectiveness: the long-standing correction of a temporary or chronic shortage;
- compatibility: no side effects; neither immediate nor in the long run;
- safety: no transfer of disease or factors causing reactions.
  Effectiveness is achieved when the blood component is:
- the appropriate component;
- fresh;
- compatible.
  Compatibility may be enhanced by:
- estimation of (in)compatibility by comparing patient and donor records;
- compatibility testing in the laboratory;
- removal of immunizing blood components.
  Safety requirements:
- sterility;
- absence of disease-transmitting micro-organisms, as established by special treatment or the results of present and previous laboratory investigations.

Steps in the preparation and transfusion of blood components

There are many stages from begin to the end:
- estimation of the demand for blood components;
- planning of blood collection sessions;
- specification of the type of blood collection for individual donors;
- checking of the donor's fitness to donate;
- identification of the donation:
    - linking the donor's identity to the donation number,
    - linking the donation number to the identity of the collection set;
- the collection procedure;
- collection of samples;
- transport, storage (quarantine);
- transfer of samples to laboratory; specification of tests requested;
- transfer of collected units to processing department;
- specification and performance of the type(s) of processing;

- taking of samples for quality checking
  - quarantine storage;
- release of blood components from quarantine storage;
- definition of the patient's need for a certain blood component;
- comparison with data on blood components in stock or in process;
- assignment of the chosen units to the patient;
- compatibility checking;
- transfer to the ward;
- transfusion to the patient;
- evaluation of the effect(s) of the transfusion.

Each step involves the following procedures: checking-in, establishment of identity, recording of time and location, the specification of the step, the test method or a result, the specification of samples for laboratory testing, checking-out, recording of the identity of the person in charge.

This amounts to a tremendous number of data, to be collected and to be available at the end of each step.

Organization and use of accumulated data

Data are useful when they are: relevant, unequivocal, reliable, complete, up to date or even up to the minute, organized and available for retrieval, scanning or processing.

Central files in the organization of data are: the patient file, the donor file and the blood component file (access codes resp.: the patient registration number, the donor registration number and the blood collection identification.)

Important data in the patient's record are:
- identity;
- history, diagnosis;
- future treatment;
- the transfusion plan;
- the transfusion history;
- hereditary and acquired factors relevant for transfusion planning (e.g. previously detected red cell allo-antibodies).

Important data in the donor's record are:
- identity;
- (donation) history;
- possible involvement in complications after transfusion;
- genetically determined and acquired factors relevant for transfusion.

Specification of a unit of blood component should comprise:
- identification of the container:
  - type and serial number of the original collection set,
  - code of the actual part of the set;
- identification of the contents:
  - specification of the component,
  - identity of the original donation.

The access codes to these files will be used numerous times for the updating of files, each time with the risk of misreading or miswriting. A recommendable way to avoid errors and at the same time to speed up data collection is to read these codes from prefabricated lables with the help of computer-assisted reading devices. This type of reading is also recommendable in specifying standard codes, e.g. blood groups and other test results, blood components, locations, collection sets, procedures and authorized personnel.

A reading station is equipped with:
- a reading device appropriate for the job to be done;
- a screen, used for messages, warnings, instructions;
- a keyboard for back-up and communication;
- a device for the storage of data and programmes for off-line processing;
- a means of communication with a central system;
- a menu sheet, with machine-readable codes for the initiation and performance of procedures;
- a manual.

If the data collection in itself is no longer a bottleneck in the total procedure, and if the accumulated data have been properly organized, then the date in the patient file, the donor file and the product file are available in helping to give to the patient the right component, as fresh as possible, with the smallest risk of incompatibility.

Apart from this good data collection the systems have proved to be of great help in quality control and in logistic problems.

Other prerequisites for the effective use of machine-readable labels are:
- reading stations at a sufficient number of locations (including the hospital);
- user-friendly programming;
- wide-spread hardware and software compatibility.

In this respect the introduction of the personal computer will prove to be a major break-through.

SAFETY AND CONTROL IN BAR-CODE SYMBOLOGY WITHIN THE BLOOD TRANSFUSION SERVICE

P.S. Skinner

To outline the use of bar codes and the latest security and control measures which are used to ensure the integrity of the system, it should first be pointed out that there are no known specifications that relate to the quality control procedures at manufacturing level. However, every manufacturer has their own particular interpretation.

What are the problems one can have with bar-code lables?

The most dangerous are:
1. Duplicate numbers.
2. A different number in the bar-code to the eye-readable interpretation.
3. Excessive amount of missing numbers.
4. Poor quality adhesive.
5. Poor reading rate and incorrect die cutting.

What can be done to avoid these known problems?

1. Duplicate numbers

There have been several fatal cases resulting from duplicate number-ed labels, or in other words two different units of blood bearing the same identification number. This error in printing eminates from the origination stage and it is now possible to eliminate this danger by creating an overriding software control which will drive the photo-typesetting generator in such a manner that each label is sequential by an increment of 1. Any other incrementation or indeed duplica-tion is automatically invalidated by the printer itself which then comes to an immediate halt necessitating operator intervention.

2. Eye-readable and bar-code interpretation

The problem of the eye-readable interpretation of the label not corre-sponding to the bar-code has been known to happen. However, if a bar-code and it's eye-readable interpretation are simultaneously generated by one central command this problem cannot occur.

3. Missing numbers

An excessive amount of missing numbers are a nuisance and create difficulties in monitoring donor sessions. Furthermore, it enhances the human error factor. Therefore, remakes should be mandatory to maintain a manageable quantity of missing numbers. As many blood transfusion centers key in missing numbers in their computer before issuing the lables, it is helpful to provide a comprehensive list of the missing numbers with their bar-code interpretation. This avoids the labourious keying in procedure as the light pen will enter this data straight into the computer.

4. Poor quality adhesive

This has always been a thorny area, however, there are reputable medical adhesive manufacturers who are only too happy to assist in the development of a product which is suitable and safe.

5. Poor reading rate of bar-code, incorrect die cutting and colour stripping

These avoidable problems can be eliminated by pre-despatch visual inspection of every roll of labels. A laser scanner will immediately warn of any readability problem with the bar-code whilst the visual inspection will detect any instances of incorrect die cutting. Colour code striping is being used more and more and will present problems if the lead in and lead out zones (also referred to as quiet zones) are not respected. That is to say there is to be a minimum space of 2 mm between the end of the colour stripe and beginning of the bar-code and likewise from the end of the bar-code to the beginning of the colour stripe.

This analysis represents an endeavour to touch upon some of the problems experienced with bar-code labels and to outline certain measures that can significantly bring more security in their use and make life easier all around. Nonetheless, there are two areas where label users can, at no extra cost, greatly help the manufacturer.

Firstly, by providing a clear outline of the specification of the label set required. That is to say:
- in what application the lables are destined to be used;
- overall size of label set;
- how many bar-coded labels are required;
- how many eye-readable only labels are required;
- which check digit routine is foreseen, if any.

Answers to the above questions help the label manufacturer to offer the industry a product which will do the job.

Secondly, by giving a sufficient delivery delay to not only manufacture the product but also to undertake all of the quality control procedures.

APPLICATION OF ROBOTICS IN BLOOD BANKING*

L.I. Friedman, S.M.L. Severns

Introduction

The word "robot" became part of the English language with the translation of Karel Capek's play R.U.R. (Rossum's Universal Robots) in 1932. In the play the robots were humanoid creations, which were developed to perform obediently in the service of mankind. The early conception was that of a mechanical man, capable of human actions and speech but having sub-human intelligence and superhuman strength. Science fiction of those years portrayed robots with sinister intentions. In the 1940's Isaac Asimov envisioned robots as benevolent servants, with fail safe circuitry to ensure that they always "keep their place". He was the first to use the word "robotics" to describe the development of mobile, intelligent machines.

Webster's Seventh New Collegiate Dictionary defines a robot as "an automatic apparatus or device that performs functions ordinarily ascribed to human beings or operates with what appears to be almost human intelligence". No currently manufactured robots have this capability. A definition which encompasses the capabilities of modern robots is that provided by the Robot Institute of America [1]. They define a robot as "a reprogrammable, multifunctional manipulator designed to move materials, parts, tools or specialized devices, through variable programmed motions for the performance of a variety of tasks".

One of the greatest assests of a robot is its ability to be configured to perform different tasks. This means that a large base of consumers can purchase the same piece of equipment and customize it for their individual applications. (Equipment which is capable of being customized in this manner is frequently referred to as "reconfigurable technology".) Since everyone is purchasing the same basic robot, the economies of scale allow it to be produced less expensively.

Robots for general laboratory use

Advances in laboratory automation have resulted from the introduction of sophisticated analytical instruments and inexpensive information management systems to analyze the resulting data. One method to further automate laboratory tasks is to use robots to prepare samples for these instruments or to move samples between instruments. Most laboratory tasks can be broken down into a series of basic operations, called Laboratory Unit Operations [2].

* Contribution No. 680 from the American Red Cross.

These operations include manipulation, liquid handling, separation, pulverization, measurement, conditioning and data management. Of these operations, manipulation and liquid handling can be handled by a robot, while the rest are performed by specialized equipment which is interfaced to the robot's controller. Therefore, a robot combined with other instruments and devices, all under computer control, (which will be referred to as a "robotic system") comprise a fully automated and integrated laboratory system. Of course, the extent of staff intervention in such a system is dependent on what is done by the individual system components.

There are, a number of potential pitfalls in the application of robotics. First, it is important to recognize that a robot is sometimes seen by management as an expensive "toy". They are frequently bought for their "high tech" image or because management decided to introduce robotics without first studying the problem. Second, robotics may not always be the best answer for meeting automation needs. Care must be taken to determine the best method of automating the task, or if the task really needs automating at all. Third, robots are not generally sold as part of a "turnkey" system. The applications engineering required to produce an integrated robotic system is not easy, and the total cost of a system to perform a task will usually amount to two to four time the cost of the robot arm. This cost includes the development of peripheral fixtures and devices and the computer programming for the robot and associated devices.

Estimates of the cost-effectiveness of robotic systems are usually based on an immediate reduction in labour costs. While this may be true in some situations, in many cases displaced staff become system operators. There may, however, be eventual labour savings as task volume increases while staff size remains constant. Immediate cost savings may still result from reduced reagent consumption, a decreased rate of retesting, more valuable output from staff, improvement utilization of equipment, and reduced paper work. Alternatively, a properly engineered robotic system may allow the user to automate several independent tasks. However, the user must determine whether this "sharing" is practical [3].

Keep in mind the fact that a robotic system generally performs a task no faster than staff. In situations where high throughput is necessary, multiple system may be called for. Finally, manual backup procedures must be available for those times when the robot is not operational.

Once a decision is made to consider the use of a robotic system, a series of steps should be undertaken to help assure a workable solution. Some of the essential steps include [4]:
1. Develop a step by step protocol for the application.
2. Determine if the task(s) can be done by a robot.
3. Complete a paper feasibility analysis, including estimates for the required fixtures, programming and facilities renovations (if required).
4. Conduct a cost analysis.
5. Review available robotic systems and select one candidate.
6. Receive management approval to proceed.
7. Purchase the robotic system, and purchase/develop fixtures.
8. Interface the system with associated devices.

9. Test and debug the system and verify that the system meets design goals.
10. Document the hardware and programming.
11. Install the system and train the operators.
12. Conduct parallel studies to insure proper operation.
13. Develop a back-up plan and maintenance schedule.

Currently, there are several different robotic systems available to automate sample preparation and other laboratory operations. For many of our prototype applications we utilized a Zymate Laboratory Automation System (Zymark Corporation, Hopkinton, MA) [5]. It consists of a robotic arm, a controller and a series of peripheral laboratory stations. The robot having an internal microprocessor, operates in a cylindrical envelope with a radius of about 60 cm. It has four degrees of freedom, dimensional repeatability of approximately 1 mm and a lifting capacity of 1.5 kg. One important feature of the robot is its ability to change hands, which include a general purpose gripper, a syringe, and a blank hand allowing attachment of accessories such as a pipette. Another microcoputer system serves as a master controller. An associated master laboratory station, having an internal microprocessor which operates under the direction of the master controller, contains three accurate and independently controlled syringes. The power and event control station, also driven by the master controller provides capabilities for connecting the Zymate to external devices. The modular design of this system makes the Zymate a very versatile system. Depending upon the peripherals needed, the Zymate system costs about US$ 30,000, exclusive of applications engineering costs.

Sample preparation for ABO/Rh testing

Severns [2] and Brennan [6] have described how the Zymate was used to automate the sample handling aspects of microplate based blood grouping. For each centrifuged blood sample, the objective was to aspirate and dispense plasma into specific microplate wells and aspirate, dilute and dispense red cells into others. One microplate can be used to hold all of the reactions for eight blood samples. After filling a microplate with plasma diluted red cells, another plate would be moved into position and filled until four plates (32 samples) were prepared. At that time an operator would remove the plates and proceed with the manual portions of the test, allowing the robot to continue filling plates with samples.

In the first system developed to carry out these steps, the robotic arm was used with two different hands: one to manipulate microplates and a second to hold the pipette used for plasma and red cell fluid handling through its connection with the automated syringes. A pipette washing station was used to prevent carryover between samples. An indexing turntable having a barcode reader held the bar-code labelled centrifuged blood sample tubes, and presented them to the robot. Both the turntable and reader were controlled by the Power and Event Controller.

The throughput of the first prototype system was 40 samples per hour. Since the spatial arrangement of the components and the programming steps had already been optimized, alternative approaches for increasing the throughput were developed. One method which was used was to process samples from several tubes simultaneously. This was done by modifying a gripper hand to hold three pipettes. By opening and closing the gripper mechanism, the spacing between pipettes could be adjusted for tubes or microplates. In addition, a new washing station was developed. A fixture was designed to hold eight bar-coded sample tubes, eight dilution tubes and one bar-coded microplate. Four of these fixtures were placed around the robot arm. It was also determined that bar-code reading was better accomplished at a separate location. A Handi Spense (Sandy Springs Instrument Co., Ijamsville, MD) was used for manual but simultaneous addition of all reagents to the microplate. With these modifications the throughput was increased to 104 samples per hour. As a result of this work, a robotic sample preparation device as part of a microplate blood grouping system has been commercially developed (MicroBank, Dynatech Laboratories, Alexandria, VA).

Quality control of bar-coded labels

Concurrent with the above project was our responsibility to assist in the evaluation and quality control of bar-coded labels. Tow of the most important parameters in this work were the determination of first pass read rates and the rate of character substitution or deletion. Both influence staff productivity. Severns [7] configured the Zymate to automate these determinations. By using the robot to move a bar-code reading wand across the labels, we hoped to increase test objectivity and accuracy. This was accomplished by standardizing wand velocity, wand angle, wand contact pressure on the label, and the number of passes per label.

For this activity the robot's gripper hand was modified so it could hold a wand. A label reading surface was fabricated, large enough to accommodate five label sets and having the compliance needed to ensure adequate but not excessive pressure between wand and label. The master controller was programmed to scan each label in the set 10 times. Visible and infrared wands were connected to a decoder (Welch Allyn, Skaneatales Falls, NY) which was in turn interfaced to a microcomputer (Applied Micro Technology, Tucson, AZ) for date capture and analysis. This microcomputer was also interfaced to the robot. As the robot arm moved, the microcomputer captures the data from the wand for a known label in the set. The captured data was then compared to the human readable data, entered via keyboard.

The robotic system provided accurate and consistent results. The first pass read rate was higher using the robotic system than the manual one, and the data analysis was improved by having the microcomputer do all comparisons and documentation. There was also a 36% reduction in labour associated with this activity. Further optimization, by reading only one label at a time led to a labour savings of 87 %, but required frequent staff involvement. However, since label quality control was done only twice per year, and then only on a small number of label sets, this was not a cost-effective system to develop. The payback period has been estimated at 20 years.

Sample preparation for HBsAg and HTLV III testing

A second type of laboratory robotic system investigated was the Tecan Sampler 505 (Tecan AG, Hombrechtikon, Switzerland). It is a dedicated liquid handling system. The robot arm, which is used to position its sampling pipette, is of the Cartesian (x,y,z) type. A level sensor connected to the pipette allows the system to detect the presence of liquid. Two computer controlled syringe pumps, connected to three way valves, allow fluids to be aspirated and dispensed through the pipette or from an external reservoir. A wash station allows cleaning of the inside and outside of the pipette. An IBM Personal Computer controls the system; programmes for the sampler were written in RatBas, a structured language preprocessor which generates standard BASIC code. The Tecan Sampler costs approximately US 30,000, depending on the options selected.

The first use of this robot was to assist in the evaluation of screening tests for anti-HTLV III [8]. One of the tests required a 900:1 dilution of the serum, which was difficult to achieve consistently by manual methods. A fixture was fabricated which held 96 sample tubes in positions corresponding to those in a microplate. The second fixture held two microplates, since the final dilution was obtained using a two step procedure. Studies using due tracers were conducted to determine dilution accuracy and repeatability, as well as carryover. Fixture design and fabrication, programming, testing and debugging took about three man weeks. In the evaluation phase, 1000 serum samples and controls were prepared. The staff time to set the system up was 2 minutes, and the Tecan took 41 minuts to prepare one microplate. A staff member doing this work manually with a Gilson Pipetman (Rainin Instrument Co., Inc., Woburn, MA) took 45 minutes. Therefore, there was a labour savings of about 95 %. Of greater importance was the improved accuracy by using the Tecan. For this dilution, the coefficient of variation for the Tecan was 4.9 % compared to 18 % for the technologist.

This work demonstrated the advantages and potential uses of the Tecan robot in an operational environment. First, it showed the relative ease of using reconfigurable technology. Second, significant labour savings and improved accuracy resulted. This allowed staff to redirect their efforts and reduce their involvement in boring and tedious tasks. Third, the need for using disposable pipette tips was eliminated. Fourth, idea were developed for incorporating positive sample identification and associated data management. Finally, the possibility of simultaneously preparing different types of samples, limited only be the robot arm work envelope, was conceived.

The success in anti-HTLV III testing led us to reconfigure the Tecan Sampler for blood center use as a centralized sample preparation robot [9].

In this application, the sampler was to dispense an undiluted plasma sample for HBsAg testing and to prepare and dispense a 441:1 dilution of plasma for anti-HTLV III testing (Abbott Laboratories, North Chicago, IL). A carousel, which held 600 sample tubes, was used to present samples to the sampler under computer control. The addition of bar code laser scanner allowed the system to positively associate each sample with a location on a bar-coded test plate. Another fixture was developed to hold two of Abbott's 60 well test plates and a disposable microplate (which was required for the intermediate dilution required in the anti-HTLV III test). Quite a bit of attention was devoted to designing a pipette washing station and associated protocol to prevent carryover. Excessive carryover could lead to false positive results in the more sensitive HBsAg assay. All fixtures were designed to be readily accessible for cleaning and maintenance. The computer programmes which ran the sampler were designed so that the system could easily adapt to differing daily operational demands, yet the user interface was simple enough for a staff person having no computer skills to use.

Extensive testing using both fluorescent tracers and HBsAg positive samples indicated that greater than a million to one reduction in contaminants adhering to the pipette could be achieved. The system prepared dilutions of plasma samples with a coefficient of variation of less than 4%. The sampler can prepare samples for anti-HTLV III and HBsAg testing at a rate of over 130 samples per hour. Field testing is underway at the Penn-Jersey Regional Blood Services of the American Red Cross. No increase in false positive rate was observed for either test during the initial 5000 samples processed.

The advantages of the Tecan Sampler are multifold. First, two manual tasks have been combined into a single automated one which operates unattended for 20 minutes at a time. Second, no disposable pipette tips are needed. Third, there has been demonstrated increased accuracy and uniformity in sample preparation, which may lead to lower costs due to fewer retests being required. Finally, the Tecan is flexible and if the testing procedures are changed, the system can be reprogrammed or refitted with new fixtures.

Robotic component laboratory automation

For a number of years, the number of components being prepared in blood centers has increased rapidly. To determine if there were specific rate limiting steps in component preparation which might be automated, we measured the time taken to complete each step in this process. Initial results indicated that no one step was significantly more labour intensive than others, but that the group of steps which took the most time were thse classed as ''data management''. While bar-code based data entry is slowly being introduced into most large component laboratories, the only automated device which is available to perform other component preparation tasks is the automated plasma expressor. Although these devices do work, there is only one which can do more than simple separate plasma from red cells [10]. Moreover, studies of their accuracy, reliability and cost-effectiveness have been inconclusive. While other individual steps could be automated with dedicated devices, an integrated approach seemed to be indicated.

With the assistance of staff at the General Motors Institute, a concept for a robotic component laboratory was developed. The system consists of an industrial robot, existing but slightly modified centrifuges, and stations to perform the bag balancing and expressing operations, all under computer control. However, processing blood bags using robots present several challenges to the field of robotics. First, the bags are flexible and have long connecting tubes which makes them difficult for a robot to handle. Second, blood bags must be handled gently or they may be punctured. If the unit of blood has been spun down, handling must be even more gentle or the red cells may become resuspended. Finally, the incoming bags are not all identical in size or weight due ot different hematocrits, fill volumes and dimensional variability.

One method of circumventing some of these problems would be to design a special fixture to hold the bags during the time that they are being processed. All necessary operations would be conducted in this fixture from time of loading until component preparation was completed. Discussions with centrifuge manufacturers had indicated that they were unwilling to undertake the design of a new rotor to meet our needs, thus one basic criteria for the fixture was that it must fit into the rotor of an existing centrifuge. Additionally, the fixture needed to hold a triple bag set and to support all of the operations necessary to prepare red cells, platelet poor plasma, and platelet concentrate, and to add an optional additive solution. This meant that it needed to have a means of being balanced, such as an isolated space to hold a liquid (so that all fixtures could be brought to the same weight) and a means of expressing from each of its three compartments. Modifying centrifuges for computer control and developing a robot hand for gripping this fixture were considered to be less complicated tasks.

A prototype fixture balancing system was fabricated and found to work. For the expressing steps, air filled bladders, rather than mechanically moved plates, were fabricated and tested. However, when all of these parts were put together, it was found that a triple bag set, with or without optional additive would not fit into a fixture which would be compatible with existing centrifuge designs. Since our attempts to persuade major centrifuge manufacturers to redesign their products met with failure, this approach was abandoned.

Discussion

As a result of this work we have reached several conclusions about the potential uses for robotics. Robotic systems work best for repetitive, high volume tasks where relatively simple operations are required. They are less expensive to produce in small quantities than dedicated equipment, making them a reasonable choice for automating tasks in specialized areas such as blood banking. Although they are not directly comparable, the automated ABO/Rh test systems which incorporate reconfigurable technology (such as the Dynatech Laboratories' MicroBank System, with its robotic sample preparation device) can be purchased for less than ⅓ of the cost of comparable "hard automation" blood grouping instruments. Additionally, systems such as the Tecan used for HBsAg and anti-HTLV III testing are available when no other automated devices exist.

Care should be taken in deciding which steps of a procedure to automate. We have found that it is more efficient to use a robot to perform the steps which are done to each sample individually, while staff should perform steps which are done to a large group of samples at once. Thus, the Tecan system is used to load samples into Abbott trays and to track data, while a staff member adds reagents and performs washing steps. Making the robotic system versatile enough to perform these additional operations slows sample throughput considerably. Keeping staff involved in the process also allows them to perform "hidden" quality control checks, such as verifying that samples were properly dispensed, or, in the case of the blood grouping system, verifying that samples are not hemolyzed.

It may be advantageous to consider novel approaches to performing a task when automating, rather than using the robotic system to mimic the steps which staff do. This may mean that procedures need to be changed completely. In general, reproducing existing steps will allow you to develop an automated system in the minimum amount of time, but this solution may not be optimum. For example, the use of a wash station eliminated the need to change pipette tips in the HBsAg and anti-HTLV III assays, reducing the overall cost per test and improving throughput, but it took over 6 months to develop.

When designing a robotic system it is needed to consider future, as well as present. Modular design techniques will allow the system to be easily expanded or changed as the processing volume increases or tests change. Do not overlook the use of available dedicated automation or devices to supplement the robotic system. The use of dedicated well washers for HBsAg and anti-HTLV III testing was more effective than developing a robotic procedure for this step.

A single robotic system will almost always have lower throughput than a human performing the same task. It will, however, perform for more than one shift without taking lunch or coffee breaks. In addition, it will be more consistent, accurate and reliable. The lowered throughput may have consequences for the integration of the robotic system into the facility as a whole, if other sections of the laboratory must wait to use the same sample tube to perform other tests, or if test results are necessary before products can be released. It may be possible, however, to allow the robotic system to run unattended during hours when conflicts of this type can be avoided.

Finally, the interface between the robotic system and staff must be designed with staff in mind. The system must be simple to operate yet flexible enough to handle day to day operational changes. Additionally, adequate quality control, backup procedures, and maintenance schedules must be part of the implementation scheme.

References

1. Engelberger JF. Robotics in practice. New York: AMA COM, 1983.
2. Severns ML, Hawk Gl. Medical laboratory automation using robotics. In: Brady M et al. (eds). NATO ASI series robotics and artificial intelligence. Berlin: Springer-Verlag, 1984:633-43.
3. Pippenger CE, Megargle RG, Galen RS. The robots are coming. Medical Laboratory Observer, 1985;February:30 – 8.
4. Hight TH. Flexible automation for the laboratory. Scientific Computing and Automation 1985;August:14 – 20.
5. Zenie FH. Trends in laboratory automation. American Laboratory 1985;17: 51 – 7.
6. Brennan JE, Severns ML. A robotic system to prepare samples for ABO/Rh testing. Proc. 37th ACEMB 1984;26:253.
7. Severns ML, Brennan JE. The use of robots in bar code label testing and evaluation. In: Hawk GL, Strimaitis JR (eds). Advances in laboratory automation robotics. Hopkinton: Zymark Corporation, 1984:323 – 30.
8. Brennan JE, Severns ML, Kline LM, Goodkofsky I, Dodd RY. A robotic system to prepare samples for HTLV III testing. Med Instr. In press.
9. Brennan JE, Severns ML, Kline LM. Centralized sample preparation using a laboratory robot. Advances in laboratory automation robotics. Hopkinton: Zymark Corportion 1985:481 – 95.
10. Loos, H. Automation in blood component preparation. In: Murawski K, Peetom F (eds). Transfusion Medicine: recent technological advances. New York: Alan R. Liss, 1986:333 – 41.

MONOCLONAL ANTIBODIES AS TOOLS FOR THE IMMUNOHEMATOLOGIST

A.E.G.Kr. von dem Borne, M.J.E. Bos, W.H. Ouwehand, J.J. Quak, P.A.T. Tetteroo

Introduction

Exactly ten years ago Kohler and Milstein [1] described their Nobel Prize winning work on the the production of murine monoclonal antibodies. The scientific and commercial value of their method was immediately recognized by themselves and by others [2]. Now ten years later it is clear that no other immunological discovery has had so much impact on biomedical sciences in general and has contributed so significantly to the newly emerging discipline of biotechnology. For immunohematologists and blood bankers monoclonal antibodies (McAb) are rapidly becoming daily tools, which will increasingly take over their familiar polyclonal antibodies. But also McAb technology will shortly lead to the emergence of new serological methods. This because nearly no protein reagent can so easily be obtained in such a high quality, specificity and purity and in such unlimited amounts as McAb.

Principles of murine McAb production [3]

Although the production of murine McAb is quite laborious and time-consuming it is simple for those who are familiar with cell culture methods. Animals (usually mice, sometimes rats) are immunized with an antigen. After a good antibody response the spleens (or lymph nodes) are taken out, and a B-cell containing suspension is prepared. These cells are fused with the cells of a murine myeloma cell line by the addition of polyethylene glycol. The fused cells are then cultured in a medium, which contains a mixture of hypoxanthine, aminopterin and thymidine (HAT). This medium is toxic for the myeloma cell line cells because they have an enzym deficiency (hypoxanthine guanine phosphoribosyl transferase deficiency) for which they were selected. Normally the metabolic block induced by the folic acid antagonist aminopterin can be by-passed by thymidine and hypoxanthine, but not when this enzyme is missing. So in culture the non-fused myeloma cells will die, as will the B-lymphocytes because of their limited life span in vitro. The fused, hybrid cells survive because they acquire immortality from the myeloma cells and the gene for the missing enzyme from the B-lymphocytes.

In the process of fusion some hybrids also acquire the capacity to produce antibodies. The cells are then further cultured and distributed into the wells of microtiter plates, in order to obtain clones derived from single cells. The supernates of these cultures are tested and selected for production of antibodies of the desired specificity. By large scale culture in vitro or growth in the peritoneal cavity of a mouse many milligrams and even grams of the desired antibody can then be obtained. The clone can be easily preserved in liquid nitrogen.

Advantages and disadvantages of murine McAb's [2]

Specificity

A monoclonal antibody is specific for one single epitope. In contrast, conventional polyclonal antisera, may contain up to 500 – 1500 antibodies with different specificities. This makes the preparation of conventional antisera difficult, because after the immunization of an animal, even with pure antigens, the resulting antiserum has to be absorbed to remove the many aspecific and cross-reacting antibodies. When McAb's are produced, aspecific or cross-reacting McAb's are identified during the screening process and discarded. Thus an additional advantage is that relatively impure antigens may be used for the generation of McAb's. On the other hand, specific McAb's can be used to purify the antigen-bearing structures, by immuno-affinity chromatography, these purified antigens may than be used to raise a second generation of McAb's or even specific polyclonal antisera.

The unique specificity of McAb can sometimes be a disadvantage. Unrelated epitopes on other antigens may sometimes unexpectedly react (so-called polyfunctional binding), although this is probably a rare event. More importantly, McAb can be too specific in that they only react with certain subtypes of the antigens or even only with certain configurations of the antigen and not or differently after conformational changes in the antigen. We found for example, that all three McAb which were prepared in our laboratory against the platelet glycoprotein IIb/IIIa complex [4] loose their reactivity at a pH above 8.5 and do not react with these glycoproteins when the platelets are treated with high concentrations of EDTA or when transferred onto nitrocellulose for immunoblotting.

Sensitivity

The sensitivity of test-system based on antibodies is determined both by their affinity and their concentration. In general, high-affinity antibodies are necessary for sensitive immuno-assays. McAb have often a low affinity, probably because mostly very sensitive selection procedures are applied to detect them in the culture supernates, but also because the mouse B-lymphocytes for fusion are often harvested quite shortly after immunization. Thus, proper adaptations can be applied to obtain antibodies with a higher affinity such as less sensitive screening methods and "affinity maturation" during immunization (longer immunization periods, other amounts of antigens, etc.).

Reproducibility

This is one of the most obvious advantages of McAb's over polyclonal anti-sera. Polyclonal antisera differ in titer, affinity and specificity between every animal from which they are obtained and even between every harvest. McAb's once identified and selected for a certain assay have always constant properties because they can be produced indefinitely and in practically unlimited amounts from one single cell clone.

Cost

The initial cost of the production of McAb's is quite high because of equipment, materials, time and skill necessary to produce them. However, once produced and used on a large scale they are practically costless.

Assay configuration

McAb's can be used to develop new types of assays. For instance two antibodies against different epitopes of one antigen, which do not sterically hinder each other, may be used for a so-called two site immuno assay. One antibody, also called the captive antibody, is used to bind the antigen to a solid phase, while the other antibody is labelled (with an isotope, an enzyme or a fluorochrome) and used in saturating amounts to measure the amount of bound antigen. This type of assay has superior specificity and sensitivity compared to the more conventional ones. Moreover, because the stoichiometry of the reaction can be studied standardization is easy to perform.

McAb's of human origin

Some monoclonal human antibodies have been around for quite a while. These are the paraproteins with antibody specificity which may occur spontaneously in the blood of some patients with a malignant B-lymphoproliferative disease. Examples are erythrocyte antibodies with anti-I, anti-i, anti-P specificity. Attempts to produce human McAb in the same way as mouse McAb has had limited success so far. The main reason is that a satisfactory homologous human fusion partner for human B-lymphocytes, a proper human myeloma cell line, is still not available. But successes have been made with other approaches. Some stabile antibody secreting human B-cell clones have been produced by Epstein-Barr virus transformation or by fusion with murine myeloma cells or xenohybrids of mixed human and murine origin thereof.

In our laboratory Zeijlemaker and co-workers [5,6] have in this way prepared human McAb's against hepatitis-B virus antigen, tetanus-toxin and recently against the Rh(D) bloodgroup antigen.

Table 1. Monoclonal antibodies for blood cell and immunoglobulin allo-antigen typing.

a. Red cells	A, A_1, B, H_1, H_2, Le[a], Le[b], Le[d], I, i, M, N, P, P[k], JMH, Wr[b], Rh(D)*
b. Neutrophils	NA1, NB1 (?)
c. Platelets	Zw[a] (?)
d. Immunoglobulins	Gm, z, a, f, n, bl, u

* human

Table 2. Polymorphic murine McAb's against HLA

HLA-Class I		HLA-Class II
HLA-A	**HLA-B**	**HLA-DR**
A2	B7	DR1
A2 short	B7 + 27	DR1 like
A2 + 28	B7 + 40	DR2
A2 + w69	B8	DR2 + 5 + short 3
A3	B8 + 14 + 18	DR3 + Ds(DQ)
A3 + 11	B8 + 37	DR4 short
A3 + 11 + 29 + 32 like	B22 + B40	DR4
A3 short All + 29	B13	DR5
A9	B14 + 18	DR7
A10 + w33 short	B14 + 38 + 39	DR7 + w15
A29	B15 + 5 + 35	DRw6 + w8
A32 + 25	B27	DRw8 + w15
	B27 + 47	DR1 + 2 + w6 like (DC1) (MT1)
	B27 + 2 + 22	DR1 + 2 + 4 + w6 + w8
	B40 + 12	DR1 + 4 + w10
	Bw4	DR1 + 4 like
	Bw6 short	DR1 + 2 – 4 + 5 + 10 like
	Bw6	DR2 + 4 + w6
		DR3 + 5 + w6 like (MT2)
		DR4 + 1 + w9
		DR4 + 5 (MB3) + 7 + 9 (MT3) like
		DR4 + 7
		DR2 + 4 + w6
		DR7 + 3 + 5 + w6
		DRw52
		MT1 + MT2
		MT3
		MB3
		DQw1
		DQw1 like
		DQw1 + 3 like
		DQw3
		DQw3 short
		DQw1 + 3

Monoclonal antibodies as blood cell antigen typing reagents

McAb's which are specific for well known human blood cell antigens are becoming increasingly available. They are listed in table 1. Most are still of murine origin. Most specific red cell McAb's are directed against polysaccharide antigens.

Apart from these, also McAb's against glycoprotein A which carries the M and N antigens, against the glycoproteins which carry the red cell Rhesus, Kell, Lutheran and LW structures, against platelet glycoprotein IIb/IIIa complex which carries the platelet antigens Bak[a], Zw[a] and Zw[b] and against the neutrophil Fc gamma receptor which carries the neutrophil antigens NA1 and NA 2 have been produced. Such "ground substance" McAb's are of great interest to isolate and characterize the glycoproteins in question and to detect genetic and acquired deficiencies of the proteins.

Although initially blood cell antigen-specific McAb's appeared to be often not satisfactory as routine typing reagents, this was frequently caused by a low affinity of the antibodies or an aberrant specificity such as for antigen subgroup or cross-reacting antigens. At present most marketed McAb's for blood cell antigen typing appear to be exquisite reagents which fulfil all criteria as typing reagents.

Also antigen typing reagents have become generally available in this way which previously were relatively scarce and difficult to obtain, such as anti-P, anti-P[k], anti JMH, anti Wr[b], anti NA1.

The most rapid advance has been made in the area of specific antibodies against HLA antigens. Those produced and available for the workers in this field are reported regularly [7]. A summary of the HLA-McAb's reported until now is shown in table 2. From the rapid advances in this field it can be predicted that in near future most, if not all, blood cell antigen typing reagents applied in the immunohematology laboratory will be of monoclonal nature. This will be certainly so once the problem of the production of human McAb's has been solved.

Basic research on blood cell antigens with McAb's

Blood cell antigen specific McAb's have boosted basic research on these structures tremendously. The McAb's are not only perfect tools to isolate the antigen-carrying glycoproteins of blood cells for chemical analysis, but also to study their function, cellular distribution and synthesis during hematopoiesis. To illustrate this, three examples will be discussed, two based on work from our own laboratory.

The bloodgroup A1-A2 problem

Recently Clausen et al. [8] produced a mouse McAb against bloodgroup A1. This McAb was applied to study the A1 antigen content of isolated and separated bloodgroup glycosphingolipids from red cells. They showed that the A1 structure is a repetitive N-acetyl-galactose-aminyl-structure present on so-called type 3 A antigen chains. It is probably synthesized only on type 3 H chains, which carry the fucosyl (alpha 1-2) galactosyl (beta 1-3) N acetyl galactosaminyl (alpha 1-3) structure by a N-acetyl galactose-aminyl transferase enzyme only produced by people with bloodgroup A1. This finding explains the genetic and immunochemical differences between bloodgroup A1 and A2 which were not so well understood before.

The cellular distribution of bloodgroup P antigen (globoside) and its pathophysiological meaning

We prepared a monoclonal antibody against bloodgroup P (globoside). This antibody reacted with red cells and a subpopulation of platelets but not with neutrophils, monocytes or lymphocytes, illustrating the expression of the P-antigen on different blood cells. In bone marrow, P-antigen was present on erythroblasts but not on their less mature precursor cells, proerythroblasts. On tissue we found that the antigen was expressed on some connective tissue cells and on vessel wall cells. This was confirmed with cultured cells. Some fibroblasts and all endothelial cells in culture were positive for the antigen. When placenta tissue was tested, the P-antigen was strongly expressed on all cells, not only from the endothelium, but also from the trophoblast and the interstitium in between.

These findings have important pathophysiological implications. A disease caused by cold auto-antibodies against P-antigen is paroxysmal cold hemoglobinuria. Patients with cold auto-anti-P in their blood, have attacks of hemolysis and hemoglobinuria, upon exposure to cold, due to red blood cell destruction. They also have cold-induced vascular symptoms, i.e. acrocyanosis or Raynaud phenomena and even gangrene of fingers, toes, nose and ears. This may be explained by damage of endothelial cells in the cold. Mothers with bloodgroup P and anti $P + P^k + P_1$ alloantibodies in their blood have often habitual abortion. This may than be explained by the destruction of the placenta by these antibodies.

Glycoprotein localization of the neutrophil antigens NA_1 and NA_2

The neutrophil specific antigen system NA consist of two allelic antigens, NA_1 and NA_2, with a phenotype frequency of 46% and 88% respectively [10,11]. The antigens may be involved in diseases such as alloimmune neutropenia of the newborn and autoimmune neutropenia of infancy, as well as neutrophil induced transfusion reaction with rigors, fever and even respiratory distress. Alloimmune and autoimmune neutropenias due to anti NA1 or anti NA2 antibodies are often accompanied by severe infections of the skin, the respiratory tract and even sepsis.

Attempts to localize the NA-antigens on specific neutrophil membrane glycoproteins have failed in the past.

Because of our interest in receptors for IgG antibodies on phagocytes, the so-called Fc-gamma-receptors, which are involved in the destruction of blood cells sensitized with IgG antibodies, we tried to prepare McAb against these structures. For the preparation of McAb against the Fc-gamma-receptor we used a protocol in which the antibodies are detected via inhibition of roset formation. In this way we obtained two McAb's with the capacity to inhibit the binding of IgG anti-D sensitized Rh(D) positive red cells to neutrophils. One of these antibodies was found to react with neutrophils of only about 50% of the donors. Studies with neutrophils of typed donors showed that this antibody was in fact directed against the NA1 antigen. Thus NA_1, and probably also the allelic antigen NA_2, is localized on the neutrophil Fc-gamma-receptor and NA polymorphism is a genetic polymorphism of this receptor. We could show that this polymorphism is accompanied by differences in the electrophoretic mobility of the receptor [10.]

Thus antibodies against NA1 and NA2 antigens affect the defence mechanism in two ways, i.e. by blocking the Fc-gamma receptor of the neutrophil and by inducing increased neutrophil destruction.

Monoclonal antibodies as antiglobulin reagents

Due to their unique properties (specificity, purity, high concentration) McAb are also ideal antiglobulin reagents. As shown in table 3, McAb against all human immunoglobulin classes, subclasses and light chain types are available, as well as against the most important complement components and their fragments.

Table 3. Monoclonal antiglobulin antibodies.

1. Immunoglobulin heavy chain class	IgG, IgM, IgA, IgE, IgD
2. Immunoglobulin heavy chain subclass	IgG1, IgG2, IgG3, IgG4, IgA1
3. Immunoglobulin light chain type	K, L
4. Complement components-fragments	C4, C3, C3b, C3c, C3d, C9

They can be used to study the nature of antibody and complement reactions with blood cells in detail, both in vitro and in vivo, and even in a quantitative way. An example is given in table 4. This shows the application of McAb's in platelet immunofluorescence. The McAb's clearly show what the immunoglobulin class of the platelet bound antibodies is and whether complement is also bound. The specificity of the reaction patterns is beyond doubt, because McAb are always monospecific. This is a great advantage in such studies over polyclonal antisera, with which the specificity of the reaction must always be proven by way of cross-absorptions.

As agglutinating antiglobulin reagents (Coombs reagents) in red cell serology, McAb's have not yet been so successfully applied. This is probably because for optimal agglutination of sensitized red cells to occur, more than one antiglobulin molecule must bind per antibody molecule. This can be realized with mixtures of McAb's directed against different epitopes, which sould not hinder each other and also have a sufficient high affinity.

Table 4. Monoclonal antibodies as antiglobulin reagents in platelet immuno-fluorescence.*

Sensitizing agent	Mc anti IgG	Mc anti IgM	Mc anti C3b**
Anti Zw$_a$	+ + + +	−	−
Anti HLA (multispecific)	+ + + +	+	±
Autoantibodies	+ +	(+)	−
Quinidine dependent antibodies	+ + + +	−	+ + + +
EDTA dependent antibodies	(+)	+ +	−
IgG aggregates	+ +	−	(+)

* McAb's not labelled, but binding detected by FITC goat-anti mouse-IgG.
** Complement binding detected after incubation with human complement.

Bispecific tetrameric complexes of McAb's as immune reagents

Lansdorp et al. [12] in our laboratory recently discovered an unique new approach to obtain McAb reagents for immuno-assays.

They produced a rat McAb directed against the Fc-part of murine IgG1, in order to link monoclonal antibodies to each other. When mixed with murine McAb's of the IgG1 class, stabile tetrameric complexes were formed i.e. complexes of two rat and two mouse McAb molecules. The mouse McAb's still had the capacity to react with the antigen, against which they were directed. In this way monospecific complexes can be prepared with one mouse McAb, but also bispecific complexes, when the rat antibody is added to a mixture of two mouse McAb of different specificity. In this way bispecific complexes of different composition can be constructed, adapted to the type of immunoassay, for which they are meant.

Examples are complexes of anti-peroxidase or anti alkaline phosphatase and anti IgG or IgM for Elisa assays, complexes of anti phyco-erythrine and anti IgG or IgM for immunofluorescence and complexes of anti-glycophorin A and anti IgG or IgM for mixed red cell agglutination tests. We applied the tetrameres for an Elisa to detect of platelet- and neutrophil-antibodies, and found them to be superior reagents in these assays.

Summary

McAb's are superior reagents for the immunohematologist. It is to be expected that they will nearly completely replace the conventional polyclonal antisera, mostly still in use at present. Moreover, McAb's will from the basic for new immuno assay methods, which will gradually replace the methods based on the conventional polyclonal antisera.

These developments will cause revolutionary changes in the coming years.

References

1. Kohler G, Milstein C. Continuous cultures of fused cells secreting antibody of predefined specificity. Nature 1975;256:495 – 7.
2. Scott MG. Monoclonal antibodies approaching adolescence in diagnostic immuno-assay. Trends in Biotechnology 1985;3:170 – 5.
3. Roitt I, Brostoff G, Male O. Immunology. Churchill Livingstone, 1985.
4. Tetteroo PAT, Lansdorp PM, Leeksma OC, von dem Borne AEGKr. Monoclonal antibodies against platelet glycoprotein IIIa. Brit J Haemat 1983;55:509 – 22.
5. Tiebout RF, Stricker EAM, Hagenaars AM, Zeylemaker WP. A human lymphoblastoid cell line producing protective monoclonal IgG1K antitetanus toxin. Europ J Immun 1984;14:399 – 404.
6. Stricker L, Tiebout RF, Zeylemaker WP. A human monoclonal IgG1lambda anti-HBs antibody: production, properties and application. Scand J Immunol 1985;22:337 – 43.
7. Colombani J, Lepage V. HLA monoclonal antibody registry: third listing. Tissue Antigens 1984;24:209 – 14.
8. Clausen H, Levery SB, Nudelman E, Tsuchiya S, Hakomori SI. Repetitative A epitope (type 3 chain A) defined by blood group A1-specific monoclonal antibody TH-1: chemical basis of qualitative A1 and A2 distinction. Proc Nat Acad Sci (USA) 1985;82:1199 – 203.
9. von dem Borne AEGKR, Bos MJE, Joustra-Maas N, Tromp JF, van Wijngaarden-du Bois R, Tetteroo PAT. A murine monoclonal IgM antibody specific for blood group P antigen (globoside). Brit J Haemat 1986 (in press).
10. Werner G, von dem Borne AEGKr, Bos MJE et al. Localization of the human NA1 alloantigen on the neutrophil Fc-gamma-receptor. Reinherz EL, Huynes BF, Nadler LM, Bernstein ID (eds). Leukocyte Typing II. Human leukocyte differentiation antigens detected by monoclonal antibodies. Springer-Verlag, New York, 1985.
11. Engelfriet CP, van Loghem JJ, von dem Borne AEGKr. Immunohaematology. Research Monographs in Immunology Vol. 5. Elsevier Science Publishers, 1984.
12. Lansdorp PM, Aalberse RC, Bos R, Schutter WG, van Bruggen EFJ. Tetrameric complexes of monoclonal antibodies. Submitted for publication, 1986.

SOLID PHASE RED CELL ADHERENCE TESTS IN BLOOD BANKING*

F.V. Plapp, J.M. Rachel, M.L. Beck, L.T. Sinor

Introduction

The immunologic technique of agglutination was first discovered in 1888 by Stillmark, when he observed that seed extracts of *Ricinus communis* strongly agglutinaed erythrocytes [1]. Durham then reported the agglutination of bacteria by serum [2]. In 1900, Ehrlich and Morgenroth reported that erythrocytes could also be agglutinated by alloantibodies [3]. Shortly thereafter, Landsteiner, using agglutination, discovered the ABO blood group system [4]. During the past 90 years, agglutination has remained the most widely used blood banking method for detecting the interaction of antibodies with red cell antigens. Today, hospital transfusion services and blood centers routinely use either manual or automated agglutination tests to perform ABO and Rh grouping, antibody screening, antibody identification, and crossmatching.

Most hospital laboratories and some blood centers continue to perform manual agglutination tests in tubes. The major advantages of this method are its simplicity, reliability, and versatility. The major disadvantages are that sample identification, reagent and sample dispensing, and the interpretation and recording of results are all performed manually. Furthermore, each serologic test requires different reagent additives and reaction conditions to enhance agglutination.

Other areas of laboratory medicine have overcome most of the disadvantages of manual testing by developing automated instruments. For instance, clinical chemistry has been revolutionized by the introduction of the continuous flow Auto Analyzer (Technicon). Automated instruments, such as the Auto Analyzer, the Auto Grouper 16C, the Groupamatic GM360 and the Mini Groupamatic (Hoffman-LaRoche, Inc.) have also successfully automated red cell grouping and typing [5 – 8]. However, they are less effective in detecting antibodies. Also, their expense and complexity have restricted their usefulness to large blood processing centers.

Because of these limitations, other methods of automating agglutination tests have been sought. In 1966, Wegmann and Smithies described the first agglutination tests for ABO grouping and Rh typing in V-bottom microplates [9]. This system provided remarkable increases in sensitivity and a

* This work was supported in part by a grant from the Victor E. Speas Foundation of the First National Bank of Kansas City.

considerable reduction in the required amount of cells and antiserum compared to conventional tube tests. Crawford et al. [10] also described a microplate system for blood grouping and antibody detection, which employed U-bottom wells pretreated with albumin or plasma. Incubation times were reduced significantly by centrifugation and the use of ficin. Increased economy of time, equipment, and reagents was realized without sacrificing senstivity. Parker and co-workers [11] described a method for ABO and Rh typing and antibody screening using flexible polyvinyl plates with V-bottom wells. They concluded that donor typing in microplates was faster, more sensitive, and more economical than manual tube methods. Warlow and Tills [12] evaluated both U- and V-bottom wells and preferred U-bottom, which required less vigorous agitation to resuspend the cells. Various modifications of these microplate methods are currently being used in many blood centers and hospital transfusion services.

Following the gradual acceptance of manual microplate blood grouping methods, several investigators attempted to automate them. In 1982, Innocenti and Nieri used microplate spectrophotometers to read agglutination tests [13]. Two years later, Bowley and colleagues [14] demonstrated that an inexpensive microplate spectrophotometer interfaced to a personal computer could read agglutination results and interpret them into blood groups. The spectrophotometer was tilted forward to displace agglutinated cells away from the optical path. An entire plate was read in about 1 minute. Automated readings correlated with visual readings in 98% of 20,000 donor samples. The 2% rejection rate was due mainly to reactions of irregular antibodies with reagent A or B red cells. These findings were soon confirmed by Severns et al. [15], who described an essentially similar system, but with slightly less impressive results. These semi-automated microplate agglutination systems represented important advances towards the ultimate automation of blood bank serology. Their major advantages was the ability to eliminate manual transcription errors and save time with relatively inexpensive and uncomplicated equipment.

Although these developments were impressive, automated agglutination methods had several inherent limitations. Problems associated with rouleaux, atypical antibodies, and exogenous additives continued to be encountered. Pigmented sera also caused problems, as noted by Severns et al. [15]. The major drawback, however, was the lack of an objective endpoint. Densitometers, like technologists, had difficulty distinguishing weak agglutination reactions from negative reactions. In order to compensate for this problem, the range of acceptable positive and negative absorbance values had to be established each day, by running a large number of cell controls in each microplate. Another drawback was that only ABO and Rh grouping tests could be successfully automated with these methods.

In view of these limitations, it was obvious that new methods were needed for the inexpensive automation of all serologic tests performed in both hospital transfusion services and blood centers. Very early in our attempt to automate microplate testing, we decided to abandon agglutination as a measure of red cell antigen-antibody interactions and develop an automated, solid phase technology that could be adapted to almost any immunologic test. Toward this end, a series of solid phase red cell adherence assays have been developed.

These solid phase assays are based on procedures first reported in the 1950s. The technique of mixed agglutination was developed by Coombs and Bedford [16] in 1955 to demonstrate the presence of blood group A and B antigens on platelets. The basis of mixed agglutination was the linking by antibody of different cell types that possessed a common antigen. The following year, mixed agglutination was used to detect A and B antigens on human epidermal cells [17]. Later, this method was used to detect other blood group antigens on platelets [18], leukocytes [19], and Hela cells [20]. It was also used to investigate the species purity of tissue cultures [21]. Although originally developed as a liquid-phase technique, mixed agglutination was later used as a solid phase method for identifying and grouping blood stains on fabric fibers [22].

In 1957, Vogel and Shelokov [23] reported that tissue culture cells infected with influenze virus adsorbed and agglutinated red cells. They called this new diagnostic test hemadsorption.

In 1959, Högman [24] combined the principles of mixed agglutination and hemadsorption to perform the first solid phase red cell adherence test for the detection of blood group antigens on cells growing in tissue culture [24]. A and B antigens were detected, but the D antigen was not. Högman later used this method to investigate the presence of blood group antigens on cultured cells from human fetal kidney, liver, spleen, heart, lung, and skin [25]. The major limitation of this method was that the cells being studied had to share common antigens with the indicator red cells. To overcome this limitation, the mixed antiglobulin reaction was introduced by Coombs et al. in 1956 [26]. By this method, the common antigen shared by both cell types was adsorbed antibody, and agglutination was induced by the addition of antiglobulin serum. The presence or absence of mixed agglutinates was assessed microscopically. They used this method to assay for anti-platelet antibodies.

In 1961, Fagraeus and Espmark [27] and Fagraeus et al. [28] described a modification of the mixed antiglobulin and hemadsorption reactions, which they called mixed hemadsorption. This technique was designed to detect the presence on cultured cell surfaces of viral antigens not capable of hemadsorption. They used sheep red cells, coated with antiglobulin specific for the species of viral antibody used, to detect rat or rabbit anti-viral antibodies adsorbed to cell monolayers. The novelty of this method was the development of the antiglobulin-coated indicator red cell. Subsequently, the mixed hemadsorption test was used to study species-specific, viral, allo, and tumor antigens as well as autoantibodies. Using this method, Franks [29] demonstrated the Tj^a antigen on several different cell lines, and Juji et al. [30] studied the antigens on platelets, immobilized on slides. Somewhat later, Shibata et al. [31] used a similar method to detect and characterize antibodies directed against platelet antigens.

The use of antiglobulin-coated indicator red cells was also advocated by Coombs and co-workers, who used chromium chloride to directly couple specific antiglobulin reagents or other proteins to red cells. These indicator cells were subsequently used in several liquid-phase assays and two solid phase assays, referred to as mixed reverse solid phase passive antiglobulin hemadherence (MrsPAH) and solid phase aggregation of coupled erythrocytes (SPACE) [32]. The MrsPAH test was designed to detect antibodies directed against bacterial or viral antigens immobilized on microplate wells. The reaction was essentially that of mixed hemadsorption, in which antibody present in test fluids was adsorbed by the solid phase antigen and detected by the addition of antiglobulin-coated red cells. The SPACE test was designed to detect viral antigens, rather than antibody. For this test, antibody directed against the antigen in question was attached to both the indicator red cells and the microplate wells. If a specific viral antigen was present in the test fluid, it bound to the immobilized antibody and was detected by the antibody-coated red cells.

Until 1977, all of the solid phase techniques for studying cellular antigens used immobilized cells as the solid phase. In 1967, Catt and Tregear [33] had made the important observation that antibodies would absorb onto polystyrene surfaces without loss of immunologic activity. Ten years later Mage et al. [34] and Wysocki and Sato [35] took advantage of this finding to separate B-lympocytes from heterogeneous spleen cell suspensions by specifically binding them to Petri dishes coated with an anti-IgG antibody. These panning experiments provided a simple and inexpensive method for the identification of specific subpopulations of cells in the peripheral blood.

Rosenfield, Kochwa, and Kaczera were the first investigators to adapt solid phase techniques to blood group serology [36]. They were convinced that, although some progress had been made, liquid phase hemagglutination procedures would never be successfully automated. Their solid phase system employed red cell monolayers attached to plastic tubes via fibrinogen and poly-D-lysine. This monolayer could then adsorb specific antibody from solution. Bound antibody was then detected in one of two ways. The first method was termed solid phase immune hemolysis. Human group AB serum was added to the sensitized monolayers as a source of complement. After incubation, cell monolayers were washed to remove serum and free hemoglobin. The remaining intact cells were then lysed with water and the A_{415} of hemoglobin was quantitated in comparison with that of a negative control. Alternatively, solid phase antiglobulin tests were used to detect adsorbed antibody. In this procedure, the sensitized monolayer was washed, then lysed with water to produce a colourless background. Antiglobulin reagent was incubated with the monolayer. Bound anti-IgG was then detected by allowing IgG or complement-coated red cells to settle out onto the monolayer. The binding of these cells was augmented by overlayering 2% K-90 polyvinylpyrrolidone. Quantitation was accomplised by lysing the bound indicator cells and measuring the absorbance of released hemoglobin. Because of unsatisfactory results this method was later modified to eliminate the need for antiglobulin. Indicator red cells were used which possessed cell surface antigens corresponding to those on the initial monolayer. These cells bound directly to antibody adsorbed onto the monolayer. Adherence was potentiated by 0.2% protamine sulfate in glycine. Although no data was shown, the authors stated that antibodies directed against Rh,

Kell, Kidd, Duffy, MNSsU, and Lewis antigens were detected. Unfortunately, these methods have never found widespread application.

In 1982, Moore and Conradie [37] reported another solid phase indirect antiglobulin test for antibody identification. They incubated serum and red cells together in U-bottom microplate wells and, after washing, transferred the cells to flat bottom microplate wells coated with sheep anti-human globulin. The microplates were centrifuged and incubated to allow antibody coated red cells to bind to the solid phase anti-IgG. Unbound cells were washed off and peroxidase reagents were added to detect bound sensitized red cells. Subsequently, this method was shown to have comparable sensitivity to conventional antiglobulin tests [38]. However, a significant number of the antibodies tested were not identified by the solid phase assay. Also, the 90 minutes protocol has precluded its use as a routine compatibility test.

Our laboratory has developed a series of solid phase red cell adherence assays for ABO and Rh typing, antibody screening, crossmatching, hepatitis testing, and platelet antibody screening and crossmatching [39]. These solid phase assays were based on the original methods described above. Forward ABO grouping and Rh typing was adapted from the panning techniques of Mage et al. [34] and Wysocki and Sato [35]. Reverse ABO grouping was a modification of Högman's tissue culture technique [24,25]. The solid phase antibody screen was based on the mixed agglutination method of Högman [24,25] and the mixed hemadsorption method of Fagraeus and Espmark [27,28]. The solid phase platelet antibody test was based on the mixed agglutination techniques of Coombs et al. [16,26], Juji et al. [30], and Shibata et al. [31]. Testing is performed in microplates, so that large numbers of samples can be handled efficiently and the results can be automatically read, interpreted, and recorded by a densitometer interfaced to a personal computer.

Methods

Solid phase ABO cell grouping and Rh typing

Anti-A and anti-B were purified from human sera using affinity columns as instructed by the manufacturer (Synsorb A and B, Chembiomed Ltd., Alberta, Canada). One gram of Synsorb A or B was suspended in 25 ml of phosphate-buffered saline (PBS), pH 7.4 and degassed. A slurry of the beads was poured into a 0.9×15 cm column and allowed to settle. Six milliliters of hyperimmune sera, containing anti-A or anti-B, were layered onto the column. The column was then washed with 60 ml of cold PBS. Bound antibody was eluted with 7.5 ml of freshly prepared 2% NH_4OH in 0.85% NaCl. The first 2.5 ml of effluent were discarded. The next 5 ml of eluate were collected into a tube containing 1 ml of cold saturated KH_2PO_4 to adjust the pH to 7.0. The eluate was immediately dialyzed overnight against 1 liter of PBS at 4°C. Murine monoclonal anti-A and anti-B were a gift (Chembiomed Ltd.). Anti-D was purified from human sera by adsorption to Rh-positive red cells and ether elution. Antibodies were diluted to 20 µg/ml protein concentration in deionized distilled water immediately prior to use.

The solid phase for ABO cell grouping was prepared by passively adsorbing anti-A or anti-B to polystyrene U-bottom microplates (Dynatech Laboratories, Alexandria, VA) according to Catt and Tregear [33]. The solid phase for Rh typing was prepared by first coating polystyrene microplate wells with affinity purified goat anti-human IgG (Cappel Labs, Cochranville, PA) and then with anti-D. Microplates were stored at 4°C prior to use. They have been stored up to 6 months without loss of activity. The solid phase assay for ABO cell grouping and Rh typing was performed by adding 1 drop (approximately 30 µl) of a 0.5% suspension of bromelin-treated donor or patient red cells to the antibody-coated wells [40]. The microplates were immediately centrifuged at 190 g for 1 minute (Model GLC 2B, Sorval, DuPont, Des Plaines, IL). A positive reaction, as defined by the effacement of RBCs over the entire surface of the well, indicated the adherence of antigen-positive RBCs to the immobilized antibody. A negative reaction occurred when RBCs lacking the antigen pelleted into a discrete button in the bottom of the wells (fig. 1).

The preceding method required the use of purified antibody on the solid phase. Beck and co-workers [41] have developed a solid phase ABO cell-grouping system which permitted use of routine serologic blood grouping reagents. The need for affinity-purified antibodies was obviated by first coating microplate wells with secretor saliva. Five milliliters of secretor saliva were placed in a boiling water bath for 10 minutes to inactivate antibodies and enzymes. The saliva was then centrifuged and the clear supernatant diluted 1 in 100 with distilled water. Diluted saliva was kept frozen until use.

The solid phase was prepared by adding 100 µl of diluted saliva to each microplate well. The plates were then incubated for 1 hour at 37°C, or for 4 hours at room temperature (23°C), or overnight at 4°C. Saliva-coated plates were washed 4 times with saline before adding 100 µl of commercially prepared anti-A or anti-B diluted 1 in 10 with distilled water. Anti-A was added to wells coated with A secretor saliva and wells coated with B secretor saliva received anti-B. Plates were incubated at room temperature for 1 hour and then washed 4 times with saline. If not used immediately, saline was left in the wells until just prior to use. Red blood cells were prepared for ABO grouping by diluting to approximately 0.2% in 1 g/l bromelin-saline solution. One drop of bromelin-treated donor red cell (40 – 45 µl) was then added to the appropriate antibody-coated wells and centrifuged at 400 g for 1 minute. Results were read as described above.

Solid phase serum grouping

The solid phase for ABO serum confirmation was prepared by passively adsorbing a 10 µg/ml solution of anti-human red cell antibody onto the wells

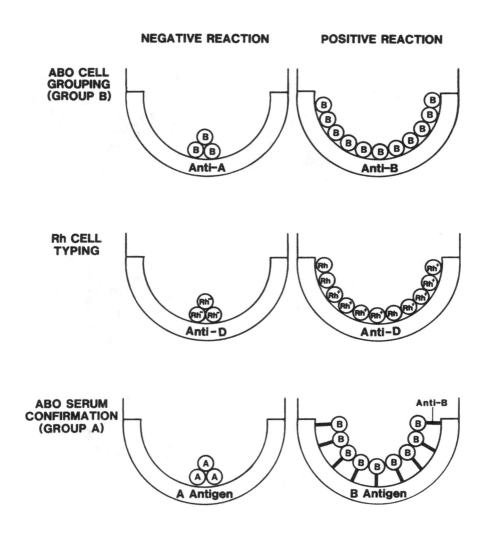

Figure 1. Diagrammatic representation of negative and positive solid phase red cell adherence assays for ABO and Rh blood grouping. (From: Plapp FV, Rachel JM, Beck ML, Coenen WM, Bayer WL, Sinor LT. Lab Manag 1984;22:39.)

[33] and then binding bromelin-treated A_1 or B red cells. The solid phase assay for serum confirmation was performed by adding 1 drop of donor or patient serum to group A_1 or B red cell coated wells and incubating for 5 minutes at room temperature. The microplate was then inverted and blotted dry on a paper towel. One drop of a 0.5% suspension of bromelin-treated A_1 or B indicator red cells was added to the appropriate wells. For example, A_1 red cells were added to wells coated with group A_1 red cell

184

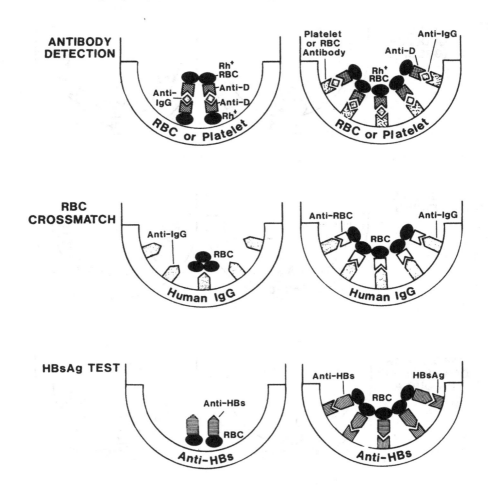

Figure 2. Diagrammatic representation of negative and positive solid phase red cell adherence assays for antibody detection (red cell or platelet), red cell cross-matching, and hepatitis B surface antigen testing. (From: Plapp FV, Rachel JM, Beck ML, Coenen Wl, Bayer WL, Sinor LT. Lab Manag 1984;22:39. With permition.)

membranes. The microplates were centrifuged for 1 minute at 190 g. Positive reactions resulted in effacement of the indicator red cells, which bound to isoagglutinins that had previously bound to the immobilized red cells. Negative reactions, in which the appropriate isoagglutinins were absent, resulted in the pelleting of indicator red cells (fig. 1).

Solid phase antibody screening

Anti-human red cell antibody (Immucor, Inc., Norcross, GA) was adsorbed passively to polystyrene U-bottom microplates [33]. One drop (approx. 30 μl) of a 0.25% (v/v) suspension of two individual human reagent red cells (Panoscreen, Immucor, Inc.) or a drop of pooled reagent red cells (Hemantigen, Immucor, Inc.) was added to antibody-coated wells. The red cells then were allowed to settle in the wells and immunologically adhere to the immobilized antibody. Unbound red cells were washed off with saline.

The assay was performed [42] by sequentially adding 1 drop of donor serum and 4 drops of 1.9% glycine solution, pH 7.0 [43], to red cell-coated microplate wells. The microplates were incubated in a 37°C water bath for 10 minutes and washed 4 times with a phosphate-glycine solution containing 1.5% (w/v) glycine, 0.16% (w/v) NaCl, 4 mM Na$_2$HPO$_4$, pH 7.3, using a Dynadrop SR-1 semiautomatic microplate washer (Dynatech Laboratories). One drop of poly-specific solid phase antiglobulin reagent (Immucor, Inc.) and 1 drop of a 0.4% suspension of IgG-coated pooled reagent red cells (Checkcells, Immucor, Inc.) were added per well. The microplates were centrifuged at 600 g for 1 minute. Positive antibody screens resulted in the binding of IgG-coated indicator red cells over the entire surface of the well. Negative antibody screens resulted in the pelleting of indicator red cells into a discrete button in the bottom of the wells (fig. 2).

Solid phase red cell crossmatch

Group O red cells of known antigenic composition were selected from reagent cell panels prepared commercially (Immucor, Inc., Norcross, GA; Pfizer Diagnostic Division, New York, NY; and Accugenics, Inc., Garden Grove, CA). Additional cell samples were selected from a frozen collection maintained by the Community Blood Center of Greater Kansas City. Red cells were washed twice with 0.85% NaCl and twice with low ionic strength solution (LISS) [45]. They were resuspended to approximately 3% (v/v) in LISS.

Sera, containing irregular antibodies of various strengths and specificities, were stored frozen. Each serum was thawed and centrifuged to remove particulate matter immediately prior to testing.

The solid phase was prepared by treating polystyrene U-bottom microplate wells with 100 μl of 2% biological grade glutaraldehyde (Polysciences, Inc., Warrington, PA) in 10 mM NaH$_2$PO$_4$ (pH 5.0), 0.14 M NaCl for 2 hours at room temperature [44]. After washing with saline, they were incubated with 100 μl of 10 μg/ml human IgG (Sigma Chemical Co., St. Louis, MO) in distilled water overnight at 4°C.

The solid phase assay was performed by adding 1 drop each (approx. 30 μl) of test serum and cells to uncoated polystyrene microplate wells [45]. Plates were mixed, incubated at 37°C for 15 minutes, and washed 4 times with 0.85% NaCl (Dynadrop SR-1, Dynatech Laboratories). Plates were centrifuged at 1600 g for 10 seconds between washes. After the fourth wash, the cells were resuspended in 3 drops of an antiglobulin reagent (Immucor, Inc.), producing a final red cell suspension of 0.5 to 1%. One hundred microliters of each cell suspension were transferred into IgG-coated wells using a multichannel pipettor (Titertek, Flow Laboratories, McLean, VA). The plates were centrifuged at 1000 g for 1 minute and read (fig. 2). Incompatible crossmatches had red cells effaced over the entire surface of the well, while compatible crossmatches had central buttons.

The sensitivity of the solid phase assay was evaluated by serially diluting sera containing antibody in nonimmune group AB sera obtained from healthy donors. Cells that were heterozygous for the test antigen were sensitized with each serum dilution. Parallel antiglobulin testing by a conventional antiglobulin method and the solid phase assay was then performed, using the same sample of sensitized red cells. Results were read independently.

Solid phase platelet antibody screening and crossmatching

The solid phase for platelet crossmatching was prepared according to the method of Catt and Tregear [33], by first coating U-bottom polystyrene microplate wells (Dynatech Laboratories) with 100 μl of anti-thrombocyte antibody (Accurate Chemicals, Westbury, NY), diluted to 20 μg/ml in distilled water. Microplates were stored at 4°C and washed 3 times with 100 μl per well of 8.5 g/l NaCl immediately before use. Solid phase platelet monolayers were prepared by adding 1 to 3 drops of donor platelet-rich plasma (PRP) to coated wells and centrifuging microplates at 35 g for 5 minutes [46]. Unbound platelets were removed by washing with 8.5 g/l NaCl. One drop of patient's or recipient's pre-transfusion serum or plasma and 3 drops of 1.9% glycine (pH 7.0) were added and mixed. After 30 minutes incubation at 37°C the wells were washed 5 times with 8.5 g/l NaCl. The binding of platelet-specific antibodies to the solid phase was detected by adding 1 drop of a 0.2% suspension of anti-IgG coated indicator red cells (Immucor, Inc., Norcross, GA) and centrifuging for 1 minute at 400 g. Incompatible crossmatches resulted in binding of indicator red cell over the entire surface of the well while compatible crossmatches had a discrete pellet of red cells (fig. 2).

The solid phase assay has also been used to diagnose neonatal isoimmune thrombocytopenia (NITP). Solid phase platelet monolayers were prepared by centrifuging platelet-rich plasma from the mother, father, or 10 – 12 random but group O blood donors onto polystyrene microplate wells coated with anti-platelet antibody. Serum from the mother, father or infant was added to the wells and incubated to allow antibody binding to the solid phase. The presence of platelet-reactive antibody was detected by addition of antiglobulin-coated red blood cells. When necessary, anti-A or anti-B was removed by absorption to allow the mother's serum to be tested against the father's platelets.

Solid phase HBsAg testing

Mouse monoclonal anti-HBsAg (Immucor, Inc.), specific for all subtypes of HBsAg was diluted to 10 μg/ml in distilled water and passively adsorbed onto U-bottom polystyrene microplate wells [33]. Plates were stored at 4°C until ready to use. Just prior to use, the plates were washed 3 times with saline and 50 ul of patient or donor serum was added to each well and incubated for 30 minutes at 25°C. The wells were then washed 4 times with saline and 50 μl of indicator red cells were added. Indicator red cells were coated with the same monoclonal anti-HBs antibody used to prepare the microplate. Microplates were immediately centrifuged at 50 g for 5 minutes. Samples positive for HBsAg were characterized by adherence of indicator red blood cells over the entire surface, while negative wells contained small central buttons . (Fig. 2).

Automated reading and interpretation

The common feature of all of the solid phase assays described above was their objective endpoint of red cell adherence or nonadherence. This uniformity permitted the easy interpretation of results, whether visually or spectrophotometrically. Positive and negative reactions were read spectrophotometrically at 405 nm (MR580 Microelisa Auto Reader, Dynatech Labs, Inc., Alexandria, VA). The light beam was offset 1.5 mm from the center of the wells so that it did not pass through the cell button in negative reactions, but did pass through the effaced red cells in positive reactions. An aborbance value of 0.253 was chosen as the cutoff to distinguish between positive and negative reactions for ABO grouping [40], Rh typing [40], and antibody screening [42]. This value was established by adding 2 SD to the mean absorbance value of 100 negative tests. There was no overlap of the absorbance values of weakly positive and negative reactions. (Fig. 3) For the red cell crossmatch [45] the instrument was zeroed on a well contained 3 drops of antiglobulin reagent as a blank. Absorbance values above 0.145, which was the mean (0.075) plus 3 times the SD (0.024) of 160 negative tests, were considered positive.

Absorbance values were interpreted into meaningful ABO groups, Rh types, and antibodyscreen results by an Apple II + computer (Cupertino, CA) with 64K RAM connected to the Microelisa reader via a RS-232 interface. Individual test results were stored onto 5.25 inch floppy disks. Software was written by Applesoft basic. Current test results were compared to past donor records stored in the blood center's Data General S140 mainframe computer via an interface with the Apple II + . Textfile data was exchanged between the two computers via Blast software (version 5.0, Communications Research Group). Inconsistencies with a donor's past record were flagged and new donors were automatically added to the existing donor file.

An automated image analysis system has also been developed to read solid phase adherence results. The computers used were an Apple II +

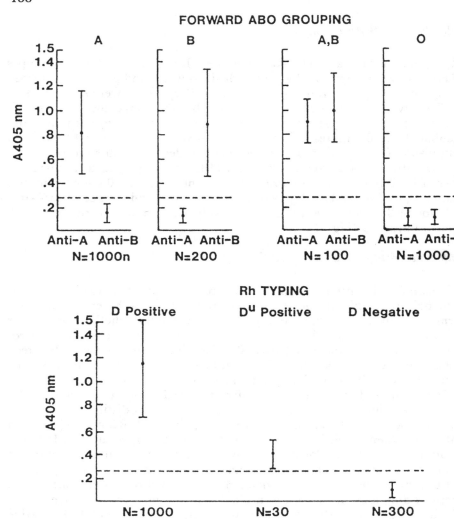

Figure 3. Range of absorbance values for positive and negative ABO cell grouping tests and RhD tests.

upgraded to 64K RAM and an Apple IIe with 128 K RAM (Apple Computer, Inc., Cupertino, CA). External devices included: 5.25 inch dual disk drives, Image writer dot matrix printer, a monochrome monitor (Apple Computer, Inc.), Computer Eyes digitizer interface (Digital Vision), Ikegami vidicon television camera model ITC-40 with 750 line resolution (Ikegami Tsushinki Co., LTD) equipped with a Computar 16-mm f/1.6 lens, and a Model LL-6515 Thermolyne light box (Sybron Corp., Dubugue, Iowa).

The Apple II + or IIe high resolution graphics mode was used to view the digitized image. The camera was positioned 31 cm above the view box containing a Sylvania fluorescent bulb covered by a white Plexiglass diffusion screen. The lens aperture was set to nearly the maximum f/2 value. Under these viewing conditions the manual Computer Eyes contrast control was adjusted so that the pellet of dark red indicator red cells in negative test wells were clearly visible, while the lightly coloured effaced red cells in positive wells were not visible on the video monitor.

The digitizer created a 280 × 180 pixel raster with 1-bit resolution – i.e, 2 grey levels corresponding to a pixel being turned on or off. In our system, a microplate well corresponded to an area of approximately 400 pixels.

Both the computer eyes software, utilized to capture a digitized image of microplates, and the optical pattern recognition software were written in Applesoft Basic and Assembly Language. Optical pattern recognition implemented by digital image processing was used to analyse and interpret the individual reactions depicted in the digitized microplates image.

Dipsticks

ABO dipsticks were prepared by binding murine monoclonal anti-A or anti-B (Immucor, Inc.) to positively charged nylon membranes [47,48]. They were stored wet at 4°C until use. The edge of the dipstick was blotted on a paper towel to drain excess liquid from the surface. On drop of whole blood from a fingerstick or a tube was added and incubated for 1 to 3 minutes at room temperature. Unbound red cells were washed off by swirling the dipstick in saline. Positive dipsticks were red due to adherence of red cells, while negative dipsticks remained white.

Direct antiglobulin dipsticks were prepared by attaching goat anti-human IgG to 13 mm nitrocellulose membrane circles or squares according to the dot immunoglobulin (dot blot) technique of Hawkes et al. [48,49]. Patient's red cells were washed 4 times with 0.9% (w/v) NaCl and resuspended to the original volume of whole blood in saline. The nitrocellulose circle was covered with 2 drops of red cells and incubated for 10 minutes at room temperature. Unbound red cells were washed off by swirling the membrane in saline. A positive reaction was characterized by a red dot in the center of the white membrane, while a negative membrane remained entirely white.

Results

The ABO groups of 2037 blood donors were determined by the solid phase forward grouping method using affinity purified antibodies and the results compared with those obtained with conventional agglutination techniques [40]. As indicated in table 1, a 99.6% correlation was obtained when the solid phase reactions were read and interpreted automatically. The ABO forward grouping results did not correlate in 8 instances. In each case, the computer programme recognized and flagged a discrepancy in the cell grouping and serum confirmation results. The cause of these discrepancies was incorrect machine interpretation due to partial collapse of the outer rim of effaced

Table 1. Comparison of conventional and solid phase results.

Test	Group	Conven-tional method	Automated solid phase	Corre-lation (%)	Visual solid phase	Corre-lation (%)
ABO forward	A	876*	870	99.3	876	100
Grouping affinity	B	143	143	100.0	143	100
Purified antibody	AB	66	65	98.5	66	100
	O	952	951	99.9	952	100
	Total	2037	2029	99.6	2037	100
ABO	A	2021	2021	100		
Monoclonal	B	504	504	100		
Antibodies	AB	171	171	100		
	O	2451	2451	100		
	Total	5150	5150	100		
ABO	A	421	420	99.8		
Serum	B	101	101	100.0		
Grouping	AB	15	15	100.0		
	O	483	481	99.6		
	Total	1020	1017	99.8		
Rh typing	D positive	1144	1144	99.9	1145	100
	D^u positive	55	55	100.0	55	100
	D negative	386	386	100.0	386	100
	Total	1586	1585	99.9	1586	100
Hepatitis	HBsAg positive	417	417	100		
	HBsAg negative	631	631	100		
	Total	1048	1048	100		

* Number tested by each method.

red cells at the point of the light path. Light passing through this area was not sufficiently absorbed to reach the limits set for positive reactions, and the wells were erroneously interpreted as negative. Visual interpretation of these tests resolved the discrepancies and resulted in a 100% correlation between the two methods.

Subsequent tests using monoclonal anti-A and anti-B for forward grouping eliminated this problem. One hundred percent correlation was achieved after testing an additional 5150 donor blood samples (table 1).

The ABO blood groups of 1063 blood donor samples were also determined using the solid phase saliva method [41]. All ABO groups were represented in the expected proportions. A correlation of 100% with a conventional agglutination technique was achieved.

Table 2. Detection of weak subgroups of A and B by solid phase testing.

Subgroups	No. tested	Automated solid phase	Visual solid phase
A_3	10	9	9
A_m	1	1	1
A_x	4	4	4
A_{bantu}	1	1	1
A_{el}	4	1	1
Weak B*	2	1	1
A_1Bm	1	1	1

* These weak subgroups of B were not further categorized.

The high degree of sensitivity obtained with solid phase ABO cell grouping was demonstrated by testing a panel of known weak ABO subgroups [40]. These samples had previously been characterized by standard serological methods including adsorption and elution studies and determination of secretor status. Monoclonal antisera were immobilized on the solid phase. The ABO groups of most of these weakly reactive samples were accurately determined, as shown in table 2. Ten examples of red cells with very weak expression of the A antigen were correctly identified. These included A_m, A_x, and A_{bantu}. Ten A_3 samples were examined, one of which failed to react in both the solid phase assay and by standard test tube hemagglutination techniques. This sample had been frozen for 6 years, which possibly resulted in diminished antigenic expression. Four examples of cells with exceedingly weak A expression (A_{el}) were examined, but only one of these proved to be detectable by the solid phase assay. A_{el} samples do not react in standard hemagglutination tests and require adsorption and elution studies for classification.

The serum (reverse) grouping results of 1020 blood donors were determined by the solid phase assay and compared to those obtained with a routine microplate agglutination method. A correlation of 99.7 % was achieved as indicated in table 1.

The Rh D blood group status of 1586 blood donors was determined by a standard microplate hemagglutination method and the solid phase assay employing automated reading [40]. Results are given in table 1. Disagreement in one case resulted in a correlation of 99.9 %. The single discrepancy was again due to partial collapse of the effaced red cell monolayer. However, visual inspection clearly indicated that the reaction was positive.

The increased sensitivity of the solid phase assay was demonstrated by testing 55 D^u donor blood samples which had required antiglobulin hemagglutination testing. As shown in table 1, each of these samples was typed as D positive by the solid phase method. Thus, the increase in sensitivity afforded by solid phase Rh typing would eliminate the need for antiglobulin testing of donor blood samples.

The ability of the solid phase assay to detect red cell antibodies in donor specimen was compared to a conventional antiglobulin test. Seventy eight

Table 3. Comparison of conventional and solid phase antibody screening results.

Antibody specificity	Donor antibodies	
	Conventional	Solid phase
Rh D	23	23
Rh C	7	7
Rh c	1	1
Rh E	15	15
K	19	19
Fy^a	3	3
JK^a	1	1
S	1	1
Lu^b	1	1
Le^a	4	1
Le^b	1	0
Le^{a+b}	1	0
Kn^a	1	0
Unidentified	0	3

irregular antibodies were detected by conventional methods in a total of 69,775 donor samples [42]. The most frequently encountered antibodies were anti-D, K, E, C, and Le^a. The strength of these antibodies ranged from 1 + to 3 + . The solid phase assay detected all of these antibodies except 3 anti Le^a, 1 anti-Le^b, 1 anti-Le^{a+b}, and 1 anti-Kn^a (table 3). None of these antibodies were considered clinically significant.

The solid phase antibody screen was subsequently simplified by the use of anti-IgG coated indicator cells. This modification improved sensitivity and eliminated the need for separate addition of antiglobulin reagent and indicator cells. An evaluation of this modified solid phase antibody screen was carried out with 84 patient sera previously found to contain antibody by conventional hemagglutination antiglobulin methods. Each of the commonly encountered specificities was represented, as indicated in tabel 4. Of the 84 sera tested, 1 anti-N, 3 anti-S, and 1 anti-P$_1$ were not detected by the solid phase assay. In each case, failure of the assay was attributed to the IgM composition of the antibody. The modified solid phase antibody screen was further evaluated by testing 101 donor sera in which antibodies had been detected by conventional screening techniques. (This series included the 78 sera tested by the original solid phase antibody screen). Again, the only antibodies not detected were the IgM antibodies missed by the original assay (table 5). Also tested by the solid phase method were 1039 donor sera expected to be free of irregular antibodies. Three of these gave consistently positive results. No evidence of specificity was observed when these sera were tested against an immobilized ten-cell panel. These reactions may have represented nonspecific adherence or indicated the presence of antibodies not detectable by conventional serology. If it is assumed that these

Table 4. Comparison of conventional and modified solid phase antibody screening results.

Antibody specificity	Patient antibodies	
	Conventional	Solid phase
D	9	9
C	1	1
Cw	1	1
c	5	5
E	5	5
e	1	1
E, c	3	3
D, c	6	6
D, Jka	2	2
E, Jkb	1	1
D, M	1	1
D, Fya	1	1
c, K	1	1
c, Fya	1	1
K	11	11
k	1	1
Kpa	1	1
Kpb	2	2
Kpa, Kpb	1	1
Fya	10	10
Fyb	1	1
Fya, S	2	2
Jka	3	3
Jkb	2	2
M	3	3
N	1	0
S	5	2
s	1	1
P$_1$	1	0
Lea	1	1
Totals	84	79

reactions were nonspecific, then the false-positive rate of solid phase antibody screening was 0.29%.

The sensitivity of the solid phase antibody screen was determined by comparing titration endpoints with those obtained by hemagglutination antiglobulin testing [42]. The solid phase assay was consistently two to four-fold more sensitive, for Rh, Kell and Duffy antibodies. The increase in sensitivity for Kidd antibodies was particularly striking (table 6).

The solid phase antiglobulin test for red cell crossmatching was performed on 113 sera, previously found to contain antibodies by a conven-

194

Table 5. Comparison of conventional and modified phase antibody screening results.

Antibody specificity	Donor antibodies	
	Conventional	Solid phase
D	21	21
C	1	1
c	4	4
E	14	14
D, C	8	8
D, E	4	4
D, S	1	1
D, C, K	1	1
E, K	2	2
E, Jk^a	1	1
K	28	28
K, Jk^a	1	1
K, Fy^a	1	1
Fy^a	4	4
Fy^a, S	1	1
Jk^a	1	1
S	1	1
Le^a	2	1
Le^a, Le^b	4	1
Kn^a	1	0
Totals	101	96

Table 6. Comparison of titration end points obtained by conventional and solid phase antibody screen.

Specificity	Conventional	Solid phase
D	1:8	1:32
C	1:8	1:16
K	1:4	1:8
Fy^a	1:4	1:16
Jk^a	1:8	1:256

tional hemagglutination antiglobulin test, which had been stored frozen [45]. Sera were thawed and retested in parallel by the solid phase compatibility test and a hemagglutination antiglobulin test. Results are given in table 7. The solid phase assay correctly identified 110 of the antibodies tested; 2 examples of anti-Lu^a and 1 example of anti-Le^a were not identified. In contrast, the conventional antiglobulin test failed to identify one example each of anti-C, -E, -c, -C^w, and -Jk^b, and three examples of anti-K. Although these antibodies had lost activity upon storage, the solid phase

Table 7. Comparison of conventional and solid phase antiglobulin testing.

Specificity	Number	Detected	
		Conventional	Solid phase
D	14	14	14
C	7	7	7
E	7	6	7
c	6	5	6
e	1	0	1
Cʷ	2	1	2
K	23	20	23
k	2	2	2
Kpª	2	2	2
Kpᵇ	2	2	2
Jkª	8	8	8
Jkᵇ	7	6	7
Fyª	10	10	10
Fyᵇ	4	4	4
S	3	3	3
s	5	5	5
U	3	3	3
Leª	2	2	1
Luª	2	2	0
Luᵇ	3	3	3
Totals	113	104	110

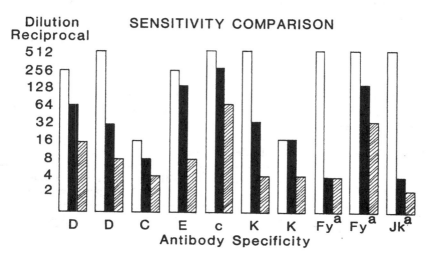

Figure 4. Results of parallel sensitivity testing, showing serum antibody titers obtained using hemagglutination antiglobulin tests ▨, solid phase antiglobulin tests read visually ■, and spectrophotometrically □. Each antibody specificity named on the abscissa respresents a single serum.

Table 8. Comparison of platelet antibody detection by solid phase (SP) and immunofluorescence.

	IF positive	IF negative
SP positive	19	15
SP negative	0	14

Table 9. Solid phase platelet crossmatch results.

	Number	Increment	No increment
Crossmatch compatible	77	52 (68%)	25 (32%)
Crossmatch incompatible	30	0 (0%)	30 (100%)

Table 10. Investigation of neonatal isoimmune thrombocytopenia by solid phase.

Number of cases	Platelets		
	Random	Father's	Auto
8	+	+	0
2	+	ND	0
1	+	+	ND
1	0	–	0

Table 11. Comparison of image analysis of solid phase results with visual interpretation of agglutination.

	ABO				Rh			AB screen	
	A	B	O	AB	Pos	Neg	Du	Pos	Neg
Agglutination	137	23	79	6	170	70	5	61	32
Immage analysis	137	23	79	6	170	70	5	61	32

Table 12. Predictive value of platelet crossmatch

Method	Sensitivity (%)	Specificity (%)	Predictive value of positive test (%)
Aggregometry	17	100	100
Lymphocytotoxicity	54	83	71
Serotonin release	40	77	67
Platelet factor 3 release	21	88	60
RIA	96	86	73
ELISA	48	78	75
Immunofluorescence	39	80	70
Solid phase*	55	100	100

* No patients were excluded from this study on the basis of pre-existing clinical conditions.

assay identified more antibodies considered to be of clinical significance than the hemagglutination antiglobulin test.

The sensitivity of the solid phase compatibility test was also evaluated by titration experiments. Serial dilutions of ten sera containing antibodies were tested by both the solid phase assay and a conventional antiglobulin technique. The endpoints of the solid phase assay exceeded those of the conventional antiglobulin test, as shown in figure 4.

The solid phase platelet antibody screen has been used for routine platelet antibody detection. The performance of this method was evaluated by comparison with a standard immunofluorescence (IF) method. Patient samples submitted for platelet antibody detection were tested by both methods in a blind study. Results are summarized in table 8. The most significant finding was that all samples positive by IF were also positive by the solid phase method. Fifteen samples negative by IF were positive by solid phase, most likely due to the increased sensitivity of the solid phase assay.

The solid phase platelet assay was also used to crossmatch single donor platelets [46]. One hundred and seven single donor paltelet preparations were crossmatched with recipients serum or plasma, and the results were correlated with transfusion outcome (table 9). Posttransfusion platelet increments greater than $15,000/\mu l$ at 2 hours or $10,000/\mu l$ at 12 hours, were considered significant. The most significant finding was the 100% correlation between crossmatch incompatibility and poor transfusion outcome. Crossmatch imcompatible transfusions never resulted in a significant platelet increment while approximately two-thirds of crossmatch compatible transfusions did produce a significant increment. It was not unexpected that one third of the compatible transfusions produced no significant response, since thrombocytopenic patients frequently have nonimmune casues of platelet destruction such as fever, sepsis, bleeding, or splenomegaly. Such patients wre not excluded from this study. The solid phase platelet antibody assay was also used to rapidly investigate 14 cases of suspected neonatal isoimmune thrombocytopenia. Maternal antibody was reactive with either random or father's platelets in 12 cases, as shown in table 10. In the two remaining cases, no maternal antibody was detected, although in one of these cases, antibody was detected in the infant's serum. When maternal antibodies were not directed against highfrequency antigens, the results with group 0 random blood donors could be used as crossmatches, to identify compatible platelets for transfusion.

The solid phase red cell adherence method has also been adapted for detection of hepatitis B surface antigen. The sensitivity of the solid phase adherence test for the detection of HBsAg was determined to be at least 0.5 ng/ml by assaying serial dilutions of specimens containing known amounts of HBsAg. Additionally, the solid phase adherence test consistently identified 417 patient or donor HBsAg positive samples, which were previously detected by 24-hour AUSRIA II testing. No false positive reactions occurred upon testing 631 negative donor samples (table 1).

The solid phase red cell adherence tests just described were read and interpreted using a Microelisa reader interfaced to an Apple II + computer. While usually adequate, false negative interpretations occasionally occurred when the light beam missed partially collapsed red blood cell monolayers. This explained why 100% correlation with agglutination methods was achieved by visual inspection, but not with an ELISA reader. Recently, we have developed an automated image analysis system to replace spectrophotometry. The performance of this system was determined by reading solid phase red cell adherence reactions and comparing the results with those obtained in parallel agglutination tests, which were interpreted visually. The results are presented in table 11. Sensitivity and specificity of the automated image analysis system matched that of visual inspection and correlated 100% with agglutination testing. Partially collapsed positive reactions were detected equally well by eye or automated immage analysis.

The performance of the ABO dipsticks was assessed by determining the blood groups of 1120 donors in parallel with our routine microplate agglutination method. One hundred percent correlation was achieved. The dipsticks correctly identified 461 group A, 480 group 0, 146 group B, and 33 group AB donors.

In preliminary experiments, the direct antiglobulin dipsticks have correctly identified 24 specimens with positive direct antiglobulin tests by conventional hemagglutination, which ranged in strength from 1 + weak to 3 + . The sensitivity of the dipsticks was determined by titration experiments to be between 100 and 200 molecules of IgG per red cell. No false positives were encountered.

Discussion

The solid phase tests thus far developed for antigen and antibody screening compared favorably with other current methods in their sensitivity and specificity. The solid phase red cell adherence method detected common ABO groups and Rh types as efficiently as agglutination methods. Spectrophotometric reading of these tests using affinity purified antibodies on the solid phase had an error rate of 0.4%, which was reduced by the use of monoclonal anti-A and anti-B (table 1). Monoclonal antibodies may give better results because a greater number of specific antibody molecules are adsorbed per unit area of a microplate well, resulting in more binding sites. Also, the monoclonal antibodies do not require purification, which may result in some inactivation and loss of affinity. Image analysis, instead of spectrophotometric reading, completely eliminated instrument reading and interpretation errors (table 11). In fact, automated video image analysis equalled the performance of the naked eye, while possessing all the benefits of an automated system. Besides its superior performance, image analysis offered several other advantages over spectrophotometry. A microplate was imaged and interpreted in 10 seconds, compared wot 4.5 minutes for a spectrophotometer. Also, the image analysis system costs less than $5,000 compared to $20,000 for a spectrophotometer system. Therefore, video image analysis should rapidly become the standard method for automated reading and interpretation of solid phase red cell adherence tests.

The solid phase ABO and Rh tests have several other advantages. Rh and ABO tests were performed identically since potentiators were no longer needed. Most importantly, solid phase assays achieved an increase in sensitivity without loss of specificity. Weak ABO subgroups that required special hemagglutination techniques were directly detected by solid phase ABO grouping (table 2). Antiglobulin Dᵘ testing could be eliminated since the solid phase method for Rh typing detected Dᵘ samples (table 1). Furthermore, anomalous reactions due to reagent additives were eliminated and those usually attributed to endogenous serum factors were not encountered. Samples containing free plasma hemoglobin, hydroxyethyl starch, or elevated levels of IgG or IgM did not interfere with the assay.

The solid phase antibody screen also compared favorably with conventional screening techniques. Good sensitivity was achieved with a single protocol designed to detect IgG antibodies (tables 3 – 6). The rate of false positivie reactions was much less than with other automated methods [50]. This was because interference from serum components and extrinsic factors, such as reagent constituents, was eliminated by the design of the solid phase system. Furthermore, enzymes, high molecular weight media, and polycations were not required. Most recently, the protocol has been simplified by the use of anti-IgG coated indicator cells, instead of separate antiglobulin reagent and IgG coated indicator cells, which seemed to slightly improve sensitivity. Also, this modification helped further standardize all solid phase adherence tests, since these are the same type of indicator cells used in the solid phase platelet antibody test and the hepatitis test.

Expansion of solid phase antibody screen techniques should greatly facilitate antibody identification in the near future. Expanded panels containing up to 90 different red cells could be immobilized on a microplate and tested just as easily as 10 or 20 cell panels. A microcomputer interfaced to a video image analysis system could readily interpret the pattern of positive and negative reactions into antibody specificities.

The solid phase antiglobulin test was developed to automate red cell crossmatches. In contrast to the solid phase antibody screen, this method was developed to perform individual crossmatches where it was not possible to prepare and store solid phase reagent red cell monolayers ahead of time. This test had increased sensitivity, without loss of specificity, compared to a conventional hemagglutination antiglobulin test. The present method was designed to detect only IgG antibodies. This explains the failure to detect a few Lutheran and Lewis antibodies, which might have been IgM (table 7). If desired, the solid phase antiglobulin test could easily be modified to detect IgM or complement-coated red cells by immobilizing IgM or complement on the solid phase and using an appropriate antiglobulin reagent. The solid phase assay required minimal reagents and was completed in less than 30 minutes. The ease and speed of handling a single microplate, rather than 96 individual test tubes were significant improvements. Washing and centrifugation steps were greatly facilitated. However, the greatest time savings were achieved by automated reading of solid phase adherence reactions. The microplate spectrophotometer reads 96 wells within 1 minute, which was much less than the time required to read 96 hemagglutination reactions manually. The solid phase antiglobulin method thus represents the first compatibility test that can be reliably read and interpreted automatically.

The need for simple tests to detect antiplatelet antibodies has attached increasing attention in recent years. The great variety of technical approaches devised to detect platelet antibodies indicates that no single method has been universally accepted. Published methods have included simple agglutination, mixed agglutination, aggregometry, lymphocytotoxicity, serotonin release, platelet factor 3 release, enzyme-labeled immunoassays, immunofluorescence immunoassays, complement fixation assays, and radiolabeled antiglobulin or *Staph.* protein A assays. Most of these methods are time-consuming, technically difficult, or require expensive equipment, which restricts their use to research or reference laboratories.

The solid phase red cell adherence test for platelet antibodies overcame these obstacles, making it ideally suited for routine use by transfusion services. The speed and simplicity were due to the use of anti-platelet antibodies on the solid phase and anti-IgG coated indicator red cells. The use of microplate wells coated with anti-platelet antibodies allowed platelets to be adsorbed selectively from platelet rich plasma, thus eliminating the time-consuming separation and washing of platelets, which is required by all other methods. The use of anti-IgG coated indicator red cells which could be centrifuged onto the solid phase platelet monolayer, in order to accelerate their interaction with bound antibodies, eliminated the need for lengthy incubations and expensive detection equipment. Solid phase assays were completed within one hour after receiving samples. This tims savings was particularly significant when performing platelet crossmatches for recipients alloimmunized to a large percentage of donors. Several hundred prospective donors could be crossmatched in a single day. The speed and simplicity of this assay also greatly facilitated investigation of suspected cases of neonatal isoimmune thrombocytopenia. Within one hour of receiving samples the diagnosis could be confirmed, allo- and auto-antibodies could be differentiated, an compatible platelets could be identified (table 10).

In addition, the solid phase assay was more sensitive than a standard immunofluorescence assay (table 8). Also, it was more likely to detect HLA antibodies than immunofluorescence, because the solid phase assay allowed each serum to be tested against a greater number of individual platelet samples. In some instances, this may preclude the need for lymphocytotoxicity testing. The preliminary results with the solid phase platelet crossmatch were also encouraging. Thus far, an incompatible platelet crossmatch has a 100% predictive value for a poor transfusion outcome, which is much higher than that observed with other methods [51 – 53] (table 9, 13). This is a significant advantage, because the ability to predict and prevent ineffective plateletphereses is cost-effective and benefits prospective donors as well as alloimmunized recipients.

The potential risk of transmitting hepatitis B virus by blood transfusion makes it necessary to screen each unit of donor blood for hepatitis B surface antigen prior to transfusion. Screening is currently performed by radioimmunoassay or enzyme-linked immunoassays. While these tests have drastically reduced the incidence of posttransfusion hepatitis B infection, they have the disadvantages of requiring expensive equipment, unstable reagents, multiple manipulations, and lengthy incubation periods. To overcome these problems, the solid phase adherence method was adapted for the detection of HBsAg [39]. The solid phase adherence assay was as sensitive and specific as current third-generation hepatitis tests (table 1), while eliminating the need for radioactive or enzyme-labeled reagents. Additionally, the assay was performed quickly (35 minutes) using inexpensive equipment common to the majority of blood banks. These features make it compatible with the protocols employed in the other solid phase red cell adherence tests.

Probably the most important advantage of the solid phase system was the objective endpoint of red cell adherence. In all assays positive reactions were characterized by effacement of test or indicator red cells over the surface of microplate wells, while negative reactions always resulted in central buttons of red cells. The clear distinction between positive and negative reactions allowed results to be read automatically much easier and less expensively than current instruments using agglutination. For instance, the initial capitalization cost of an AutoAnalyzer or Groupamatic instrument varies from $115,000 to $420,000. In contrast, the solid phase method can be automated for less than $20,000. If video image analysis is utilized, instead of spectrophotometry, this cost is further reduced to less than $5,000.

The solid phase system is really a modular system which can be individually tailored to the needs of small and large laboratories. Laboratories with low volumes can perform the assays manually and read and interpret the results visually. Alternatively, the reactions can be read automatically. The further addition of a personal computer interfaced to the reader provides automated reading, interpretation, and storage of results, which reduces manual transcription errors. To further automate the system, the personal computer can be interfaced to a blood center's mainframe computer. This interface allows current test results to be compared to past donor histories. Discrepancies between current and past records are automatically flagged, signalling the need for further investigation. New donors are automatically added to the existing donor file. Semiautomated pipettors and washers can also be employed as the need arises. This modularity allows a laboratory to purchase only the equipment it requires, which reduces capitalization costs and allows the purchase of additional backup equipment. This redundancy allows laboratories to reduce staffing. In addition to the savings in capitalization and labour, the costs per test are also less. It has been estimated that an ABO and Rh test costs between $0.83 and $1.23 with current automated instruments. In comparison, solid phase ABO and Rh tests cost less than $0.65 per test.

Solid phase red cell adherence assays in microplates are ideally suited for batch processing in hospital or blood center laboratories. The application of these same methods to dipsticks greatly expands their potential use. Since these dipsticks are accurate, fast, simple, and do not require any equipment they are especially useful for testing individual samples outside of the laboratory. Possible uses include blood donor mobiles, doctors' offices, emergency care situations, home transfusions, military operations, and underdeveloped countries. Also, they can be used at the hospital bedside to confirm ABO groups prior to transfusion.

The excellent performance of these dipsticks is not surprising since nitrocellulose and nylon membranes have much higher protein binding capacities than polystyrene. At the concentrations usually employed in coating microplates, polystyrene will maximally bind 10 μg of protein per cm^2. In contrast, nitrocellulose has a protein binding capacity of 90 μg/cm^2 and charged nylon has a capacity of 500 μg/cm^2. Furthermore, labile proteins actually become more stable after binding to nylon or nitrocellulose. This enhanced stability allows dipsticks to be stored without impairing their antibody activity. These excellent protein binding properties probably explain why the ABO dipsticks were as sensitive, specific and fast as the solid phase microplate test, without requiring enzyme treatment of red cells or centrifugation to accelerate antigen-antibody binding. The flat testing surface allowed dipstick to be thoroughly washed by merely dipping them in saline, instead of repeated filling and decanting. Also, the flat white surface provided an excellent background to read positive and negative reactions. Even weak positive reactions were distinctly red, while negative reactions remained clearly white. Because of this clearly visible endpoint, instrumentation was not needed to read dipsticks. However, we have read and interpreted blood grouping dipsticks by video image analysis. This may prove especially useful for automatically interpreting multi-dot cell phenotyping dipsticks in the near future. We have already been able to phenotype a drop of blood for the ABO, Rhesus, Kell, MNSs, Kidd and Lewis antigens within 10 minutes.

In view of these properties, the performance of the direct antiglobulin dipsticks was not surprising. Tests could be completed within 15 minutes after recieving the sample. The sensitivity of the dipstick was two to four fold greater than routine antiglobulin tests and equaled the red cell ELISA technique [54]. In one instance, the dipstick was clearly positive with a patient sample, which was negative by routine hemagglutination testing, but had 94 molecules of IgG per red cell by ELISA. This dipstick method is presently being modified to directly determine IgG subtypes. Dipsticks for ABO reverse grouping and antibody screening of serum are also under development.

Summary

Solid phase red cell membrane assays offer many advantages over conventional methods. A similar, simple protocol is employed for each of the tests. Their sensitivities are at least as good as conventional assays, without compromising specificity. The objective endpoint of red cell adherence allows results to be read quickly and reliably, either visually or by relatively inexpensive equipment. Simple, fast protocols and automated reading result in significant labour savings.

The use of these assays is not limited to blood banking. Many investigators have described solid phase red cell adherence assays to detect IgM antibodies to rubella [55,56], mumps [57], parainfluenza [58], respiratory syncytial virus [59], Toxoplasmosis [69], and fimbriated Hemophilus influenza [61]. They have been used to detect allergen-specific IgE antibodies [62], rheumatoid factor [69], and antibodies to collagen [64], gliadin [65], Schistosoma mansoni [66], and islet cells [67]. They have also been used to screen for monoclonal antibodies to cell surface antigens [68,69] and to quantitate Rotavirus in feces [70] and human chorionic gonadotropin in serum [71]. These assays are faster and as sensitive as currently existing immunofluorescent, enzyme-linked and radioimmunoassays. The only obstacle preventing their widespread use has been the inability to automatically read and interpret results. Application of the video image analysis system developed for our blood banking tests should readily solve this problem. Also, the adaption of red cell adherence tests to dipsticks will optimize individual testing, as well as batch testing, and allow tests to be performed in the field.

References

1. Stillmark H. Über Ricin, ein giftiges Ferment aus den Samen von *Ricinus Communis* L. and einigen anderen Euphorbiaceen. Thesis. Dorpat 1888.
2. Durham HE. On a special action of the serum of highly immunized animals. J Pathol Bacteriol 1896;4:13 – 44.
3. Ehrlich P, Morgenroth J. Über Haemolysine. Dritte Mitteilung. Berl Klin Wschr 1900;37:681 – 7.
4. Landsteiner K. Zur Kenntnis der antifermentativen, lytischen und agglutinierenden Wirkungen des Blutserums und der Lymphe. Zbl Bakt 1900;27:357 – 62.
5. McNeil C, Helmick WM, Ferrari A. A preliminary investigation into automatic blood grouping. Vox Sang 1963;8:235 – 41.
6. Sturgeon P, Cedergren B, McQuiston D. Automation of routine blood typing procedures. Vox Sang 1963;8:438 – 51.
7. Muller A, Garretta M, Hebert M. Groupamatic System: Overview, history and development and evaluation of use. Vox Sang 1981;40:201 – 13.
8. Knight RC, Slater NGP. Automated blood grouping in a hospital laboratory with the Minigroupamatic. Med Lab Sci 1983;40:7 – 13.
9. Wegmann TG, Smithies O. A simple hemagglutination system requiring small amounts of red cells and antibodies. Transfusion 1966;6:67 – 73.
10. Crawford MN, Gottman FE, Gottman CA. Microplate system for routine use in blood bank laboratories. Transfusion 1970;10:258 – 63.
11. Parker JL, Marcoux DA, Hafleigh EB et al. Modified microtiter tray method for blood typing. Transfusion 1978;18:417 – 22.
12. Warlow A, Tills D. Micromethods in blood group serology. Vox Sang 1978;35:354 – 6.
13. Innocenti P, Nieri A. Micrometodi in immunoematologia: laIettura automatica-esperienze presso il centro transfusionale dell' opedale di treviso. Transfus Sang 1982;27:65 – 9.

204

14. Bowley AR, Gordon I, Ross DW. Computer controlled automated reading of blood groups using microplates. Med Lab Sci 1984;41:19 – 28.
15. Severns ML, Schoepner SL, Cozart MJ, Friedman LI, Schanfield MS. Automated determination of ABO/Rh in microplates. Vox Sang 1984;47:293 – 303.
16. Coombs RRA, Bedford D. The A and B antigens on human platelets demonstrated by means of mixed erythrocyte-platelet agglutination. Vox Sang 1955;5:111 – 5.
17. Coombs RRA, Bedford D, Rouillard LM. A and B blood-group antigens on human epidermal cells demonstrated by mixed agglutination. Lancet 1956;1: 461 – 3.
18. Ashurst DE, Bedford D, Coombs RRA. Examination of human platelets for the ABO, MN, Rh, Tjª, Luteran, and Lewis systems of antigens by means of mixed erythrocyte-platelet agglutination. Vox Sang 1956;1:235 – 40.
19. Gurner BW, Coombs RRA. Examination of human leukocytes for the ABO, MN, Rh, Tjª, Lutheran and Lewis systems of antigens by means of the mixed erythrocyte leukocyte agglutination. Vox Sang 1958;3:13 – 22.
20. Kelus A, Gurner BW, Coombs RRA. Blood group antigens on Hela cells shown by mixed agglutination. Immunology 1959;2:262 – 7.
21. Coombs RRA, Daniel MR, Gurner BW, Kelus A. Species characterizing antigens of L and ERK cells. Nature (London) 1961;189:503 – 4.
22. Coombs RRA, Dodd BE. Possible applications of the principle of mixed agglutination in the identification of blood stains. Med Sci Law 1961;1:359 – 77.
23. Vogel J, Shelokov A. Adsorption-hemagglutination test for influenza virus in monkey kidney tissue culture. Science 1957;126:358 – 9.
24. Högman C. The principle of mixed agglutination applied to tissue culture systems. A method for the study of cell-bound antigens. Vox Sang 1959;2:12 – 20.
25. Högman C. Blood group antigens A and B determined by means of mixed agglutination on cultured cells of human fetal kidney, liver, spleen, lung, heart, and skin. Vox Sang 1959;4:319 – 32.
26. Coombs RRA, Marks J, Bedford D. Specific mixed agglutination: mixed erythrocyte-platelet antiglobulin reaction for the detection of platelet antibodies. Br J Haematol 1956;2:84 – 94.
27. Fagraeus A, Espmark A. Use of a mixed haemadsorption method in virus infected tissue cultures. Nature (London) 1961;190:370 – 1.
28. Fagraeus A, Espmark JA, Jonsson J. Mixed haemadsorption: a mixed antiglobulin reaction applied to antigens on a glass surface. Immunology 1965;9: 161 – 75.
29. Franks D. Antigenic markers on cultured human cells. 1. Li, Tjª, Donath-Landsteiner and "non-specific" auto-antigens. Vox Sang 1966;11:674 – 85.
30. Juji T, Kano K, Milgrom R. Mixed agglutination with platelets. Int Arch Allergy 1972;42:474 – 84.
31. Shibata Y, Juji T, Nishizawa Y, Sakamoto H, Ozawa N. Detection of platelet antibodies by a newly developed mixed agglutination with platelets. Vox Sang 1981;41:25 – 31.
32. Coombs RRA. Assays utilizing red cells as markers. In: Voller A (ed). Immunoassays for the 80's. Lancaster: MTP Press 1981:17 – 34.
33. Catt K, Tregear GW. Solid phase radioimmunoassay in antibody-coated tubes. Science 1967;158:1570 – 2.
34. Mage MG, McHugh LL, Rothstein TL. Mouse lymphocytes with and without surface immunoglobulin: preparative scale separation in polystyrene tissue culture dishes coated with specifically purified anti-immunoglobulin. J Immunol Methods 1977;15:47 – 56.

35. Wysocki LJ, Sato VL. Panning for lymphocytes: a method for cell selection. Proc Natl Acad Sci (USA) 1978;75:2844 – 8.
36. Rosenfield RE, Kochwa S, Kaczera Z. Solid phase serology for the study of human erythrocytic antigen-antibody reactions. Proc 15th congr Int Soc Blood Transfusion, Paris 1976:27 – 33.
37. Moore HH, Conradie JD. Solid phase indirect anti-human globulin test for identification of red blood cell antibodies in human sera. Transfusion 1982;22:540.
38. Moore HH. Automated reading of red cell antibody identification tests by a solid phase antiglobulin technique. Transfusion 1984;24:218 – 21.
39. Plapp FV, Rachel JM, Beck ML, Coenen WM, Bayer WL, Sinor LT. Blood antigens and antibodies: solid phase adherence assays. Lab Manag 1984;22:39 – 47.
40. Sinor LT, Rachel JM, Beck ML, Bayer WL, Coenen WM, Plapp FV. Solid phase ABO grouping and Rh typing. Transfusion 1985;25:21 – 3.
41. Beck ML, Sinor LT, Rachel JM, Plapp FV. Solid phase ABO grouping using saliva. Med Lab Sci 1985;42:86 – 7.
42. Plapp FV, Sinor LT, Rachel JM, Beck ML, Coenen WM, Bayer WL. A solid phase antibody screen. Am J Clin pathol 1984;82:719 – 21.
43. Rosenfield RE, Shaik SH, Kaczera IZ, Kochwa S. Augmentation of hemagglutination by low ionic conditions. Transfusion 1979;19:499 – 510.
44. Place JD, Schroeder HR. The fixation of anti-HBs antigen on plastic surfaces. J Immunol Methods 1982;48:251 – 60.
45. Rachel JM, Sinor LT, Beck ML, Plapp FV. A solid phase antiglobulin test. Tranfusion 1985;25:24 – 6.
46. Rachel JM, Sinor LT, Tawfik OW et al. A solid phase red cell adherence test for platelet crossmatching. Med Lab Sci 1985;42:194 – 5.
47. Gershoni JM, Palade GE. Electrophoretic transfer of proteins from sodium dodecyl sulfate-polyacrylamide gels to a positively charged membrane filter. Anal Biochem 1982;124:396 – 405.
48. Towbin H, Gordon J. Immunblotting and dot immunobinding-current status and outlook. J Immunol Methods 1984;72:313 – 40.
49. Hawkes R, Niday E, Gordon J. A dot-immunobinding assay for monoclonal and other antibodies. Anal Biochem 1982;119:142 – 7.
50. Moore BPL. Automated antibody detection. In: Sandler SG, Nusbacher J, Schanfield MS (eds). Immuno-biology of the erythrocyte. New York: Alan R. Liss, 1980:271 – 89.
51. Unger JL. Platelet crossmatch techniques: how good are they? Diag Med 1984;7:59 – 71.
52. Kickler TS, Braine HG, Ness PM, Koester A, Bias W. A radiolabeled antiglobulin test for crossmatching platelet transfusion. Blood 1983;61:238 – 42.
53. Kakaiya RM, Gudino MD, Miller WV et al. Four crossmatch methods to select platelet donors. Transfusion 1984;24:35 – 41.
54. Bodensteiner D, Brown P, Skikne B, Plapp F. The enzyme-linked immunosorbent assay: accurate detection of red cell antibodies in autoimmune hemolytic anemia. Amer J Clin Pathol 1983;79:182 – 5.
55. Krech U, Wilhelm JA. A solid phase immunosorbent technique for the rapid detection of rubella IgM by haemagglutination inhibition. J Gen Virol 1979;44:281 – 6.
56. Denoyel GA, Gaspar A, Peyramond D. Diagnosis of recent rubella virus infection by demonstration of specific immunoglobulin M antibodies: comparison of solid-phase reverse immunosorbent test with sucrose density grandient centrifugation. J Clin Microbiol 1981;13:698 – 704.

57. Van der Logt JTM, Heessen FWA, van Loon AM, van der Veen J. Hemadsorption immunosorbent technique for determination of mumps immunoglobulin M antibody. J Clin Microbiol 1982;15:82 – 6.
58. Van der Logt JTM, van Loon AM, van der Veen J. Detection of parainfluenza IgM antibody by hemadsorption immunosorbent technique. J Med Virol 1982;10:213 – 21.
59. Cranage MP, Coombs RRA. An indirect haemadsorption procedure (MrsPAH) for detecting antibodies to respiratory syncytial virus. J Virol Meth 1982;5:119 – 208.
60. Remington JS, Elmstod WD, Araujo FG. Detection of IgM antibodies with antigen-tagged latex particles in an immunosorbent assay. J Clin Microbiol 1983;17:939 – 41.
61. Connor EM, Loeb MR. A haemadsorption method for detection of colonies of haemophilus influenza type B expressing fimbriae. J Infect Disease 1983;148:855 – 60.
62. Scott ML, Thornley MJ, Coombs RRA. Comparison of red-cell linked anti-IgE and ^{125}I-labelled anti-IgE in a solid phase system for the measurement of IgE specific for castor bean allergen. Internatl Arch Allergy Appl Immunol 1981;64:230 – 5.
63. March RE, Reebock JS, Holborrow EJ, Coombs RRA. MrsPAH: a simple microtitre plate test for rheumatoid factors of different classes. J Immunol Meth 1981;42:137 – 46.
64. Coombs RRA, Gurner BW, Oldham G, Barnes MJ, Kieffer M. Antibodies to type II collagen measured by mixed reverse (solid phase) passive antiglobulin heamadsorption. Internatl Arch Allergy Appl Immunol 1982;67:377 – 9.
65. Kieffer M, Frazien PJ, Daniels NWR, Ciclitira PJ, Coombs RRA. Serum antibodies (mesured by MrsPAH) to alcohol soluble gliadins in adult coeliac patients. J Immunol Meth 1981;42:129 – 36.
66. Stek M. Erythroadsorption and enzyme linked immunoassays (EAIA and ELISA) for specific circulating antibodies and antigens in schistosomiasis. Ann Immunol (Inst Pasteur) 1984;135:13 – 23.
67. Maruyama S, Suguira M, Nakazawa M et al. Detection of islet cell surface antibodies by an indirect rosette assay, using islet cells and protein A-labeled sheep red blood cells. J Immunol Meth 1984;73:173 – 80.
68. Wyatt DM, Rylatt DB, Bundesen PG, Parish CR, Street GD. Rapid screening of monoclonal antibodies by spin adherence double immunosorbent test (SADIST). J Immunol Meth 1985;76:273 – 82.
69. Clark MR, Cobbold SP, Waldmann H, Coombs RRA. Detection of monoclonal antibodies against surface antigens: the use of antiglobulins coupled to red blood cells. J Immunol Meth 1984;66:81 – 7.
70. Bradburne AF, Almeida JD, Gardner PS, Moosai RB, Nash AA, Coombs RRA. A solid phase system (SPACE) for the detection and quantitation of rotavirus in faeces . J Gen Virol 1979;44:615 – 23.
71. Gupta SK, Guesdon JL, Avrameas S, Talwar GP. Solid-phase competitive and sandwich-type erythro-immunoassays for human chorionic gonadotropin. J Immunol Meth 1985;80:117 – 87.

A PRELIMINARY REPORT ON THE EVALUATION OF THE KONTRON MICROGROUPAMATIC

J.M. Sangster

Introduction

A preliminary evaluation of the Kontron Microgroupamatic was performed at the London Hospital, Whitechapel during the month of January 1985. The system was evaluated for reading of results of ABO, D typing and antibody screening.

Description of the instrument

The Microgroupamatic system consists of a microplate photometer, a Digital Equipment Corporation microcomputer for data processing (floppy disc based), a video terminal, a printer and optional codabar reader, and automatic plate loader.

The instrument interprets micro well hemagglutination reactions by taking several readings from different positions in each will. Interpretation is made from the central reading and the contrast value which is the difference between the highest and lowest readings. The operator can select the three best steps for obtaining the photometric readings of each well by the standardization procedure. This is required for each new batch of antisera, or if the manufacturer of the microtitre plate is changed.

One microplate containing eight patient samples can be read in approximately one minute. The blood group and antibody screen interpretation and parameter settings are software controlled by the operator. There is also a graphic data analysis for daily quality control of cell concentrations and antisera performance.

The option of the barcode reader can be used for plate identification and the correlation of reactions to each sample. Alternatively each individual row in the plate can be given a laboratory number via the software programme prior to reading the plate. There is also a communications package for data transmission to a host computer, but this function could not be evaluated.

Work throughout time as based on photometric reading, interpretation and ''on line editing of results'' is approximately 5 minutes per plate, consisting of 8 samples. The cost of the system is approximately £20,000 depending on which optional extras are required. The system can be incorporated into a bench space of 20 square feet.

Evaluation

A total of 600 samples were tested in duplicate with routine microhemagglutination techniques, and a further 825 were tested with the Microgroupamatic incorporated into the routine work.

The Microgroupamatic was initially calibrated as per instruction manual, with slight changes to the threshold values as a broad spectrum of samples were tested. The analysis and interpretation tables were set up to operator specifications, and the following set of analyses were selected: ABO, Rhesus D, antibody screen, auto reaction.

An interpretation table was set up for each individual analysis. The symbol 0 is used where the results of that particular well are not to be included in the interpretation. Positive or negative reactions are indicted by + or − symbols. The symbol M can be incorporated if an interpretation using weak positive reactions was desired.

The cycle and threshold tables were set up with the same microtitre plates, cell concentrations, and dilutions of antisera used throughout. Two manufacturers of microtitre plates were tested i.e. Nunc and Kontron, both gave similar results. All plates were soaked in 0.1% albumin/saline and shaken dry before use to reduce problems of static electricity. The plates were reused three or four times after soaking in a nuetral detergent and rinsing in distilled water. The plates were discarded if any wells were badly scratched or occluded.

Blood Group Reference Laboratory (BGRL) antisera was used throughout, incorporating monoclonal anti-A and anti-B which could be diluted for use 1:5 and 1:32 respectively. Human anti-A + B was diluted to 1:2 and the two human IgG anti-D's were used undiluted. A cell concentration of 3% was used throughout. The standard A1, A2, and B cells were made up to an accurate 3% in 0.1% bromelin/saline. The patient's cells were diluted to approximately 3% by visual comparison. The recommended use of anticoagulated samples was not followed because of the extra expense incurred of having two samples i.e. one clotted and one anticoagulated, and the inevitable increase in sampling error.

Antibody screening consisted of two screening cells issued by the BGRL cells 1 and 11, suspended in 0.1% bromelin/saline. The indirect antiglobulin technique was performed in the microtitre plates but was read visually because the type of agglutination produced is not suitable at present for reading by the photometer.

Test and standard cells were premodified for 10 minutes in the bromelin before testing. All tests were performed with 25 μl volumes and incubated for 20 mintues at R.T. before spinning at 110 g for 40 secondes. The plates were then agitated using a Titertek plate shaker based on orbital movement, until the negative reactions were evenly resuspended. In practice gentle agitation for 2 minutes was required, followed by the lowest speed rotation to keep the cells suspended before reading. It is important that the reactions are not allowed to settle prior to reading and for this reason it was found impractical to use the automatic plate feeder which takes a stack of 10 plates.

The plates are easily loaded into the plate reader individually, from the plate shaker.

Results

The first 600 samples were set up independantly (table 1) of the routine testing, which involves a microhemagglutination technqiue using the "stand and stream" method, visual reading and recording. The percentage of "no type determined" (% NTD) was calculated from the first run prior to "on line editing". These were then broken down into causes of rejection. An acceptable level of rejection should be established for each individual laboratory. The use of "on line editing" reduces the number considerably, there is also room for a typed comment from the oeprator. This does require that the operator must be sufficiently experienced to perform on line editing.

1.5 % of the samples tested were from premature infants and cord blood, the majority of these will not contain ABO antibodies and therefore will be rejected by interpretation.

The presence of cold reacting atypical antibodies will also give false positive reactions in the serum group and therefore lead to no interpretation. These samples will require further investigation, and in practice 2.5 % of samples tested were rejected for this reason which correlates will with samples requiring further investigation by manual techniques. A 3 % saline suspension of standard cells was used for the 150 samples tested during week 3, with no apparent loss in sensitivity as compared to a bromelin/saline diluent. But the number rejected due to cold reacting clinically insignificant antibodies was reduced.

Rapid settling of cells leading to false positive readings is a problem that reduces with operator experience. Adequate mixing followed by gentle agitation until the plate is read, eliminates this problem. The automatic plate loader was not found to be useful for this reason.

Rejection due to weak agglutinates tended to be confined to the anti-A, anti-D and the A2 cells. These gave visual + reactions which were spread evenly over the base of the well, giving a low contrast value and therefore a negative reaction. A common cause of poor agglutination with the anti-D was due to several anemic patients requiring an increased volume of blood to obtain a 3 % suspension of cells and a resultant loss in the effect of bromelinisation.

Two samples gave false D negative reactions due to the formation of a large monolayer of positive cells over the base of the well giving a low contrast value. On repeating the reactions a good positive result was obtained. Routine D^u testing of all D negatives would eliminate this problem. One example of an Ax and a Db were tested several times and found to give a weak positive or M reading which would be flagged for the operators attention.

Samples with knwon Rhesus antibodies gave good correlation with the antibody screening channels, enzyme reactions are readily adaptable to the automated reader.

Table 1. Correlation of ABO and Rhesus D results using the Microgroupamatic.*

Number of samples	Number of samples rejected	% Rejection	Correlation with visual reading %	
			ABO type	Rh D type
600	53	8.8	100	99.7

* All testes were performed in duplicate with routine microhemagllutination techniques and visual reading of results.

Table 2. Causes of rejection of results by the Microgroupamatic.

			Causes of rejection (% of samples tested)								
Number of samples	Number rejected	% rejected (without editing)	Cord sample	Atypical anti-bodies	Pre-mature settling/ inade-quate mixing	Weak ABO reactions cell	Weak ABO reactions serum	Weak Rh D reactions	False Rh D negatives	Large agglu-tinates	Lysis
Week 1 338	40	11.8	1.5	1.4	0.5	0	2.5	1.7	0.6	2.9	0.2
Week 2 334	39	11.6	1.2	3.5	0.1	1.2	1.8	0.2	0	2.4	0.2
Week 3 150	9	6.0	2.0	2.0	0	0	1.3	0.6	0	0	0
Total 822	88	10.7	1.5	2.3	0.3	0.4	1.9	0.8	0.2	1.7	0.13

Conclusions

The overall rejection rate of 10.7% (table 2) can be considereably reduced using "on line editing". Cord samples and atypical antibodies are legitimate reasons for rejection, the remaining problems could be overcome by visual appraisal of the plates and concurrent on line editing. This became relatively easy for the operator with experience, all rejected results are halted on the VDU for operator attention.

The floppy disc can store the data from approximately 175 plates or 1400 patient samples, which can be used for permanent storage. The ability to assign an individual number per patient coupled with a plate identification number via a codabar system or manual input reduces transcription error. The manual input of the plate identification number is required after the plate has been read, and can be rechecked by the operator at this point.

The claim of the company referring to great savings in antisera is of course an advantage of the microtitre methodology over standard tube technique, and not one of the automated reader. The versatility of the programme allows the interpretation and analyses tables and threshold setting to be under the control of the laboratory. Graphic analyses of each channel allows instant access to quality control of antisera and cell concentrations.

Comments on the software are mostly favourable, but some suggested improvements for a hospital blood bank would be:

1. The ability to print a single group from a plate rather than having to have on file all the results from the plate including the empty wells;
2. The ability to delete obsolete batches from the results disc;
3. The ability to edit results after recording when using the ''no correction function'' where the results are printed as read. Approval of these results could be done at leisure.

One minor fault led to two identical breakdowns in the 4 week period. The prongs for retrieving and positioning the plate in the reader failed to work.

The system proved a successful and acceptable method of reading, interpreting and recording blood group data, removing a great deal of cumbersome clerical work. Two medical technicians required to read, record interpret and report the results could be reduced to a single operator on the Microgroupamatic. Initial experience would not preclude the use of this system from a routine hospital blood bank.

CMV ANTIBODY TESTING OF BLOOD DONORS

R.L. McShine, G. Sinninge, P.C. Das, C.Th. Smit Sibinga

A variety of methods has been developed to detect CMV antibodies including the indirect flueorescence assay (IFA), the fluorescent immunoassay (FIA), the complement-fixation test (CFT), the enzyme linked immonosorbent assay (ELISA) and the indirect hemagglutination assay (IHA). Although most test procedures produce essentially the same results, there are marked variations in convenience and ease of use. The test chosen should be as practical, specific, sensitive, reproducible and as cost-effective as possible. Although the IFA has proven to be the most sensitive, for routine blood banks where large scale testing will be done an ELISA, an IHA or a Latex test are probably most appropriate.

When our Blood Centre decided to make CMV antibody negative blood and blood products available for seronegative patients at risk, we were faced with the dilemma, which test to choose. Most comparative reports in the literature [1,2] spoke favourably of the IHA. In September 1984 we did a comparative study between three commercial ELISA kits (Abbott, Organon, Ismunit) and the IHA kit from Cetus Corporation, California.

Of 80 donor serum samples tested, three gave discrepant results. These three samples were also tested for us at the Division of Clinical Immunology of the University Hospital Groningen. The best concordance was obtained between the IHA and one of the three ELISA techniques (table 1).

Table 1. Cetus CMV-IHV versus ELISA.

	Cetus IHA	ELISA	
Sensitivity	97.9%	95.9%	concordance 96.2%
Specificity	93.8%	96.8%	

When a pool of CMV antibody positive sera was titrated in both tests (dilutions being made in a pool of CMV antibody negative sera), the titre in the Cetus CMV IHA test was >100 while the titre in ELISA was 40.

The final choice for routine testing was the Cetus CMV IHA. However, because of the high cost of the kit, a modified technique was developed which could make testing less expensive and still retain sensibitivy and specificity. The method we use is a modification of the microtechnique described by Henry et al. [3]. Using this method, from the standard 500 test kit about 6,000 tests could be performed. A short description of the test is as follows:

1. Reconstitute the lyophilised test and control cells both with 3 ml of the Cetus dilution buffer and leave to stand at room temperature for two hours;
2. Centrifuge at 800 g for 60 seconds;
3. Remove the supernatant and resuspend the sediment in 3 ml of the dilution buffer. Keep at ± 4°C until needed;
4. Resuspend the cell suspensions properly and pipette 5 μl of the CMV test cells in rows 1, 3, 5, 7 and 9 of a Terasaki plate* and 5 μl of the control cells in rows 2, 4, 6, 8 and 10;
5. Keep the cells in suspension by placing the plates on a shaker at speed 800 per minute;
6. Dilute the serum samples 1 and 6 in diluting fluid (0.5 ml Tween 20 in 1 litre phosphate buffered saline pH 7.4);
7. Add 5 μl of each diluted sample of the test cells and to the control cells. Mix by taking up and releasing twice with an automatic pipette. The control sera are treated the same way;
8. Place on a shaker, speed 800 for 1 minute;
9. Set the plate on a non-vibrating level surface and incubate at room temperature for a minimum of 10 minutes;
10. Centrifuge the plate at 25 g for 15 seconds;
11. Set the plate at an angle of 45° in a non-vibrating surrounding and leave at this angle for at least 15 minutes. A Rhesus view box is very useful for this purpose;
12. Read the angled plates on a lighted box.

In a preliminary study 222 samples were tested in parallel in both the standard Cetus IHA method and the modified (micro) technique. The concordance was 99%. Four pools of CMV positive sera were also titrated in pooled CMV antibody negative sera and tested in both methods. No significant differences in the titres were observed.

References

1. Phipps DH, Grégoire L, Rossier E, Perry E. Comparison of five methods of cytomegalovirus antibody screening of blood donors. J Clin Microbiol 1983;18: 1296 – 1300.
2. Hunt AF, Allen DL, Brown RL, Robb BA, Packett AY, Entwistle CC. Comparative trial of six methods for the detection of CMV antibody in blood donors. J Clin Pathol 1984;37:95 – 7.
3. Henry SM, Ramirez AM, Woodfield DB. Micromodified cytomegalovirus antibody screening test. J Clin Pathol 1985;38:111 – 3.

* Terasaki plate is pretreated as follows to remove any static electricity: rinse the plate and cover in a solution of 0.05% Tween 20 in distilled water and leave to dry in air at room temperature.

STANDARDS AND QUALITY ASSURANCE

R.E. Klein

It is realized that the subjects of standards and quality assurance are not new. Some have had these activities for several years, but perhaps not all. It was stated at a meeting at the World Health Organization about five years ago that less than 25% of WHO member nations had any national standards or regulations pertaining to blood banking. Probably there has been some change in that figure because in most nations the numbers of patient care physicians has preogressively increased and most reporting nations are spending more money on health services based on WHO literature. So, it can be stated that regarding standards pertaining to blood banking it is "old hat" for some of us but futuristic for those in many nations.

Is there a need for national blood banking standards? Yes. Assuredly yes. While some medical directors may argue that standards are restrictive to their modes of operations this is usually minor and infrequent. Such problems usually arise in established blood banks or hospital transfusion services in large institutions. In these situations procedures were long ago established and those in authority resist change. However, the benefits far overwhelm those objections. The majority imparted by the standards helps to elevate and maintain the level of medical, technical and nursing performances in blood banks and transfusion services where the standards are followed.

It is highly preferable that the standards in each nation be authored by directors of blood banks and hospitals transfusion services, those who are knowledgeable in the art, active in the field. They are the most qualified for the task. The process of initial preparation and annual or biennial revision should be by consensus. Before finalization of initial and revised editions prepublication is recommended to obtain comments and criticisms from those who must implement the new standards.

The primary purposes of standards are to protect donors, patients and personnel from harm and to assure the therapeutic needs of patients. The standards should be minimum requirements and embody all aspects of blood banks and transfusion services from donor selection to post transfusion. It is preferable that standards be goal directed and state "what do" but not include technical advice, often referred to as "how do". This then allows medical directors and others of authority in each facility some freedom in technique selection so long as those selections meet the minimum requirements. The words "minimum requirements" do not mean the least possible level; rather they are realistic goals beneath which we should not operate.

The standards of one nation should not be adopted in toto by another nation unless the demographics, climates, populations, language and so forth are very similar. The use of standards of other nations as guides to subject matters is appropriate.

The standards should relate to criteria for donors and those items which cause deferral of blood donations. Such criteria are designated to protect the donor or the recipient or both. These donor criteria can not be the same in all nations. For example, in countries non-endemic for malaria there must be safeguards against accepting donors who rencently have been in a malarial endemic area. This more nearly assures the disease is not transmitted to recipients. On the other hand, in some malarial endemic countries to apply that same malaria standard would exclude all prospective donors. The same may be true of other endemic diseases. Another example is the total volume of blood to be drawn from donors routinely. It can not be the same in all nations because body size, therefore, circulating blood volume of the average prospective donor will differ. The amount whould not exceed 15% of the circulating volume of the smallest acceptable donor, including samples for testing of the donor blood.

The criteria for testing the units of donor blood must differ from nation to nation. If the native population is 100% $Rh_0(D)$ positive there is no reason for routine Rh testing of donor or patient bloods. Also, testing donor and patient bloods for unexpected antibodies to red cell antigens is not always possible because in some nations there are no reagent red blood cells available for that purpose. Likewise, testing for antibodies to HTLV-III/LAV can not be required in some nations because equipment and reagents are not available or there are no funds for purchase of the kits or there are no trained personnel.

If components are prepared from whole blood donations there should be criteria in the standards. Such criteria should declare minimum contents of cells or coagulation factors for which the components are intended. However, the criteria can not be the same in every nation because as previously stated the volume of blood drawn from donors is not the same.

The standards would be written with brevity and, based on those, each medical director, with the help of staff, should prepare a procedure manual unique for that blood bank or transfusion service (collectively called facilities). The facility procedure manual should detail all assigned personnel activities. A part of that manual should be details of quality assurance testing of personnel, reagents, equipment and blood components. The quality of any facility should be measurable by the recorded results and interpretations of the quality assurance programme. Rightfully such a programme begins with competency and proficiency testing of personnel. Personnel competency to perform assigned tasks should be assured when first employed prior to beginning assigned duties and subsequently before assigning new tasks. It is a means to assure that each person can perform as expected. Additionally, a proficiency testing programme should be utilized. This tests not only the individual performers but also the facility procedures. Proficiency testing is usually of extramural design while competency is usually of intramural origin. Proficiency is comparison of test interpretations from several facilities, evaluating each of those against reference facilities and the group of participants. To proceed with other aspects of quality assurance without first assuring the personnel and procedures may lead to unexplicable results in reagent, equipment and component quality assurance tets. The medical director should know what is expected of nursing, technical, and clerical employees and assure their knowledge and abilities.

But it should not end there. It is essential that the personnel are motivated properly. Those who participate must be cognizant of why quality assurance is essential to their work. If personnel do not appreciate the meanings and purposes of the quality assurance testing it becomes drudgery and done by rote, if at all.

Recent trends in reagent and equipment quality assurance testing is toward reduced volume and frequency with the intent to increase quality and meaningfulness of results. For example, if serologic centrifuge testing has been done at monthly intervals and review of past records reveals no problems for several or more months then consideration should be given to testing at 3 or 4 month intervals. Testing of reagent anti-A, anti-B and anti-D each day of use should be minimized as to scope. Mixing anti-A with B cells and anti-B with A cells is unnecessary each day of use and where large numbers of donor bloods are batch tested only a review of the recorded test results is sufficient to detect malfunctioning reagents. On the other hand, testing of reagent red cells and antiglobulin serum need to be assured each day of use, albeit the scope need be only very limited, because these reagents have the propensity of diminished reactivity. It seems appropriate to say that if you have not a quality assurance programme for reagents, equipment, components and personnel it is most advisable; conversely, if you do have a quality assurance programme it is recommended it be reviewed periodically to reduce excessiveness.

In summary, there are needs in many nations for blood banking standards. These should be prepared by consensus of knowledgeable medical directors, covering all apsects of blood banks and hospital transfusion services. Based on those brief, goal directed standards each facility medical director needs to provide a unique procedure manual for the nursing, technical and clerical personnel. A very important part of that manual is quality assurance testing of personnel, reagents, equipment and blood components. Each facility employee should appreciate the value of that quality assurance programme because it measures the quality of that facility.

DISCUSSION

Moderators: H.F. Polesky and R.L. McShine

H.F. Polesky (Minneapolis): Dr. Prins, one of the problems we have seen in the United States with barcoding is the failure for the hospital base systems and the Blood Bank systems to get together. I wonder what you have done to encourage uniformity. I still think our major problem is misidentification of the patient. The fact that there are two different kinds of barcode systems could potentially lead to some troubles.

H.K. Prins (Amsterdam): I took the example of Sweden, where they did the work so well. I know that also in The Netherlands people are beginning to try to connect patient files and donor files. There are two types of incompatibility, hardware and software incompatibility. The hospital system is different from the Blood Bank system; and the attitude in the hospital is different from that in the Blood Bank. But I think, and I hope, that people will come together, attitude-wise, hardware-wise, software-wise.

H.F. Polesky: I think it is extremely important that we in the Blood Bank, at least in the United States, adopt the uniform Barcode system. The hospitals have gone a different way. Perhaps with a microchip in the readers that are available, one can read two different ones, which will solve the problem. I still think it is important that we integrate from the Blood Centre to the bedside in some way, because that is where these barcodes have a great advantage.

C.F. Högman (Uppsal): I have a comment to Dr. Polesky's question. I think that the reason why the development concerning the patient's side has been rather slow is really hardware costs. There will be quite a change when we switch to micro-computers which are really inexpensive. When the software is there, we will see quite a change as well.

J.P.H.B. Sybesma (Dordrecht): Dr. von dem Borne, you pointed out very clearly the advantages of monoclonal antibodies. Will there be no disadvantages, too?

A.E.G. Kr. von dem Borne (Amsterdam): What are the advantages and disadvantages of monoclonal antibody immuno-assays?
   The advantages are the specificity (singel epitope) and the pure antibody. Impure antigen can be used because the antibody is so pure. However, the problem sometimes can be that the antibody is too specific and recognizes only subgroups of antigens. An important other problem is that the reaction of the antibody can be configuration-dependent.

Monoclonal antibody assays are very sensitive, provided that you have a high concentration, but that is always so with monoclonal antibodies. There should also be a high affinity; often monoclonal antibodies are selected in such a way that they have a low affinity. One can cope with that simply be selecting out monoclonal antibodies that have a high affinity for assays. The reproducibility is a unique feature, of all monoclonal antibodies, because you always have an identical antibody and it is available in a truly unlimited quantity. Everyone can use therefore the same antibody for the assays.

There are many advantages in the assay configurations in that you can alwaus apply an antibody excees, which cannot be done with polyclonal antibody immuno-assays, simply because the antibody titres are too low. You can use different epitopes to bind antigens; that gives you the two-sided immuno-assays. But the problem is that they are bad cross-linkers, because they only recognize one epitope; they are condition-sensitive and that is because the reaction may be configuration-dependent. But this is again a matter of selecting out the really good monoclonal antibodies for your assays.

The cost at present for monoclonal antibodies is quite high, and that is a disadvantage, but inflation will help us to solve this problem.

H.F. Polesky: Dr. von dem Borne, you talked about reproducibility in unlimited quantities, but is that really true when you go into commercial production? Have there not been some problems particularly in the non-mouse system of clones changing with time?

A.E.G. Kr. von dem Borne: The huan monoclonals?

H.F. Polesky: Right! The other question would relate to the issue of storage. How well will these store? I think that becomes another problem for the Blood Centre.

A.E.G. Kr. von dem Borne: I think that was a problem with the initial clones of human antibodies, because they were not stable and they were actually not monoclonal. The clones we have now are stable and for some years have produced the same antibodies, same class, same specificity – they do not change. Sometimes an interesting switch occurs of antibodies in monoclonal clones. What you see then is that some cells switch from one class to another, but the variable part of the antibody remains the same time. So, the properties and their capacity to bind complement may change, but the variable part remains the same.

C.Th. Smit Sibinga (Groningen): Dr. Friedman, your presentation was exciting as usual. I noticed from what you said that we are definitely going to see a shift in the workload and the training of the staff in the laboratory. That is one point. The other point is that once robotic equipment is operational, what do you think the impact will be on laboratory personnel?

L.I. Friedman (Bethesda): I think you will see some of the same changes you have seen in hospitals. A physician of today is not what a physician of ten years ago was. The physician of today may know some engeneering or computer science and relies on biomedical engeneering departments which have developed within hospitals. I think in the Blood Centre you will see a similar kind of shift. Physicians and technologists will have to become more familiar with micro-computers and automation, and centres may need to hire or consult with specialists more frequently. While instruments will replace many of the tedious aspects of a technologist's work, they will still be needed for specialized tests where instruments will not work. Instruments will not replace technologists, they will allow them to do more 'exciting' work. However, retraining or upgrading skills will be essential on a periodic base.

H.J. Loos (Amsterdam): Dr. Friedman, one of the things which I noticed was that, in your robot for loading and unloading the centrifuge, one of your major diffculties was that you had to handle multiple blood bags. In this respect, I wonder whether the solution of sterile connection devices would solve part of your problems in this instance, because in that case you could be collecting the blood in single bags and later on connecting them to a prepared pack of other bags. Would this not be a solution to your problems?

L.I. Friedman: One approach to solve the problem is, indeed, the use of sterile docking devices. The problem with sterile docking devices, as Dr. Prins indicated, is if we use them we have to ensure that labelling is transferred from the intial pack to the satellite packes.

Also sterile docking devices have been talked about for a number of years. They are not inexpensive, they may not be 'fail-safe' and I think it will be another several years before we see them commonly used.

But what we are trying to do is take our existing blood bag system and adapt instruments to it, rather than redesigning our blood bag system to be automated. If we want automation, just as the car industry has found out, you design the car to be automtically manufactured. So we all have to get together and design a blood bag system which can interface to automated instruments.

T.J. Greenwalt: Dr. Plapp, you pointed out that your problem with Rh-typing was a folding over, I believe, of a positive. It seemed to me that in the TV-monitor reading, you would still see a solid button towards the centre, or have you tried to reproduce folding over to see what happens, so that you do not get positive readings when you use the video scan?

F.V. Plapp (Kansas City): Yes, what happened in that one was actually a folding down of a positive reaction. It never does fold down enough that you get a small button as you do in a negative reaction. Therefore, the video camera does not call that a false negative.

H.F. Polesky: Is there a possibility of an intermediate reading on the video scan?

F. V. Plapp: The present system is not really black or white; it is on or off. We now have the software alsmost completed on our phase II of this system, where we will actually measuring gray levels within the well. We can do sixteen gray levels with the present computer system. This allows us to easily grade agglutination reactions as well as get intermediate readings in solid phase reactions. Phase III that we are developing, as soon as we get the funds to buy a more powerful computer, it will expand our capability to 256 gray levels. This will allow the same camera to read ELISA reactions, agglutination reactions and solid phase reactions.

H. F. Polesky: By using the gray scale, you think you can differentiate the colours in ELISA reactions.

F. V. Plapp: The human eye has a capacity for reading 40 gray levels. If you can read 200 gray levels with a computer, then you can have a very sensitive ELISA detector.

C. Th. Smit Sibinga: Dr. Plapp, the dipstick is, of course, a very exciting development. As you quite rightly pointed out, there might be a potential specifically in those countries who have a poor access to the more high-powered technology, which you presented in the first part of your presentation. The question I have in that respect is: Could you put the dipstick in the perspective of reagent use? How much does it reduce? Is it durable, can it last a long time? Is it easy to store? For instance, I have had an experience – Dr. Woodfield asked me several years ago: "Could we get access to a dry reagent for blood grouping?"; because he has a good friend of Sir Edmund Hillary, who regularly goes up to the Himalayas to support a hospital up there. But all reagents and all equipment must be carried up by man. It is freezing there and all reagents usually freeze and cannot be used – specifically cells. How about these dipsticks and their use up in the hills and mountains of Nepal? Could you say something about that?

F. V. Plapp: The stability of proteins – and specifically in this case antibodies – bound to these dipstics is much greater than it is in microplates. For some unknown reason, when you bind proteins to nylon or nitrocellulose membranes, even very labile proteins become very stable. So, it is possible to store antibodies on these dipsticks for months. At the present, I have stored these in a damp solution, but we know it is also possible to dry the dipsticks and keep them at room temperature for at least 6 months. The only requirement is that you wet the dipstick in saline before you add the red blood cells. As far as the cost, we buy large sheets of membranes which are 33 cm wide by 330 cm long and cut it into little 1.0×1.0 cm^2. So, the cost of the nylon membrane is less than a penny a test. One million of the monoclonal antibody makes over 2000 dipsticks; so the cost to make these dipsticks is about 2 US cents.

P. C. Das (Groningen): Dr. Plapp, you showed that there is a very good relationship with the recovery of the platelets, when you do the crossmatching.

It takes 45 minutes. That means, if you find a donor who is not compatible, the donor has to wait 45 minutes and go back home while you call another one.

F. V. Plapp: That is true. What we try to do now, since we are also having to do HTLV testing, is request the donors to come the day before. We draw a sample of blood and do our HTLV testing and the crossmatching, and call the most compatible donor back that day. We have that person come in to be scheduled for the next day. On an emergency basis, they do have to sit there and wait an hour before we know which donor is the best suited.

P. C. Das: Could you do that test with frozen platelets? If you freeze the platelets in advance with DMSO and put in liquid nitrogen and take them out before you call the donor the day before, could you crossmatch them?

F. V. Plapp: We have not done that, but other people say that you can freeze platelets on the microplate as a monolayer, and actually do ELISA testings. So I suspect you could the same type of testing with our tests on frozen platelet monolayers; but we have not tried it. I think it is a good idea.

J.P.H.B. Sybesma: Mr. McShine, how high is the percentage of the CMV negatives in Groningen and how is it changing with age?

R.L. McShine (Groningen): We have in Groningen 52% positive, 48% negative. We have not looked into the age distribution as yet.

C. Th. Smit Sibinga: Dr. Klein, your very first remark was that the implementation and the organization of standards, and writing them, is something which certainly is a future development in many nations. You mentioned the 25% of some years ago of the WHO. That number has perhaps increased a bit. As we learned from Dr. Ala's presentation, there are a number of nations that are developing and setting their strategies for the future, specifically in blood banking as part of the national health care. Not many nations have an organization like in the United States: An AABB. If there is an organization, that organization is not always so active or so powerful as the almost 40 years old AABB. Do you think going for standards, writing them, getting a consensus, and implementating them, should be within the jurisdiction of health authorities? Would that be a solution to getting things started? Should it be stimulated by the health authorities and referred to the professionals to write these standards and obtain consensus on them? What is your view on this?

R.E. Klein (Winston Salem): Voluntary participation I think is the answer, wherever possible, through peer review of those authors of the standards to their colleagues in the smaller facilities would be preferable. If at some point along the way, the program does not progress as you would hope, then you have to put teeth into it and ask for some kind of ecouragement 'from your governing bodies', so that they will participate; that they are actually promulgate their own standards, as they did in our country. I wonder if it really is necessary. At least there ought to be cooperation there, as there is now in our own nation. A much closer cooperation between the federal government and the blood bankers. I would say: It would be nice to be a voluntary program with encouragement from government, but if that does not work then I think that those in the hinterland should be encouraged a little bit more.

H.F. Polesky: One response to Dr. Smit Sibinga's question is that perhaps there is a role for a group like the ISBT, for example, through thier guideline mechanism. I think one of the problems one needs to address in underdeveloped countries is that you do not have in the government or even in the Blood Service the necessary technical expertise to put together such standards. Having just come from the ISBT retrovirus workshop in Washington – where we in fact tried to write some guidelines on this issue – I clearly recognize that there is a great difficulty in applying what we, in the developed countries, see as important criteria and what might be practical for the underdeveloped countries. Nevertheless, the expertise is there within that organization (ISBT)

C. Th. Smit Sibinga: I fully agree on that, and the reason why I asked Dr. Klein the question is not per se to have an answer in the field of voluntarism in the professional area, but in many developing countries it is a matter of economics, of budgeting. If one develops blood banking, which is just a minute share of the cake, then the amount of money put into the developments of Blood Banks and Blood Transfusion Services in these countries is of great value. I noticed in my travals that involvement of the government is more or less a must, to see that the money spent on this planning is being spent well, and that once one has organized Blood Transfusion Services and National Centres one has to be sure that they do function according to a standard.

H.F. Polesky: Dr. Klein, it seems to me that one of the deficiencies in the standards that we have in the United States is that we have never tackled the issue of blood utilization criterion. I wonder if, certainly in the developed countries, this is an area we ought to be venturing into. Would you comment on this.

R.E. Klein: In our standards there are quite a few peripherals. Testing of blood warmers and neonatal transfusions which are often done by the neonatologists, and outpatient transfusion commonly under the supervision and control of internists – and there are more. So, we have a fair number of peripherals in our standards. Once it is part of the standards, we have to inspect to be sure. It would not surprise me a bit to see them encroaching on in-house transfusion therapy before long.

H.F. Polesky: For example, the Joint Commission on Accreditation of Hospitals, which is an organization that inspects hospitals in the United

States, requires that every transfusion done in the hospital be reviewed unless you establish that the blood is properly utilized. It seems to me that we ought to be leading in assuring that blood is appropriately used.

IV. Clinical aspects

RECENT CHANGES IN PATIENT POPULATION: A MISSION FOR BLOOD BANKS

C. Coffe, P. Hervé, Y. Couteret, M. Masse, B. Lamy, E. Racadot, A. Peters

Introduction

In 1975, the mission of blood banks was above all transfusion safety. We had three main activities: the collection of blood, the control and the quality of blood products and their distribution. Concurrently cytapheresis, plasma exchanges and cryobiology of red blood cells were created.

In the last five years, numerous changes in the activities of blood banks have occurred. The Regional Blood Centers provide a network through which a wide variety of clinical research and development programmes can be undertaken:

1. They attempt to provide specific transfusion products for each clinical indication (leukocyte poor red blood cells or platelets). They only deliver patients the cells needed. Thus there is more efficient use of the available resources and a reduction in outdating (also partly related to the longer shelf life of products collected).
2. The focus has been on the development of products which are not only effective but also safe. Blood banks attach importance to transfusion safety for both immunological (compatibility, immunisation prevention and so on) and infectious (disease transmission) reasons.

These changes of techniques or activities have three main origins:

1. In some cases, blood banks themselves have increased the quality of blood products delivered (for example, preservation of some products such as red blood cells or platelets).
2. In other cases, patient treatment has forced blood banks to adapt to new requirements (for example irradiation of blood).
3. In still other cases, medical teams have asked blood banks to take the responsability of new activities because blood banks were already implicated in technique very close to these new activities (for example processing of bone marrow, cryopreservation of tissues).

The purpose of this paper is to present all the new changes which have occurred recently in blood banking and the future developments.

Obtaining specific products for each clinical indication

A. Red blood cells

(1) Leukocyte poor red cells: Before 1984, in France frozen red cells were the product of choice to decrease the risk of immunization and especially severe and/or repeated febrile non hemolytic transfusion reactions. Since this date, the use of filters to obtain leukocyte poor red cells has increased because they are cheaper, the ease of production and the use few materials [1]

The results of a comparative study of 6 filters in our blood bank on whole blood stored for six to ten days are shown in table 1. The frozen red cells which have lower levels of residual leukocytes are kept for recipients with aplastic anemia or who are undergoing bone marrow transplantation in mismatch situation, for highly sensitized recipients in kidney transplantation, and for patients who have some reactions with the leukocyte poor concentrates prepared by filtration or centrifugation. The future will show if the leukocyte poor red cell concentrates are as efficient as the frozen red cell concentrates, in the reduction of the immunization rate or in the decrease of unwanted immunization of leukocyte antigens.

(2) The neocytes are relatively young red cells with a mean cell age of 30 days and a potential survival of 90 days. They may be obtained either from packs of donor blood, or with blood cell separators. They enable a decrease of 20% in transfusions in patients requiring chronic transfusions, to reduce iron loading and to increase red cell circulating half life [2]. But this approach now is expensive and time consuming. In the future, two ways of research must be developed: the first is the obtaining of a greater hemoglobin level in the bag of neocytes and the second is the decrease of cost.

Table 1. Preparation of leukocyte poor red cells, comparative study of 5 filtration techniques.

	Erypur G2	Imugard	Maco-pharma	Miropore L	Sepacell 500
Composition	Cellulose acetate	Cotton wool	Cellulose acetate	Cotton wool	Cellulose acetate
Technique	Manual use or mechanical device	Manual use	Manual use	Manual use	Manual use
Leukocyte removed (%)	98	97	93	97	98

B. Platelet concentrates

(1) *Single donor platelet:* The need for platelet concentrate from single donors has increased. We only deliver this type of platelet concentrates either to patients who are immunized (crossmatching with a microcytotoxicity technique) or to patients in need of future transfusion support (for example: allogenic bone marrow transplant recipients). Platelets obtained by cytapheresis may be stored for only 24 hours if the method of preparation utilizes an open collection system and if the concentrte contains a white blood cell count greater than 1×10^9. A storage of 5 days is possible for platelets collected within a completely closed system with a blood cell separator providing leukocyte poor platelet concentrates (Haemonetics V50 and Fenwal CS 3000). Moreover, it is necessary to leave an appropriate volume of plasma (platelet function and pH), to agitate platelet concentrate appropriately during 22°C storage, and to use new platelet storage bags (Polyolefin plastic: Fenwal PL 732 or polyvinylchloride plastic with tri-2-ethylhexyl trimellitate: Cutter CLX, Fenwal PL 1240) [3,4,5].

This new possibility has changed the management of the frozen platelet bank. We onlyt keep in the liquid nitrogen phase autologous platelets from patients who are immunized and allogenic HLA typed platelets according tot he phenotype of the patients who undergo bone marrow transplantation (BMT). The latest application is to keep some PL[A1] negative units for newborns with isoimmune neonatal thrombocytopenia (the incidence of this condition is estimated at one out of 3600 live births).

(2) *Leukocyte poor platelets:* Leukocyte poor concentrates may be prepared by filtration of platelet suspension through cotton wool filters [6]. This method removes 95 to 100% of leukocyte ($<1.10^8$) and the platelet loss is less than 10% but does not remove red blood cells (necessity to keep ABO compatibility). A comparative study of 4 filters carried out in our blood bank is shown in table 2.

Table 2. Leukocyte poor platelet concentrates, comparative study of 4 filtration techniques.

	Sepacell R500 Asahi medical	Erypur G2 Organon Teknika	Imugard IG500 Terumo	Miropore L Travenol SA
Processing time (mn) Range	5 (4 – 6)	12 (11 – 13)	25 (22 – 29)	16 (13 – 20)
Platelet loss (%)	16 (8 – 22)	14 (9 – 24)	11 (5 – 20)	11 (9 – 33)
% of removed leukocytes	92.8 ± 1.6	96 ± 2	95 ± 2	92.5 ± 2.5

C. Leukocytes concentrates

Since 1982 in Besançon, we have decreased the use of such concentrates in pancytopenic patients because:
1. we have been able to improve response to antibiotic therapy, by using newer and better antibiotics and new protocols of antibiotics with closer and better monitoring of antibiotic regimens and by an earlier introduction of empiric antifungal therapy on patients in sterile rooms or laminar air flow rooms [7];
2. of the high incidence of alloimmunization and of transmissible diseases (CMV infection is in close relationship with the number of white cell transfusions in seronegative recipients).

At present prophylactic granulocyte transfusions cannot be recommended. For the curative indication of leukocyte concentrates, the daily dose is the most improtant point (5 to 7×10^8 granulocytes per kg per day) [8].
In the future:
a. explorations into enrichment of one cell type or another should improve the product because the current collection is a combination of granulocytes, monocytes and lymphocytes (for example with regards to monocytes, some investigations are currently undertaken in the United States);
b. ways of reducing antigenicity would be of particular value to reduce the impact of histocompatibility factors. A safer product is desirable in particular to reduce reactions and to eliminate the transmission of disease [9]. The technology for long term culture of human granulocytes could also be explored.

D. Hemopoietic stem cells

Autologous and/or allogenic bone marrow transplantations play a more and more important role in blood banks. Seven years ago, this activity was not an integral part of our dedicated expertise. But being in the position of performing cell separation, we were led to investigate and carry out various methods of hemopoietic stem cell concentration because of the basic equipment, environment, and technical skills available. From our own experience concerning bone marrow harvesting (120 autologous and 52 allogenic bone marrow transplantations), we will expose all changes and new activities that we have developed.

The first point is that BMT provides us with an interesting opportunity to manage a new category of patients. Although, the need for blood and components to support BMT patients has generally increased, these needs are relatively modest as shown in figure 1.

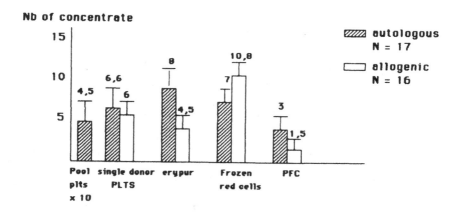

Figure 1. Blood transfusion supportive care during the bone marrow transplantation (CRTS Besançon 1985).

1. Stem cells from bone marrow

(a) Processing of the bone marrow

The necessity to reduce the volume of bone marrow for freezing or further in vitro treatment before transplation has led us to use several methods for the concentration of stem cells. The main goals of all procedures are to recover the majority of stem cells, to redcue the volume, to eliminate red blood cells (which could have an anti complementary activity and in the case of ABO incompatible transplantation to avoid plasma exchanges), polymorphonuclear cells (which fix on specifically monoclonal antibodies and also have an anti complementary activity) and platelets [10]

Table 3 shows the results obtained by the different teams in France, with different methods. The technique with Ficoll IBM 2991 appears to be the best one. Our experience has led us to propose a definition of product to be obtained after processing with a volume lower than 200 ml. a hematocrit lower than 1%, a granulocyte cell contamination lower than 10% of initial value, a CFU GM higher than 60 to 10×10^6 per kg with a final recovery higher than 70% [11]. In the future, the most important point to develop is the search for a technique enabling the obtainign of a product with less than 1% hematocrit and good yield without ficoll hypaque gradient.

(b) Ex vivo manipulation:

1. In autologous situations: The BMT programme requires the development of new procedures for the ex vivo manipulation of harvested stem

Table 3. Processing of bone marrow results of different teams in France with 6 methods.

Manipulations		H30 CNTS Paris 30	V50 CTS St.Louis Paris 56	Dideco Vivacell Hotel Dieu Paris 30	Ficoll IBM 2991 CRTS Besançon 90	IBM 2997 Besaçon, Strassbourg 15	CS 3000 CTS Bordeaux 10
Volume ml							
	Initial	760 ± 129	1120 ± 530	714 ± 192	419 ± 122	1159 ± 282	1000 ± 100
	Final	163 ± 31	118 ± 41	242 ± 68	94 ± 2.3	129 ± 4	190 ± 10
	%	22 ± 7	11 ± 5	34	24 ± 9	11 ± 5	19 ± 2
RBC × 10^9							
	Initial	2800 ± 900	3120 ± 980	2230 ± 730	1775 ± 39	3419 ± 1335	3120 ± 1000
	Final	252 ± 70	91 ± 51	47 ± 19	5.8 ± 2.3	68 ± 58	260 ± 180
	%	9 ± 9	3 ± 2	2.1	0.32 ± 0.5	1.8 ± 0.9	8.3 ± 3.5
Platelets × 10^9							
	Initial	49 ± 24		154 ± 113	68 ± 24	173 ± 84	
	Final	19.6 ± 5	49 ± 23	72 ± 60	29 ± 13	7 ± 34	
	%	41 ± 23		46.7	44 ± 12	43 ± 15	
Nucleated cells × 10^9							
	Initial	14.1 ± 10	17 ± 11	21.2 ± 7.9	16 ± 5	27.7 ± 8.8	
	Final	9.2 ± 6.5	7 ± 3	3.7 ± 1.6	3.2 ± 1	5.6 ± 2.2	46.3
	%	65 ± 9	48 ± 4	18 ± 6	20 ± 4	20.2 ± 6.8	
Mononucleated cells × 10^9 (1)							
	Initial	2.6 ± 1.2	2 ± 0.9	3.3 ± 1.3	2.6 ± 1	4.0 ± 1.6	
	Final	1.9 ± 1.0	1.5 ± 0.8	1.9 ± 0.7	2 ± 0.5	3.0 ± 1.5	
	%	73 ± 23	74 ± 25	58 ± 14	73 ± 17	75.0 ± 16	93.2 ± 17.1
Granulocytes × 10^9 (2)							
	Initial	10.5 ± 7.8	12.7 ± 9.7	13.5 ± 6	11.2 ± 4.1	14.5 ± 6.8	7.6 ± 2.8
	Final	6.1 ± 4.8	4.6 ± 3.3	0.9 ± 0.6	0.3 ± 0.2	1.3 ± 0.86	0.9 ± 0.9
	%	58 ± 18	46 ± 28	7 ± 3	2.5 ± 1.5	8.9 ± 4.98	11.8 ± 13.6
CFU GM × 10^5 (3)							
	Initial	9 ± 10	18.6 ± 14.8	23.2 ± 13	13 ± 8.2	16.2 ± 10.9	
	Final	7.6 ± 8.4	14.4 ± 8.1	18.2 ± 12	10 ± 6.3	12 ± 5.6	
	%	84 ± 18	78 ± 19	75.8 ± 22	74 ± 16	74 ± 30.2	63.6 ± 22.5
Procedure time (mn)		150				90	90

cells. In autologous grafts, four methods are mainly used in attempting the removal of contaminating tumor cells before cryopreservation: the use of chemical agents such as 4-hydroperoxcyclophosphamide (4-HC), mafosfamide-cyclohexylamine (Asta Z-7557), mafosfamide-L-lysine (Z-7654) and etoposide (VP-16-213), complement-mediated cytotoxicity using anti CALLA or anti T monoclonal antibodies, immunotoxin (T 101-Ricin, A or A + B chains), immunomagnetic removal have demonstrated their feasibility [12,13]. The combination of chemical agents with cytotoxic monoclonal antibodies is under investigation in some laboratories. If the feasibility of most methods has been demonstrable in open pilot studies, we do not have reliable and reproducible techniques to assess the efficiency of in vitro treatments.

2. In allogenic situations, T cell depletion is required to prevent graft versus host disease (GvHD). Many ex vivo methods are applied to T cell depletion. Methylprednisolone was a failure. Elutration was employed with success in The Netherlands. E-rosetting in combiantion with soybean agglutinin can deplete marrow of T lymphocytes, because these cells were shown to reveal the receptor for soybean agglutinin while stem cells did not.

Cytotoxic monoclonal antibodies covalently linked to toxins are currently being applied to deplete human marrow of T lymphocytes. The cellular immunoadsorption and immunomagnetic removal have not yet been applied to human models.

In our pilot study of 45 patients who received a T cell depleted bone marrow allograft, two pan T antibodies were used: OKT11/CD2 with OKT3/CD3. We only observed two actue GvHD grade II and no graft failure or late rejection occurred [14]. Te evaluate the efficacy of T cell depletion, we dispose a panel of in vitro methods: for example the flow cytometry [15], the double labelling of immunofluorescence, and the limiting dilution assay.

Another new mission for blood banks in BMT is the quality control of animal reagents (baby rabbit complement, monoclonal antibodies) used for ex vivo and pilot clinical in vivo studies and perhaps also, in the future, blood banks, might produce their own reagents.

(c) Thirty to thirty five percent of patients have an HLA identical donor in siblings. For the others, donors have to be parental haploidentical persons or volunteers. These volunteers will be chosen from a national bone marrow volunteer donor panel in which blood banks will be implicated. They will participate in the selection of donors, education and information campaigns, HLA typing and the establishment of listing by computers.

2. Stem cells from peripheral blood

At present, many teams are working on the posibility of obtaining an adequate number of peripheral stem cells by leukapheresis either from donors or from patients with AML after the induction of chemotherapy in view of autologous BMT during the complete remission.

234

E. Plasma and plasma derivatives

(a) We think that future well-conceived studies will further clarify the specific needs for fresh frozen plasma and other plasma derivatives because the majority of patients who receive these components could be managed more effectively with other and safer forms of treatment [16,17].

(b) Another way of development is the increase of yield in factor VIII or von Willebrand factor. For example, heparin [18] and, as recently proposed by a Swedish team, the stimulation of plasma donors with a vasopressin analogue (DDAVP stimate) that could increase the normal level of factor VIII and Von Willebrand factor three times [19].

(c) In the future, new products could be improved such as biological glue for surgery, fibronectin concentrate (infections, acute respiratory detress syndrome), antithrombin III (large scale preparation of highly purified antithrombine III concentrate) [20].

(d) The need for preventing cytomegalovirus (CMV) infection is a new mission for blood banks. Blood banks must participate in CMV prevention by providing CMV hyperimmune globulin which has an activity eight times superior to that of polyvalent intravenous immunoglobulins. Blood banks must also deliver blood products collected from CMV negative donors or frozen blood products to patients who are CMV negative and immuno-deficient [21,22]. The indications for CMV negative blood product are shown in table 4.

Table 4. Indication for blood product collected from CMV negative donors.

---

1. Absolute indications:
   - sero negative patient with transplantation (bone marrow, or liver)
   - sero negative low birth weight premature infants (< 1200 g)
   - congenital immune deficiency syndromes

2. Relative indications:
   - intra uterine transfusions in sero negative mother
   - neonatal exchange transfusion
   - sero negative AIDS
   - pregnancy

F. Irradiation of blood products

Table 5 summarizes the doses from which there will be radiation side effects on red cells, platelets and granulocytes. Future studies are necessary to specify what radiation dose will be recommended as safe and effective between 2000 and 4500 rads for the prevention of posttransfusion GvHD. The indications for blood product irradiation are the following: patients at highest risk of developing post transfusion GvHD include patients with aplastic anemia, children with severe congenital immune deficiences and recipients of allogenic or autologous bone marrow grafts. Of lesser risk of

Table 5. Radiation side effects on blood products.

Red cell	exposure > 10,000 rads
Platelet	exposure > 5,000 rads
Granulocytes	exposure > 5,000 rads
Lymphocytes	exposure > 2,000 rads
	(is likely to eliminate lymphocyte mitotic ability and to prevent GvHD)

GvHD are infants receiving intra uterine and exchange transfusions and patients receiving immuno suppressive chemotherapy for treatment of lymphoma and acute leukemia. The routine use of irradiated blood is not recommended for solid tumors except for patients heavily treated and for patients with acquired immune deficiency syndrome (AIDS). These last indications need to be specified in the future [23,24].

Blood bank and organ transplantation

(A) For kidney transplantations, many studies are ongoing to prove the role of transfusion before transplantation from family donors. The frequency of first rejection episodes in patients that received transplants of sibling HLA identical grafts was not influenced by blood transfusions done prior to transplantation. In patients receiving one haplotype mismatched graft, significantly more rejections were seen in the non transfused group (85% with rejection) compared with the transfused group (58%) [25].

(B) In liver and heart transplantations, blood banks are involved. Liver transplantation is associated with factors tending to increase the difficulty in providing adequate blood products (RBC, platetes). Time between donor organ harvest and transplantation must be less than 12 hours, and the procedure takes 6 to 12 hours to perform, bleeding may be very important as a result of poor hemostatic recipient capabilities and technical difficulty in the surgical procedure for liver transplantation making unusual demands on the blood bank. P. Butler [26] has recently shown:

a. the frequency distribution of per-operative red cell use;
b. the strong correlation between units transfused and patient outcome;
c. the relation between intra-operative blood use and the patient's primary diagnosis. Sclerosing cholangitis and cirrhosis require greater quantities of red blood cells.

When the recipient is immunized, additional planning is required. A satisfactory approach is to use cross-matched negative red cells for the antibody specificity for the first 10 to 20 units. If bleeding continues, only ABO-compatible blood is given. Administration of antigen negative blood is then resumed for the estiamted final 10 to 20 units.

(C) Role of blood banks in cryobiology. This activity was developed because much of the physical and administrative machinery required was present in blood banks. The cryobiology unit keeps its activity of preservation of blood cells and samples of leukemic cells obtained at the time of the initial diagnosis of leukemia for the retrospective analysis of immunological diagnosis, or to establish the immunological phenotype in view of the selection of monoclonal antibodies for in vitro treatment, and so on. This unit has two other main roles: tissue banking and research of new methods of cryopreservation. Blood banks participate in donor selection, tissue procurement, tissue processing and storage. At present, blood banks cryopreserve corneal tissue (for emergencies or for keratoplastia), skin (in patients with traumatic dermal denudations or major thermal injuries), bone (for treating fractures, filling bone cysts, for cervical spine fusions). Fascia, arteries and nerves are also frozen.

Two new methods of cryopreservation are to be developed in the very near future:

1. Freeze drying which avoids the surface tension effects, maintains the biochemical integrity and solubility and enables the storage of specimen at room $T°$. Some success has been obtained with fascia and nerves.
2. Vitrification has led to success with monocytes and embryos [27,28]

New laboratories and changes in the others

(1) In immunohematology, there has been both a general increase activity and a need for some special red cell serologic procedures. There has been an increase in routine serologic tests to determine red cell compatibility and also in the typing of red blood cells or in the research of sex chromonsome chimerism to distinguish donor from patient cells enabling the determination of engraftment after bone marrow transplantation.

(2) In immunology, there has been a increase in the HLA typing for cytapheresis donors, bone marrow recipient and recipient family; for HLA mismatch graft and in the phenotype of donors in view of bone marrow graft in unrelated situations. given the increased understanding of the D/DR locus, the histocompatibility laboratories have at their disposal new methods for exploring the HLA phenotype in mismatched situation.

(3) Laboratories for detection of transfusion transmissible disease: Recently, an increasing activity has developed for the detection of CMV negative HTLV-III/LAV negative donors. In the future, numerous investigations must be undertaken in order to try:

a. to discover new assay in the detection of hepatitis B virus genome or of non-A non-B hepatitis and so on;
b. to improve the sensitivity of anti HTLV-III/LAV tests to identify all false reactives (false negative and false positive).

(4) Production of monoclonal antibodies: Some blood banks will develop production of monoclonal antibodies against red blood cell antigens, intact human platelets or specific T (or B) cell antigens for diagnostic use [29,30].

The production of human monoclonal antibodies (conjugated with drugs, toxins, or isotopes to improve their target effectiveness) should prove useful for the prevention and treatment of disease (in the treatment of leukemia, lymphoma, neuroblastoma). This technology is beginning to develop clinical applications.

(5) The quality control laboratory will become more and more important with the development of all the laboratories and the above-mentioned activities. This laboratory must enable the demonstration of the quality of products, their biological efficacy and eventually their acceptable tolerance and their harmlessness.

(6) Robotics: With further modifications, a completely robotized preparation of blood components will soon be possible. Numerous investigations are trying to demonstrate the feasibility of automatic devices:

a. for producing from centrifuged blood a cell poor plasma, a buffy coat and leukocyte poor red blood cells;

b. for dispensing and preparing samples in some laboratory techniques (anti LAV/HTLVIII and HBsAg testings) thereby avoiding risks of contamination for technicians [31].

Other activities

(1) *Preservative solutions:* (to extend the storage time for whole blood) [32]. The primary goals of these solutions are to maintain viability and function of red cells and to prevent physical changes detrimental to red cells. They should prevent clotting and provide proper nutrients for continued metabolism of cells during storage. One of the first optional additive solutions was SAGM (saline, adenine, dextrose and mannitol) which enabled the storage of blood for up to 35 days [32]. Numerous researchers are trying to discover new solutions to enable storage for up to 52 or 49 days, for example in ADSOL AS-1 (additive solution with saline, adenine, dextrose and mannitol: Fenwal laboratories) and PAGGSS (phosphate, adenine, guanosine, glucose, saline: Biotest laboratories). With these last solutions, 82% of cells are viable 24 hours after the transfusion and the percentage of initial value of ATP is more than 75% [33].

(2) *Therapeutic apheresis:* Speculation seems to focus mainly on greater specificity. Progress is expected:

a. in the research of fundamental pathophysiology;

b. in the definition of the modalities (for a given patient how much plasma exchanges must be practiced, with what frequency, at what volume, and what treatment must be associated?).

In the future, many indications must be confirmed or specified. Techniques, enabling the removal of specific proteins from plasma while the remainder are returned to the patient, will soon become available. One of the available machines permits the removal of cold precipitable immune complexes while preserving the patient's plasma albumin and coagulation factors. Similar machines are readily applicable to affinity column perfusion. Columns may be coated with a variety of substances which have a specific affinity. For example, protein A which removes IgG from plasma, or DNA collodion which reduce DNA antibodies, immune complexes. Columns coated with monoclonal antibody will be able to remove specific subsets of T lymphocytes from the blood [34].

(3) *Red cell substitutes:* The usefullness of various human blood substitutes, such as fluosol DA 20% and polymerized hemoglobin must receive increasing scrutiny [35].

Conclusion

In the future, the development of additional missions of blood banks, in order to assure the clinical treatment of new patients, is to be envisaged. The revolution in the activity of blood banks as begun in the 1970s, will continue in the next 5 to 10 years. Particularly in genetic engineering (recombinant DNA technology to commercially produce several proteins such as factor VIII, insuline, plasminogen activator), large scale human hematopoietic cell culture (human long term marrow on cell culture as a source of human stem cells for clincial purposes obtaining of an in vitro growth technique of pure human multipotential stem cells, such as the one already obtained in experimental models by Van Bekkum in 1984), monoclonal antibody production, in vitro manipulations of cells for avoiding platelet immunization (modification with cyclosporin or ultraviolet light), suppression of the recipient's immune response before transfusion. Thus, we can conclude on an optimistic note of future development in our blood banks.

Acknowledgement

The author is indebted to Mrs. M.C. Bichet for typing the manuscript.

References

1. Mijovic V, Brozovic B, Hughes ASB, Davies TD. Leukocyte-depleted blood. A comparison of filtration techniques. Transfusion 1983;23:30 – 2.
2. Marcus RE. The preparation and use of young red cells. Apheresis Bulletin 1983;1:125 – 31.
3. Murphy S, Kahn RA, Holme S, Phillips GL, Sherwood W, Davisson W, Buchholz DH. Improved storage of platelets for transfusion in a new container. Blood 1982;60:194 – 200.
4. Lamy B. La conservation in vitro des plaquettes dans les nouveaux plastiques utilisables en transfusion sanguine. In: CRTS (ed) Rapports des séances plénières du congrès national d'Hématologie et de Transfusion sanguine, Bordeaux 1985:154 – 66.
5. Simon TL, Nelson EJ, Carmen R, Morphy S. Extension of platelet storage. Transfusion 1983;23:207 – 12.

6. Sirchia G, Parravicini A, Rebulla P, Bertolini F, Moralati F, Marconi M. Preparation of leukocyte free platelets for transfusion by filtration through cotton wool. Vox Sang 1983;44:115 – 20.

7. Greene WH. The role of the newer beta-lactam antibiotics in the treatment of infection in compromised hosts. Bull NY Acad Med 1984;60:426 – 38.

8. Wright DG. Leukocyte transfusions thinking twice. Am J Med 1984;76: 637 – 44.

9. Herzig RH. Granulocyte transfusion therapy: past, present and future. In: Garratty G (ed). Current concepts in transfusion therapy. Arlington VA, AABB 1985:267 – 94.

10. McCullough J. Role of blood bank in bone marrow transplantation. In: Weiner S (ed). Bone marrow transplantation. Arlington VA, AABB 1983: 101 – 22.

11. Lopez M, Andreu G, Beaujean F, Ehrsam A, Gerota J, Hervé P. Human bone marrow processing in view of further in vitro treatment and cryopreservation. In: Hervé P, Gorin NC (eds). Recent advances in autologous bone marrow transplantation in oncohematology. Librairie Arnette Paris Publishers, 1986:200.

12. Hervé P, Cahn JY, Plouvier E, Tamayo E, Leconte des Floris R, Peters A. Autologous bone marrow transplantation for acute leukemia using transplant chemo-purified with metabolite of oxazaphosphosines (ASTA Z 7557, INN mafosfamide). First Clinical Results. Investigational New Drugs 1984;2: 245 – 52.

13. Hervé P, Tamayo E, Cahn JY, Plouvier E, Flesch M, Peters A. Attempts to eliminate residual acute myeloid leukemia from autologous bone marrow grafts through in vitro chemotherapy. A review. In: Löwenberg B, Hagenbakc A (eds). Minimal residual disease in acute leukemia. Martinus Nijhoff Publishers, Dordrecht, Boston, Lanchaster, 1986 (in press).

14. Hervé P. Methods for ex vivo purging of bone marrow of residual tumor cells or GvHD producing T cells. A review. Plasma Ther Transfus Technol 1985;6:359 – 64.

15. Laerum OD, Farsund T. Clinical application of flow cytometry: a review. Cytometry 1981;2:1 – 13.

16. Smit Sibinga CTh, Das PC. Uses and abuses of single donor plasma. In: Plasma products: uses and management. Arlington VA, AABB 1982:29 – 31.

17. Oberman HA. Uses and abuses of Fresh Frozen Plasma. In: Garratty G (ed). Current concepts in Transfusion Therapy. Arlington VA, AABB 1985: 109 – 24.

18. Smit Sibinga CTh, Das PC. Heparin factor VIII. Scand J Haematol 1984; 33(suppl.40):111 – 22.

19. Mikaelson M, Nilsson IM, Vichardi H, Wiechel B. Factor VIII concentrate prepared from blood donors stimulated by intranasal administration of a vasopressin analogue. Transfusion 1982;22:229 – 33.

20. Wickerhauser M, Williams C. A single-step method for the isolation of antithrombin III. Vox Sang 1984;47:397 – 405.

21. HO M, Dowling JN. Cytomegalovirus infection in transplant and cancer patients. In: Remington JS, Schwartz MN (eds). Current clinical topics in infectious diseases. New York: Mc Graw Mill, 1980:45 – 67.

22. Winston DJ, Ho WG, Howell CL. Cytomegalovirus infections associated with leukocyte transfusions. Ann Inter Med 1980;93:671 – 75.

23. Letiman SF, Holland PV. Irradiation of blood products: indication and guidelines. Transfusion 1985;25:293 – 304.

24. Button LN, DeWolf WC, Newburger PE, Jacobson MS, Kevy SV. The effects of irradiation on blood components. Transfusion 1981;21:419 – 26.

25. Solheim BG, Flatmark A, Halvorsen S, Jervell J, Pape J, Thorsby E. Effect of blood transfusions on renal transplantation: Transplantation 1980;30: 281 – 4.

26. Butler P, Israel L, Nusbacher J, Jenkins DE, Startzl TE. Blood transfusion in liver transplantation. Transfusion 1985;25:120 – 3.

27. Meryman HT. Principles of cryopreservation and the current role of frozen red blood cells in blood banking and clinical medicine. In: Glassman AB, Umlas J (eds). Cryopreservation of tissue and solid organs for transplantations. Arlington BA, AABB 1983:1 – 12.

28. Rall WF, Fahy GM. Ice free cryopreservation of mouse embryos at – 196°C by vitrification. Nature 1985;313:573 – 5.

29. Salmon Ch. Monoclonal antibodies in immunohematology. In: Abstracts of the 18th Congress of the ISBT Munich (GFR), July 22 – 27, 1984:14

30. Bron D, Feinberg M, Teng N, Kaplan H. Production of human monoclonal IgG antibodies against Rhesus (D) antigen. Proc Nat Acad Scie (USA) 1984;81:3214 – 8.

31. Friedman LI. Applications of robotics in blood banking. In: Smit Sibinga CTh, Das PC, Greenwalt TJ (eds). Future developments in bloodbanking. Martinus Nijhoff Publishers, Dordrecht, Boston, Lancaster, 1986.

32. Hogman CF, Aekerblom O, Hedlund K, Rosen I, Wiklund L. Red cell suspensions in SAGM medium. Further experience of in vivo survival of red cells, clinical usefulness and plasma-saving effects. Vox Sang 1983;45:217.

33. Hessian O, Noel L, Fabre G, Saint Blancard, Saint Paul B. Determination du taux de recirculation à 24 h d'hématies autologues conservées au dela de la durée légale (42 – 49 jours). Un double marquage est-il nécessaire. Journal de biophysique et biomédicine 1985;9:188 – 92.

34. Pineda AA. Future directions of apheresis. In: Kolins J, Jones J (eds). Therapeutic apheresis. Arlington WA, AABB 1983:99 – 109.

35. International forum. Which is the foreseeable clinical application and impact of oxygen carrying blood substitutes (fluocarbons and hemoglobin solutions)? Which impact they likely to have on the activity of blood services? Vox Sang 1982;42:97 – 109.

PERSPECTIVES IN SUPPORTIVE HEMOTHERAPY

C.Th. Smit Sibinga

Introduction

The principle perspective in supportive hemotherapy should lie in ongoing efforts to minimize sofar unavoidable risks together with sincere endeavours to optimize clinical efficacy as a fundamental goal in patient care. The continuing process of recognition of both risks and benefits of hemotherapy encourages a better understanding of the role of the Blood Bank in clinical transfusion practice. Blood transfusion as a clinical discipline is well on its way to be fully respected. The profession develops the understanding and respect grows, its position in the clinical team becomes more circumscript, evident and accepted.

Developments in clincial transfusion practice

Developments in therapeutic approaches to chronic and acute diseases needing supportive hemotherapy, demand an anticipative attitude from the Blood Bank as well as a balanced symbiotic relationship between clinician and blood banker. There is an ongoing need for more specific support in hemotherapy, fulfilling criteria of increased safety, purity and potency, resulting in optimization of clinical efficacy. Clinical transfusions practice part of patient care and strategy.

The most relevant fields of development, deserving a perspective discussion are oncology, transplantation, neonatology and hemophilia care. Besides, surgical procedures and hemapheresis are of importance when discussing perspectives in supportive hemotherapy.

1. Oncology

Developments in public education and diagnostic approaches have their impact on increased efforts to develop therapeutic strategies, aiming for complete eradication of the cancer process. These strategies usually are effected through intense total body irradiation and ablative cancer chemotherapy, and unavoidably lead the patient into a transient but very dangerous period of severe immunocompromittence and often total bone marrow aplasia. It is apparent that the benefits of this approach in terms of cancer treatment efficacy are totally dependent on the possibilities for a balanced hemotherapy support and adequate infection prevention. The latter can be achieved through selective gut decontamination and adequate disinfection regimes. Balancing the hemotherapy support is a more complex issue, depending very much on the knowledge of and insight in the specific clinical problems. The patient's condition of immunocompromittence does increase the risks, both immunologic and infection, of blood transfusion.

On the other hand the need for optimal functional behaviour of cells and proteins is of paramount importance to safeguard the clinical efficacy of the hemotherapy support on oncology patients.

2. Bone marrow transplantation

Both in the solid organ and hematological oncology bone marrow transplantation has reached the state of accepted routine. However, the motives for and the place in the strategy of therapy are different. In solid organ oncology, bone marrow transplantation of autologous type has a rescue function. The ablative cancer chemotherapy and irradiation therapy unavoidably do eradicate the patients own bone marrow stem cells. By harvesting autologous stem cells before the eventual ablative therapy, rescue material of optimal compatibility can be obtained. Following the therapeutic scheme, autologous bone marrow transplantation is then done. The hemotherapy support will then be needed over the period of grafting and repopulation, until the patient becomes self-supporting again in this respect. In leukemia's and other hematological cancers affecting the bone marrow, transplantation plays an immediate therapeutic role. Sofar, most cases have been treated with allogeneic bone marrow stem cells, although increasingly purged and treated autologous marrow is being used [1]. Again, there is a period of aplasia and severe immunocompromittence to be covered by high-quality hemotherapy. In both types of bone marrow transplantation, autologous and allogeneic, Blood Banks do play a role in the purification and preservation of bone marrow stem cells.

Recently, the harvesting and preservation of stem cells collected from peripheral blood has been reported as a potential means for bone marrow transplantation [2]. Here the harvesting procedure is done through machine apheresis techniques.

3. Organ transplantation

The transplantation practice of solid organs like liver and heart-lung is rapidly developing. Increasingly centres become involved in this advanced medical care for end-stage non-malignant parenchymal diseases. Technically, these operations are now accepted as fullgrown, being not anymore experimental practice. However, the hemotherapy support for these procedures still is not a day-to-day routine type of exercise in the Blood Bank involved. The support of specifically a liver transplantation programme has two dimensions. First the cover of the usually unpredictably long standby period, where a minimum of red cells and platelets need to be available around the clock. Second, the support during the actual transplant when there is an additional need for support with CMV negative blood components and specific red cell antigen selection, the perspectives for maintaining an adequate stock and the guarantee of an optimal supply once the transplantation is in action, are not always so clear. The logistics therefore are not only of quantitative but also of qualitative magnitude. This urges Blood Banks and transplant teams to carefully prepare the possibilities for adequate hemotherapy support before implementing a programme, as there are definitely limits to the availability of human blood [3].

4. Neonatology

Neonatology has developed into a separate and mature speciality within the discipline of pediatrics. Special knowledge and expertise have been gained in the pathophysiology of very low birth weight premature infants. The borders of life have been successfully diverted. Here, very specific quality criteria and metabolic requirements apply to the necessary hemotherapy support. Premature newborns show a complexity of problems in organ function, immune function and susceptibility to infections, such that blood transfusion becomes a dangerous practice and needs to be balanced carefully against the desired efficacies.

Blood components need to be functionally as optimal as possible. This usually means 'very fresh' or to be transfused as quick as possible following donation. However, to guarantee an absolute minimal infection transmission, time is needed to quality control the blood. Besides, there are periods of the year where logistics clash with availabilities, for instance Christmas and other long weekend type of holidays. It is not so much the quantity but very outspoken the quality of the components needed for hemotherapy support in neonatology, which defines the perspective.

5. Hemophilia

Hemophilia, as an inherited disease, needs a life long hemotherapy support. The institution of home therapy has definitely increased the quality of life and shifted life expectancy to almost normal. The development of more purified and freeze-dried clotting factor concentrates has made possible these fortunate developments.

However, chronic exposure to still an enormous amount of foreign and in essence not needed proteins and other materials from thousands of individuals has shown to have an effect on depressing the immune system of the hemophilia patient. Besides, there is a definite relation between transmission viral diseases and the magnitude of exposure of the pool size of the source plasma.

The development of rDNA clotting factors, the reduction of pool sizes by reducing the sofar unavoidable losses of functional proteins during fractionation and the introduction of virus inactivating techniques to be applied to finished product, certainly will have a positive and favourable effect on patient safety [4].

However, in many countries the availability of therapeutic material for hemophilia care is still limited to a great extent. The development of a well organized and optimal functioning blood supply system should be a major perspective in the ongoing endeavour to optimise clinical efficacy and minimise the risk factors.

6. Surgical procedures

The hemotherapy support needed in surgery depends very much on the type of surgery, for instance use of extracorporeal circuits, extend and cause of blood loss, i.e. in multiple complicated trauma or liver transplantation, and the pre-operative condition of the patient, i.e. orthopedic surgery in hemophilia patients.

Increasingly pre-operative autotransfusion is used to avoid unnecessary wastage of blood lost in body cavities. The technique, however, is limited to the salvage of red cells. So, when blood loss is extensive and blood coagulation diminished or hampered, further supportive hemotherapy might be needed.

Another approach is in the predeposit of blood for hemotherapy support during surgical procedures. By tradition this is limited to patients with multiple red cell antibodiees, although in autologous bone marrow transplantation there is a place for predeposition of autologous platelets to be stored in frozen condition.

An additional advantage of predeposition of blood and pre-operative autotransfusion is in the avoidance of transmissible diseases like hepatitis, CMV and LAV/HTLV-III infection.

7. Hemapheresis

A newly developed and specific dimension in hemotherapy support is the technique of hemapheresis. The major application of hemapheresis is in the removal of unwanted substances from the blood, usually present in the plasma. Hemapheresis mostly focuses on plasma exchange. Removal of unwanted cells such as red cells in sickle cell crisis, platelets in thrombocythemia and white cells in hairy cell leukemia or multiple sclerosis has been applied with some success using machine hemapheresis techniques.

Developments are ongoing in the attempt to more specifically remove plasma constituents by adsorption, precipitation or cascade filtration techniques [5].

Sofar, the technique of hemapheresis has been of value in the support of a variety of diseases such as paraproteinemia's, autoimmune diseases affecting the kidneys, lung and central nervous system. Since the introduction of cyclosporin in the prevention of renal allograft rejection, vascular rejection episodes have increased. In the acute phase of vascular rejection therapeutic plasma exchange has shown to have a beneficial effect on prolongation of allograft viability [6].

These developments can only progress when at the same time the Blood Bank does develop mechanisms and techniques to produce the appropriate blood component, improve their safety, purity and potency as to allow supportive hemotherapy to be given in adequate quality and quantity in the clinical practice. These considerations need an active policy in donor motivation and management, as well as collection, processing and preservation technology. Quality assurance and continuous professional education and motivation are fundamental in this respect. Developmental work to reduce sofar inevitable losses in cell function and protein characteristics is needed to further improve both safety and efficacy of clinical transfusion practice.

Specific blood components – cells

In optimizing clinical efficacy, blood component production should focus on techniques to minimise the risks of transfusing these components. This comprises efforts to improve the safety, purity and potency of the respective components to be produced and preserved.

Red cells	a.	development of techniques to further purify red cell concentrates from contaminating white cells and platelets;
	b.	the harvesting of neocytes for the support of patients chronically in need of red cells, like thalassemic, sickle cell and aplastic anemia patients.
Platelets	a.	development of techniques to purify platelet concentrates from contaminating white cells by elutriation and filtration principles;
	b.	extension of in vitro shelf-life by improving storage techniques;
	c.	development of techniques for harvesting and long-term preservation of autologous platelets.
Nucleated cells	a.	harvesting and preservtion of monocytes;
	b.	development of techniques for harvesting pluripotent stem cells from peripheral blood using hemapheresis principles;
	c.	improving techniques for purging and purifying stem cells from bone marrow and subsequent preservation for elective bone marrow transplantation programmes.
Infection prevention	a.	selection of CMV-negative donors and the organization of a CMV-negative Blood Bank for red cell and platelet transfusion;
	b.	screening for HTLV-I and LAV/HTLV-III antibodies.
Graft vs host disease	–	irradiation of poentially white cell contaiminated blood components to eliminate the progenitor function of lymphocytes.

Specific components – proteins

Here too the main emphasis is in optimizing safety and purity as to achieve an optimal clinical efficacy.

Factor VIII   a. reduction of pool size to be achieved by further developing high-yield purification techniques such as continuous thaw principle, controlled pore glass chromatography and heparin double cold precipitation technique;

                                   b. the development of a monoclonal antibody adsorption chromatography for the production of an extremely highly purified factor VIII;

                                   c. further exploration of rDNA production technology;

                                   d. the development and implementation of virus inactivation technology both for retroviruses, hepatitis B virus and other transmissable viruses.

IV-immunoglobulines a. harvesting and purification of specific immunoglobulins for intravenous use;

                                   b. improvement of techniques to safeguard optimal molecular composition of immunoglobulins during the purification procedures.

Development of purification methods for the production of fibronectin, transfer factor, interferons and interleukins. Application of fibrin glue, a combination of cryoprecipitate and human thrombin, in elective surgery of the ear and plastic surgery.

Conclusion

Blood as a living tissue is not a pharmaceutical source material. It deserves an entirely different approach, philosophical as well as practical, both at the Blood Bank and the clinical level. The perspective in in supportive hemotherapy should be delineated by qualitative rather than quantitative reflections.

References

1. Löwenberg B. Is the basis of cleaning autologous bone-marrow transplants in leukemia strong enough? In: Smit Sibinga CTh, Das PC, Opelz G (eds). Transplantation and blood transfusion. Martinus Nijhoff Publishers, Dordrecht, Boston, Lancaster, 1984:161 – 4.
2. Körbling M, Fliedner ThM. Autologous transplantation of blood derived hemopoietic stem cells. In: Smit Sibinga CTh, Das PC, Opelz G (eds). Transplantation and blood transfusion. Martinus Nijhoff Publishers, Dordrecht, Boston, Lancaster, 1984:199 – 203.

3. Smit Sibinga CTh, Achterhof L, Waltje J, Swieringa J, Das PC. Blood Bank logistics in liver transplantation. In: Gips CH, Krom RAF (eds). Progress in liver transplantation. Martinus Nijhoff Publishers, Dordrecht, Boston, Lancaster, 1985:85 – 9.
4. Smit Sibinga CTh. A scheme for the future. Scand J Haematol 1984;40(suppl.): 535 – 44.
5. Pineda AA. Future directions of apheresis. In: Valbonesi M, Pineda AA, Biggs JC (eds). Therapeutic hemapheresis. Wichtig Editore Milano 1986:187 – 94.
6. Allen NH, Dyer P, Geoghegan T et al. Plasma exchange in acute renal allograft rejection: A controlled trial. Transplantation 1983;35:425 – 8.

LIVER TRANSPLANTATION WITH CMV NEGATIVE BLOOD AND ITS PRODUCTS

A. Maas, K. Timmermans, J. Waltje, J. Swieringa, P.C. Das, C.Th. Smit Sibinga

Introduction

Although orthotopic liver transplantation (OLT) is carried out in a few specialized centres, the numbers are incresing. In Groningen 50 liver transplantations have been done over the last five years. OLT requires the support of a considerable amount of blood and blood products [1,2]. The commitment of a regional Blood Bank to support an OLT programme means a 24 hours obligation for 7 days a week, since it is not known when the organ will be available for transplantation. Such an intense commitment should not adversely affect the routine care for other patients; in Groningen this means about 5,000 acute beds.

In addition, implementation of an OLT programme in the Blood Bank must be done smoothly and optimally without changing much of the donor call-up programme or wasting valuable blood products. Our routine logistics for liver transplantation support has been previously described [3,4]. During the entire period of 'green' light, when a patient has been selected but is waiting for a suitable donor liver for transplantation, the agreed protocol stipulates that a minimum of 10 RCC's, 20 units of modified whole blood and 12 units of platelets per patient are in stock. During the operation these blood components are the minimum amount safeguarded by the Blood Bank.

With improved surgical techniques and skill the outcome of OLT has improved over the last years. However, it seems that the morbidity and mortality following OLT may be influenced by CMV infections. One of the routes of such an infection is blood transfusion. This paper raises the question whether a regional Blood Bank could support an OLT programme with CMV-negative blood products, specifically, in those cases where the donor liver as well as the recipient of the organ are CMV-negative.

The study attempts to answer the complex question involving overlapping areas. It concentrates on the logistic of platelets, because plasma products can be frozen and red cells have a longer shelf-life. Platelets can be kept only for five days maximally.

Materials and methods

For the OLT-patient group requiring CMV-negative support it was decided that Rhesus positive or negative patients should receive compatible group

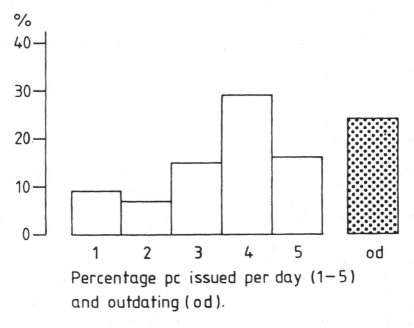

Figure 1. Percentage of platelets issued per day and outdating.

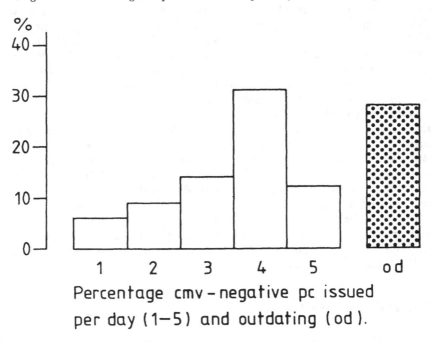

Figure 2. Percentage of CMV negative platelets issued per day and outdating.

O blood which are routinely screened. The blood products like modified whole blood, RCC and platelets were prepared according to the AABB manual [5]. Details of the test for CMV antibody have been described elsewhere [6].

Study design

The study was divided into two parts. The first in which the CMV negativity of the platelets was identified only, and the second part in which the identification was followed by reservation of the platelets for a specific patient. In this second period we consented in supporting an OLT with CMV negative blood and its products. During this two-phase study several parameters were studied: the CMV antibody reactivity and its distribution in our donor population, the day to day variation in the inventory of the CMV negative platelets, the shelf-life of the platelets when issued to the clinics and the percentage of outdating of the platelets.

Phase I results

Phase I is an observation period ascertaining our strength and weakness before commitment to a pilot study in an OLT patient.

In this phase 46% of the donations were found CMV negative, but the day to day distribution of their negativity varied widely from 8 – 78%. Figure 1 shows the percentage of platelets issued each day in our region covering the requirements of all acute patients. Most platelets are issued at day 4. It was therefore decided that CMV negative platelets should be identified and reserved for an OLT patient for three days. Then they should be returned to the routine inventory for issuing to other patients, thus minimizing unnecessary outdating.

Figures 2 and 3 show the results of this policy applied to CMV negative and CMV positive platelets. Although the outdating in the CMV negative group was higher (28%) than the CMV positive group (24%) the overall outdating was comparable to our routine outdating which has been 25% over the last year.

Figure 4 shows that the 12 units of platelets guaranteed for OLT are available for 80% of the days considered over a month time.

Phase II results

Phase II represents a pilot study to support a selected OLT with CMV negative blood and blood products. Platelets were identified as CMV negative and kept separately for this patient. During the waiting period before the patient was transplanted, again 80% of the time a minimum of 12 units of CMV negative platelets were present in our stock. Outdating of CMV positive platelets was 14%, of the CMV negative group 12%.

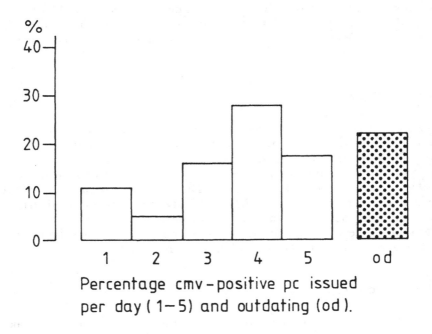

Figure 3. Percentage of CMV positive platelets issued per day and outdating.

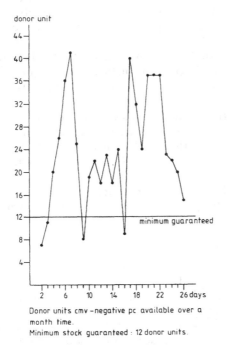

Figure 4. Units of CMV negative platelets in stock over a month time.

The liver transplantation was carried out after two months waiting. For the Blood Bank it meant the screening of 631 donors over that period to maintain the CMV negative platelets' stock. During the actual liver transplantation operation an additional amount of platelets (12) was required. The phase I study suggested that only over 40% of our waiting time this amount would be available, and it is a matter of coincidence that the extra 12 units of CMV negative platelets were available for the patient.

Discussion

The clinical indications for CMV negative blood and its products are limited and this includes CMV negative bone marrow and renal transplantation, premature low birth weight neonates delivered from a seronegative mother. Once the CMV donor screening test had been introduced successfully at the Blood Bank, the above clinical demands are not difficult to meet. However, the logistic of CMV negative blood support in OLT are somewhat different, because of the enormity of the task. More importantly such a support has to be guaranteed continuously for weeks to months on a 24 hours basis. The fact that over 600 donor screenings were necessary for an OLT ultimately requiring 35 units of blood and 24 units of platelets illustrates this point.

The other alternative is to screen and reserve the CMV negative products for the OLT patient to the end of its shelf-life. In a regional Blood Bank responsible for 5,000 acute beds such an extraordinary status given to the CMV negative OLT is not recommended. The support of an OLT with CMV negative blood may be complex and unique to each centre, nevertheless, it seems feasible. The Blood Bank has to play a dynamic role within the OLT team, where a senor staff member of the Blood Bank should continuously be in touch with the team and assess the trends of events. With experience and proper sense of anticipation one could adapt and change the system continuously in order to perform better at the current and next operations.

References

1. Butler P, Israel L, Nusbacher J, Jenkens DE, Starzl TE. Blood transfusion in liver transplantation. Transfusion 1985;25:120 – 3.
2. Newton DEF, Wesenhagen E. Supportive therapy for liver transplantation. In: Das PC, Smit Sibinga CTh, Halie MR (eds). Supportive therapy in haematology. Martinus Nijhoff Publ. Boston, Dordrecht, Lancaster 1985:217 – 8.
3. Gips CH, Sloof MJH, Wesenhagen H, van Goor H, Bijleveld CMA, Krom RAF. Organisation of livertransplantation. In: Gips CH, Krom RAF (eds) Progress in liver transplantation. Martinus Nijhoff Publ. Boston, Dordrecht, Lancaster 1985;:229 – 38.
4. Smit Sibinga CTh, Achterhof L, Waltje J, Swieringa J, Das PC. Blood Bank logistics in liver transplantation. In: Gips CG, Krom RAF (eds). Progess in liver

transplantation. Martinus Nijhoff Publ. Boston, Dordrecht, Lancaster 1985: 85 – 92.

5. Technical manual AABB 9th ed. Widmann FK (ed), 1985.

6. McShine RL, Sinninge G, Das PC, Smit Sibinga CTh. CMV antibody testing of blood donors. In: Smit Sibinga CTh, Das PC, Greenwalt T (eds). Future developments in blood banking. Martinus Nijhoff Publ. Boston, Dordrecht, Lancaster 1986.

FACTORS AND MECHANISMS INVOLVED IN RENAL ALLOGRAFT REJECTION IN MAN

J.D.L. Schot*, G.F.J. Hendriks **, R.K.B. Schuurman*

Introduction

Except for transplantation between identical twins, irreversible rejection is a continuous threat for the recipients of renal allografts. The survival of organs and tissues in allogeneic hosts is dependent on a series of factors, most of which are involved in the humoral and cellular immune response of the host to the foreign antigens present in the graft. Allograft survival is determined by an interaction between the immunogenicity of the allograft and the strength of the immune response of the host. Many factors, determining either the immunogenicity of the graft or the strength of the immune response, have been identified. Factors reported to be polymorphic in their effect have been given priority for such studies, especially those factors which can be evaluated before transplantation. The final goal of these studies is to obtain a so called 'transplantogram' on which donor-recipient selection and treatment protocols can be based. The first attempts to obtain relevant factors for such a transplantogram were retrospective analyses. In this way the influence of HLA- and ABO-determinants on renal allograft survival has been demonstrated [1,2]. A major problem encountered in such statistical analyses however was the presence of confounding factors. Although several factors each might demonstrate an influence on allograft survival, multiple regression analyses should be performed to determine their final impact on allograft survival.

Rejection of renal allografts is suppressed by drugs such as corticosteroids, alkylating agents and cyclosporin A. Especially cyclosporin A has improved renal allograft survival rates. Consequently the influence of some relevant factors on graft survival might disappear. However, as long as immunosuppressive drugs do not interfere with the mechanisms by which particular factors exert their influence, those factors will remain relevant. Therefore it is important to investigate their mechanisms to find out whether those factors still influence allograft survival. Unfortunately the very effective immunosuppressive regimens used today hamper such investigations. In particular factors which are involved in the regualtion of the immune response of the host to the graft can hardly be investigated, in con-

* Division of Immunobiology, Department of Immunohaematology, University Medical Center, Leiden, The Netherlands.
** Eurotransplant Foundation, Department of Immunohaematology, University Medical Center, Leiden, The Netherlands.

trast to factors involved in the induction of rejection. Immunomodulatory factors are: the number of pretransplant blood transfusions and, possibly, the duration of hemodialysis. Both have been associated with a suppressed immune response after transplantation [3,4].

Consequently, identification of factors which might modulate the host's immune response should be performed before transplantation when no immunosuppressive drugs are administered. Preferably, in vivo tests should be applied which evaluate the immune response induced by new antigens. A simple and very suitable method is the use of the DNCB skin test in which a neo-antigen (dinitrochlorobenzene) elicits a cutaneous cell mediated immune (CCMI) response in vivo [5].

As long as the mechanisms behind most factors, known or postulated to influence allograft survival, are elusive, all those factors should be investigated for their effect on CCMI. Apart from the fact that HLA antigens appear to function mainly as immunogenetic determinants in the induction of allograft rejection, HLA encoded genes are postulated to play a role in the regulation of the immune response [6]. Individual differences in the strength of the immune response to the graft are observed in the population of renal transplant patients. Since these differences would be encoded by genes which are polymorphic in their effect such genes could be encoded by the very polymorphic HLA system.

In this report we focus on the effects of the various factors which influence allograft survival and CCMI. By comparison of their effects on graft survival and CCMI we were sometimes able to indicate whether they exert their main influence on the immune response of the host or have their influence as immunogenetic antigens in the allograft. Special care was taken to avoid confounding effects.

Materials and methods

Patients

All patients with end stage renal failure were on regular hemodialysis, had no treatment with immunosuppressive drugs and were awaiting first kidney transplants. One hundred and forty patients from eleven regional dialysis centers were investigated.

Patients with glomerulonephritis were regarded as having an immunopathological basis of their kidney disease, whereas all other patients with end stage renal failure were not.

The HLA-A, -B, and -DR typings had been performed with the standardized Eurotransplant AB- and DR-serum sets. The serological definition of HLA-DRw6 was based on several groups of oligospecific sera [7]. Patients with at least one HLA-DRw6 positive allele were designated HLA-DRw6 positive.

The duration of hemodialysis was defined as the time between the first date of hemodialysis and the date of the DNCB sensitization.

DNCB skin test

Patients were sensitized by the application of 2 mg DNCB, dried onto 2 cm² felt pads, to the skin of the upper arm for 24 hr. The sensitization and the measurement of the DNCB response upon challenge were performed by the same investigator to avoid interobserver bias. Sixteen patients showing no reactivity upon sensitization were excluded from the analysis because of the possibility that the required contact with DNCB had not been sufficient. Challenge dosages of 30, 15, 7.5, 3.7, and 1.8 μg of DNCB on 1 cm diameter felt pads were applied to the skin of the forearm two weeks later. After three days each of the 5 test areas was assigned a score: 0 = no reaction or erythema only; 1 = erythema and induration confined to the patch area; 2 = erythema and induration extending beyond the patch area; 3 = 2 plus blistering. The total DNCB score was the sum of the responses to each of the 5 challenge tests (range 0 – 15).

Statistical analyses

Normalization of the distribution of the DNCB scores was reached by pooling the patients with negative (score 0), low (score 1 – 2), intermediate (score 3 – 5) and high (score 6 – 11) DNCB responses into four classes which encompassed 33, 46, 26, and 19 patients respectively.

The distribution of the number of blood transfusions was normalized into five classes with 0 – 1, 2, 3 – 5, 6 – 11, and 13 – 67 transfusions, which encompassed 26, 27, 24, 23 and 24 patients respectively.

The duration of hemodialysis was normalized into six classes with 0 – 5, 6 – 10, 11 – 16, 17 – 24, 25 – 46, and 47 – 136 months of hemodialysis representing 20, 22, 24, 19, 21, and 18 patients respectively.

Correlation coefficients were determined between the DNCB score and four DNCB response classes, the number of blood transfusions and five blood transfusion classes, the duration of hemodialysis and six hemodialysis classes had the age of the patients to validify the normalization applied. Nine-non-transfused patients were regarded as missing values in the analysis of the relation between transfusion free interval and other factors.

To analyse which of the variables or which combinations of variables gave the best estimate of the corresponding DNCB value, multiple regression equations were performed utilizing the forward and enter method of the SPSS[x] regression programme. By the 'forward' method the programme selected the variable which had the largest contribution, followed by an analysis of the contribution other variables still had to the DNCB response, given the effect of the first variable. In the 'enter' method we choose a variable, analysed the contribution of the other variable(s).

The significance of the differences in the distribution of the ABO bloodgroups, pathogenesis of renal disease, HLA-DRw6 and sex among the patients in the four DNCB response classes was determined by Chi squares' (Tables 2a, 6a, 7 and 8a) and the p values in tables 2b, 6b and 8b were derived from two tailed student's t-test for two means.

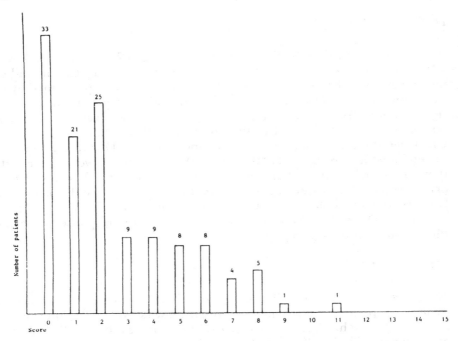

Figure 1.   Distribution of the DNCB scores in 124 hemodialysis patients.
DNCB scores, see materials and methods.

Results and discussion

High and low responder status and HLA encoded immune response regulators

Inbred mouse strains have been distinguished as high or low responders to particular antigens. High and low responder strains carried distinct histocompatibility determinants encoded by the mouse MHC complex [8]. It was proposed that the human MHC complex, the HLA system, not only encoded histocompatibility determinants but also encoded polymorphic immune response regulators [9]. Such an HLA-associated immune responsiveness was recently observed in renal transplant patients. HLA-DRw6 positive recipients reject non HLA-DRw6 renal allografts more rapidly and vigourously than non HLA-DRw6 recipients receiving DR mismatched allografts [6]. HLA-DRw6 carrying helper T lymphocytes have also been found to be more easily stimualted by streptococcal antigen than lymphocytes not carrying HLA-DRw6 [10]. These data suggest that the HLA-DRw6 gene codes for a high responder phenotype probably expressed at the level of T helper cells. To test this hypothesis we investigated the cellular immune response by means of the DNCB skin test. The distribution of DNCB scores obtained in 124 patients was gradual and not bimodal (fig. 1). Thus no high or low responders could be distinguished.

Thirty three patients (27%) did not respond to the DNCB challenge, whereas the DNCB dosage applied (2 mg) at sensitization was amply sufficient to obtain a 100% response in healthy persons [11]. This indicates that the immune response of these patients was suppressed.

The patients were divided into four classes according to their DNCB scores of 0, 1 − 2, 3 − 5 and more than 5 respectively. This division was validified by a high correlation coefficient between DNCB scores and DNCB response classes (table 1).

The distribution of HLA-DRw6 positive and negative patients did not differ significantly within these DNCB response classes (table 2a). We concluded that HLA-DRw6 was not correlated with a high responder status in CCMI. This result might be due to the method of investigation which is apparently more suitable to investigate suppressive effects. If the postulated

Table 1. Correlations between the DNCB response, blood transfusions, transfusion free interval and duration of hemodialysis.

	DNCBResp	**NB1dtr**	**Intvl**
DNCB	.95	− .26	− .02
NB1dtr	− .31		− .22
DurDia	− .18	.42	.03

DNCBResp = DNCB response classified into four groups (see methods).
NB1dtr = Number of blood transfusions.
DurDia = Duration of hemodialysis.
Intvl = Time between last blood transfusion and DNCB sensitization.

260

Table 2a. Distribution of patients according to HLA-DRw6 within the four DNCB response classes.

HLA-DRw6	DNCB response class			
	1	2	3	4
Positive	9	17	11	7
Negative	24	29	15	12
	$X^2 = 1.56$		p = ns	

Table 2b. Confounding effects in the analysis of the HLA-DRw6 associated effects on CCMI.

HLA-DRw6	n	Number of transfusions	Duration of hemodialysis
Positive	44	5.6 ± 8.9 #	16.9 ± 15.7 # *
Negative	80	9.9 ± 13.5	28.3 ± 27.6
		p = ns	$p < 0.02$

\# = mean ± SD; * = in months

HLA-DRw6 associated immune response regulator operates exclusively in the induction of helper T cell activity a differential effect may not be observed as a sensitization dosage of 0.5 mg already induced a response in 100% of healthy volunteers [11].

The suppression found in the hemodialysis patients, as compared to healthy controls, also indicates that other factors interfered with the results. These other factors, i.e. number of blood transfusions and, possibly, the duration of hemodialysis (see further) were analysed in the HLA-DRw6 positive and negative patients. We found no significant difference between the two groups in respect to the number of blood transfusions, but HLA-DRw6 positive patients had a significant shorter duration of hemodialysis (table 2b). However, if hemodialysis had any effect on the DNCB skin test, it was an immunosuppressive effect which was stronger in patients with longer duration hemodialysis. This should thus have led .to an increased DNCB score in the HLA-DRw6 positive group, which was not found (table 2a).

Thus we conclude that the postulated HLA-DRw6 associated high responder status is not observed in the effector phase of the CCMI response.

Blood transfusion induced immunosuppression

Administration of blood transfusions before renal transplantation has been shown to improve the allograft survival rate, which is likely due to immuno-suppression [3]. The exact mechanism of this immunosuppressive effect is still evasive. Leukocyte free blood has no suppressive effect [1]. Administration of leukocytes to patients before transplantation may induce the formation of leukocyte antibodies. These antibodies can lead to positive crossmatches between the organ donor and the recipient. The percentage of patients sensitized by blood transfusions has been shown to reach a fraction of 0.3 of the patients having a positive reaction to more than 80% of a random panel of leukocytes [12]. Some authors have postulated that the blood transfusion effect on allograft survival is largely due to selection of crossmatch negative donor-recipient pairs [13]. Many authors did not agree that selection was the only explanation for the blood transfusion effect [1].

It would provide further insight if it could be demonstrated that blood transfusions indeed effectuate immunosuppression. The DNCB evoked CCMI test is a very attractive test as selection is excluded. Moreover this test evaluates immunomodulation only.

A correlation was found between the CCMI response and the number of blood transfusions but the number of blood transfusions was also correlated with the duration of hemodialysis. There is however no perfect correlation ($r = 0.42$, table 1) which is explained by the observation that almost all patients had already received blood transfusions before entering the hemodialysis programme. The numberof blood transfusions given before hemodialysis varied between 0 to 10.

A second point is that our patients received only $1 - 5$ containing red blood cell suspensions as part of the pretransplant blood transfusion protocol to effectuate blood transfusion associated immunosuppression. Most blood transfusions given to correct anemia during hemodialysis were cotton wool filtered. These red blood cell suspensions will hardly contain leukocytes if fresh whole blood is used. If isolated from whole blood taken 48 hours before, it is very likely that these suspensions will contain leukocyte fragments. Although these leukocyte fragments still can induce anti-leukocyte antibody formation they are thought to the patients before and during hemodialysis were red blood cell suspensions which contained only small amounts of leukocytes and thus could have had only a small immunosuppressive effect. In this respect it is remarkable that we observed a relation between the number of blood transfusions and immunosuppression in CCMI.

It is still a matter of dispute how many leukocyte containing blood transfusions should be given to hemodialysis patients awaiting transplantation. Our findings are in agreement with the findings of some authors who reported about the additonal enhancing effect of pretransplant blood transfusions [14]. We also studied the duration of the blood transfusion effect by an analysis of the influence of the time interval between the last blood transfusion and the time of the DNCB sensitization.

Despite a range of 0.5 to 48 months, no influence of the time interval on the CCMI response was found (table 1). Therefore we concluded that blood transfusions have a long lasting immunosuppressive effect and that blood transfusions have an additive effect.

Table 3.   Duration of hemodialysis amongst the four DNCB response classes.

DNCB response	Duration of hemodialysis
DNCB response class	
1	34.0 ± 26.8 #
2	19.4 ± 15.4
3	24.8 ± 35.4
4	17.9 ± 15.7

= mean $\pm$ SD of duration of hemodialysis in months.

Table 4.   Multiple regression analysis of the effects of blood transfusion and hemodialysis on the DNCB response.

Method	First variable	p value	Other variable	p value
Forward	NBldtr	0.001	DurDia	ns
Forward	NBldtr	0.001	DiaCl	ns
Forward	BldCl	0.015	DurDia	ns
Forward	BldCl	0.015	DiaCl	ns
Enter	DurDia	0.049	NBldtr	0.004
Enter	DiaCl	0.016	NBldtr	0.008

BldCl = Number of blood transfusions classified into five classes (see methods)
DiaCl = Duration of hemodialysis classified into six classes (see methods)
For other abbreviations see table 1.

The effect of hemodialysis

The duration of hemodialysis was found to be correlated with the DNCB response (table 3). However, because hemodialysis and blood transfusions were interdependent (tabel 1) we analysed both effects by multiple regression analysis. Using the forward method (see methods), it was found that blood transfusions had the major effect and that hemodialysis had no effect on the CCMI response (table 4). Using the enter method by which the duration of hemodialysis was first entered into the programme, an effect of hemodialysis was found, however still with a major contribution of blood transfusions. Because the enter method does not exclude a concomitant blood transfusion effect, it was concluded that the duration of hemodialysis had only a minor effect, if any.

There is circumstantial evidence for an effect of hemodialysis [15]. Immunosuppressive factors have been found in uremic patients. These factors were reported to be polypeptides with a molecular weight of 600 – 2000 daltons. It is unknown whether these factors accumulate during the hemodialysis programme. Our results on CCMI demonstrate that the question whether or not the duration of hemodialysis influences the level of

H.D. = Duration of hemodialysis in months; N = Number of patients.

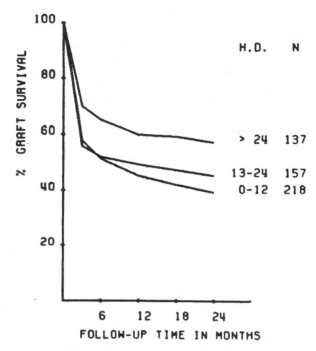

Figure 2. First renal allograft survival in non-transfused recipients (Euro-transplant file 1967 – 1979).

immunosuppression can only be answered by eliminating the associated blood transfusion effect. Since the majority of patients had already recieved blood transfusions we could not perform such an analysis. However, the Eurotransplant data base contains patients who had not received blood transfusions prior to renal transplantation. A retrospective analysis of the influence of hemodialysis on graft survival was performed in these non-transfused patients (fig. 2). This analysis revealed that first kidney graft survival rates are significantly higher in patients who had been dialysed longer before ther transplantation. All data taken together suggest that longer duration of hemodialysis is associated with increased immunosuppression.

The relationship between sex and the immune response

Females have a significantly higher mean serum IgM level than males [16]. Whether this reflects a better or faster humoral immune response to various pathogenic agents is not clear. It has been suggested that regulation of IgM levels is encoded by X-linked genes and that the female serum IgM level just reflects a gene dosage effect.

Females appear to be more easily immunized to allogeneic leukocytes in blood suspensions given to the patients before transplantation. The sera of 2488 patients awaiting first transplantation were screened for the presence of leukocyte antibodies. Sixty percent of the 'highly immunized' patients, i.e. positive serum reactivity with more than 85% of the panel leukocytes, were females [17]. In the group of patients without leukocyte antibodies only 30% were females. The one-year graft survival rates in males, nulliparous females and multiparous females does not differ significantly despite their differences in the sensitization by blood transfusions.

Table 5. Degree of immunization to leukocyte antigens amongst the four DNCB response classes.

Leukocyte panel reactivity	DNCB response class			
	1	2	3	4
≥ 20%	5	6	3	2
< 20%	28	40	23	17

The sera of patients with higher DNCB responses contained less alloantibody reactivity (table 5). Since the DNCB response was correlated with the numberof blood transfusions, the lower sensitization rate observed in the higher DNCB response group is most likely due to less blood transfusions.

We found no difference between males and females in respect to the strength of the CCMI respons (table 6a). There was a confounding effect.

Table 6a. Distribution of males and females within the four DNCB response classes.

Sex	DNCB response class			
	1	2	3	4
Males	13	29	16	14
Females	20	17	10	5
	$X^2 = 7.23$ P = ns			

Table 6b. Mean number of transfusions and mean duration of hemodialysis in males and females.

Sex	n	Number of transfusions	Duration of hemodialysis
Males	72	5.4 ± 7.7 #	22.4 ± 24.8 # *
Females	52	12.4 ± 15.7	26.7 ± 24.4
		p < 0.02	p = ns

= mean ± SD; * = in months

The male patients had received significantly less blood transfusions than the female patients (table 6b). This suggests that males are more easily suppressed in their cell mediated immune (CMI) respons than females. Males might also be more easily suppressed in their humoral immune response by blood transfusions, which could explain their lower degree of sensitization by leukocyte antigens.

The effect of the underlying renal disease

Glomerulonephritis is a heterogenous group of diseases. Most of them are based on an immunopathologic process in which disturbances in the immune system are found. Consequently patients with glomerulonephritis might have a different immune response to renal grafts. Indeed the renal allograft survival rate is lower in patients with glomerulonephritis than in patients with e.g. pyelonephritis [18]. We investigated the CCMI response in both groups of patients and found that patients with glomerulonephritis had a higher DNCB response than patients with other pathogenesis of their renal disease. However, when we compared both groups with respect to the distribution of the number of blood transfusions it turned out that patients with glomerulonephritis had received significantly less blood transfusions. This again was an example of a confounding factor in the analysis, which made

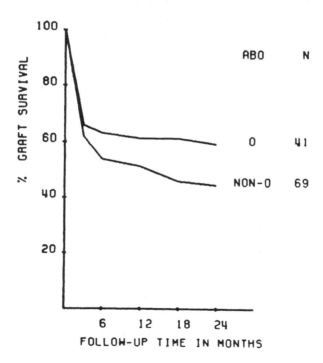

Figure 3. Survival of HLA-A, B identical first renal allografts in non-transfused blood group O and non-O recipients (Eurotransplant file 1967 – 1979).

us finally conclude that no increased CCMI response was observed in hemodialysis patients with end stage glomerulonephritis.

The effect of the ABO blood groups

Transplantation across an ABO blood group barrier usually leads to a strong immune response against the graft, except for O kidneys into A, B and AB recipients and for O/A or B kidneys into AB recipients. Successful transplantation of A_2 kidneys into O recipients has been reported because O recipients fail to make anti-A_2 agglutinins [19]. An analysis of the survival rates observed in recipients of first renal allografts, which were transplanted between 1967 and 1979 at the Eurotransplant institutions, is shown in figure 3. All patients had received HLA-A and -B matched renal allografts and had not received blood transfusions. Non-O recipients have a lower graft survival rate than O recipients, independent of the ABO type of the donor. The data suggest that non-O recipients, if not transfused, mount a stronger immune response to renal allografts.

We analysed transfused O and non-O hemodialysis patients for their level of CCMI to DNCB (table 7a) and found no significant difference. A confounding effect of blood transfusions was excluded (table 7b). However the duration of hemodialysis was found to be significantly longer in the O group than in the non-O group. This could have suppressed the immune response of the O patients and thus have masked an inherent higher response. Since the suppressive effect of hemodialysis on CCMI appeared to be marginal, if any, we conclude that the O patients did not expose a high responder status in CCMI.

Table 7a. Distribution of patients according to O versus non-O blood groups within the four DNCB response classes.

Blood group	DNCB response class			
	1	2	3	4
O	22	20	15	10
non-O	11	26	11	9
	$X^2 = 4.33$		p = ns	

Table 7b. Mean number of transfusions and mean duration of hemodialysis in the blood group O and non-O patients.

Blood group	n	Number of transfusions	Duration of hemodialysis
O	67	8.8 ± 12.2 #	30.1 ± 28.4 # *
non-O	57	7.8 ± 12.2	17.3 ± 16.9
		p = ns	$p < 0.01$

= mean $\pm$ SD; * = in months

Conclusions

None of the polymorphic genes discussed here, i.e. HLA genes, sex and ABO types, as well as polyphorphic pathogenic mechanisms, i.e. glomerulonephritis versus other renal diseases were shown to have an effect on CCMI. Nevertheless such effects on CCMI may exist as our method was possibly inadequate to test the afferent phase of CCMI. The efferent phase of CCMI was not influenced by these factors. Moreover we could not identify high and low responders. This suggests that high or low responders do not exist in the efferent phase of the immune response, at least not in the (outbred) human population of patients with end stage renal disease.

Sex had an effect on humoral immunity as measured by lymphocytotoxins induced by leukocyte containing blood transfusion(s). Part of this effect was dependent on previous pregnancies. It would be demonstrated that females were less easily suppressed in CCMI by blood transfusions. It is likely that the higher degree of sensitization for leukocyte antigens will be accompanied by selection based on positive crossmatches before transplantation. The most relevant effect on CCMI was found to be mediated by blood transfusion. This effect was long lasting and increased with the number of blood transfusions. As the degree of immunization to leukocyte antigens is known to increase, to a maximum of 40% of the patients, with increased numbers of blood transfusion, the conclusion of these results still favours a restricted use of blood transfusions. There was also a small effect of the duration of hemodialysis which was not large enough to be of clinical significance. However it is relevant to pursue further studies on the suppressive factors associated with uremia because these factors are endogenous and thus likely far less toxic than immunosuppressive drugs. Blood transfusions and hemodialysis exert their main effect in the CCMI response of the allograft recipients. If the present-day immunosuppressive drugs operate by the same mechanisms one might consider to neglect the effects of blood transfusion and hemodialysis with the advantage of less sensitization to leukocyte antigens. However, we propose to pursue studies on the mechanisms behind their effects because this will ultimately expose endogenous immunosuppressive agents. Such endogenous suppressive factors are a very attractive alternative, as the long term goal in kidney transplantation is to limit the side effects of the immunosuppressive drugs and thus to restrict their application as much as possible.

References

1. Persijn GG, Hendriks GFJ, van Rood JJ. HLA matching, blood transfusion and renal transplantation. In: Clinics in Immunology and Allergy 1984;4: 535 – 65.
2. Joysey VC, Roger JH, Evans DB, Herbertson BM. Kidney graft survival and matching for HL-A and ABO antigens. Nature 1973;246:163 – 5.
3. Opelz G, Mickey MR, Terasaki PI. Blood transfusions and unresponsiveness to HL-A. Transplantation 1973;16:649 – 54.

4. Fehrman I, Groth C-G, Lundgren G, Magnusson G, Möller E. Pretransplant dialysis and blood transfusion – Correlation with cadaveric kidney graft survival. Transplant Proc 1979;9:152 – 5.
5. Bleumink E, Nater JP, Schraffordt Koops H, The TH. A standard method for DNCB sensitization testing in patients with neoplasms. Cancer 1974;33: 911 – 5.
6. Hendriks GFJ, Claas FHJ, Persijn GG, Witvliet MD, Baldwin W, van Rood JJ. HLA-DRw6-positive recipients are high responders in renal transplantation. Transplant Proc 1983;15:1136 – 8.
7. Schreuder GMT, Parlevliet J, Termijtelen A, van Rood JJ. Reanalysis of the HLA-DRw6 complex. Tissue antigens 1983;21:62 – 74.
8. McDevitt HO, Chinitz A. Genetic control of the antibody response: relationship between immune response and histocompatibility (H-2) type. Science 1969;163:1207 – 8.
9. Snell GD. T cells, T cell recognition structures, and the major histocompatibility complex. Immunological Rev 1978;38:3 – 69.
10. Lehner T. The relationship between human helper and suppressor factors to a streptococcal protein antigen. J Immunol 1982;129:1936 – 40.
11. Friedman PS, Moss C, Shuster S, Simpson JM. Quantitative relationships between sensitizing dose of DNCB and reactivity in normal subjects. Clin Exp Immunol 1983;53:709 – 15.
12. Opelz G, Graver B, Mickey MR, Terasaki PI. Lymphocytotoxic antibody responses to transfusions in potential kidney transplant recipients. Transplantation 1981;32:117 – 83.
13. Möller E. Conditions for optimal transplant survival in man. In: Yamanura Y, Tada T (eds). Progress in Immunology V. Academic Press, London 1983: 1477 – 89.
14. Opelz G, Terasaki PI. International study of histocompatibility in renal transplantation. Transplantation 1982;33:87 – 95.
15. Goldblum SE, Reed WP. Host defenses and immunologic alterations associated with chronic hemodialysis. Ann Int Med 1980;93:597 – 613.
16. Grundbacher FJ. Human X chromosome carriers quantitative genes for immunoglobulin M. Science 1972;176:311 – 2.
17. Hendriks GFJ, de Lange P, D'Amaro J, Schreuder GMT, Claas FHJ, Persijn GG, van Rood JJ. Eurotransplant experience with highly immunized patients. Scand J Urol Nephrol Suppl 1985;92:81 – 6.
18. Perdue ST, Terasaki PI, Cats S, Mickey MR. Kidney transplantation trends from UCLA registry data, 1975 – 1982. Transplantation 1983;36:658 – 65.
19. Brynger H, Rydberg L, Samuelsson L, Blohmé I, Lindholm A, Sandberg L. Renal transplantation across a blood group barrier – A_2 kidneys to O recipients. Proc Eur Dial Transpl Assoc 1982;19:427 – 31.

BEDSIDE PRACTICE OF BLOOD TRANSFUSION TO BE DEVELOPED?

K. Mayer

Traditionally transfusions served to replace the blood cells or components that are reduced in the peripheral blood and constituted a triggered response to a low or 'abnormal' count. Such abnormality has traditionally been defined as falling outside two standard deviations of the mean (fig. 1).

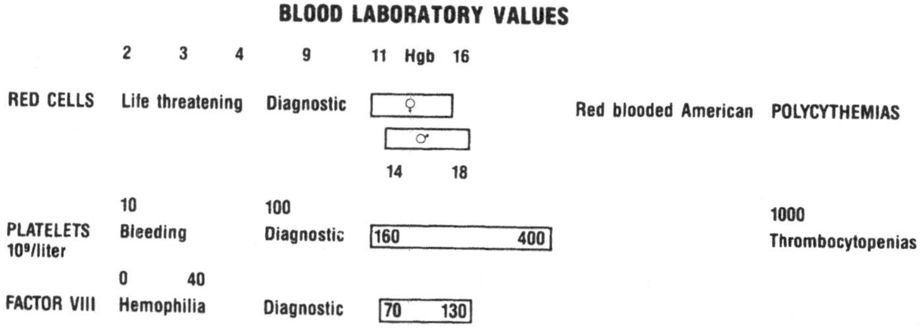

BLOOD LABORATORY VALUES

Figure 1.

Although such values have diagnostic significance they do not necessarily require therapeutic intervention. In fact were such individuals transfused the evidence might be obliterated making a hematologic diagnosis difficult or impossible. They may also be counter productive in that red cell transfusion can be shown to reduce marrow erythropoiesis and reticulocytosis in the peripheral blood. In addition, transfused normal cells will normalize cell morphology and cell indices such as mean corpuscular volume or hemoglobin. The same is true for platelet transfusions which inhibit megakaryocytosis and, therefore, platelet production.

When limits are reached which cause serious morbidity or are life threatening something needs to be done but again transfusion is not necessarily the answer.

The major diagnostic question in hematology is whether the pathology is due to lack of production or increased destruction (fig. 2). The peripheral blood values are always the balance between what enters the circulation and that which leaves. The latter may be frank blood loss or hemolysis. This process is analogous to the balance in a bank account, the delta (difference) between deposit and withdrawal.

ABNORMAL BLOOD PARAMETERS

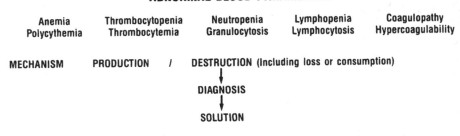

| Anemia | Thrombocytopenia | Neutropenia | Lymphopenia | Coagulopathy |
| Polycythemia | Thrombocytemia | Granulocytosis | Lymphocytosis | Hypercoagulability |

MECHANISM   PRODUCTION   /   DESTRUCTION (Including loss or consumption)

DIAGNOSIS

SOLUTION

CORRECTION OF UNDERLYING CAUSE

CORRECTION BY REPLACEMENT OR REMOVAL

Figure 2.

The transfusionist must be a hematologist who is willing and capable in helping to determine the mechanism of altered production and destruction. If the anemia is due to defective hemoglobin synthesis because of iron deficiency then iron replacement is more appropriate, more cost effective and safer. Iron dextran can be given in large doses to correct chronic blood loss. We have maintained for many years a patient with familial telangiectasia, Osler-Weber-Rendu disease, who hemorrhaged a measured average of 2 litres per week on intravenous iron dextran. This patient with a reticulocyte count always in excess of 40% was comfortable at a very low hemoglobin in the 4 to 5 gm/dl range. In fact her red cell 2-3 diphosphoglycerate (2,3 DPF) was at all times 2 to 3 times normal. Such patients need not and, therefore, should not be transfused. It is entirely appropriate for the transfusion service director to make suggestions, to influence behaviour and thereby to improve medical practice.

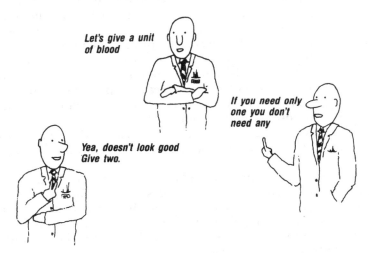

Figure 3.

Once the indications for transfusion are established the component and quantity are again medical judgements (fig. 3). Because of the ill conceived criterion that single unit transfusion is immoral or not justified, two units are requested where one would do. This misuse of transfusion can be avoided by the transfusion service director's intervention to hold off on transfusion until one unit is needed and then to transfuse only one unit, at least at a time. In fact for medically anemic patients, not those incurring trauma, surgical or otherwise, single unit transfusions are encouraged. It reduces transfusions and it certainly makes our life easier in follow up of transfusion reactions.

The same problems exist for platelet transfusions. The only indications for transfusion is to stop or prevent bleeding. The clinician should be aware that in idiopathic thrombocytopenia purpura (ITP) there is destruction of circulating platelets causing a shift to the left or a skewing of the cell age distribution.

Younger platelets like younger people are better and function better. An ITP patient with a platelet count of 40,000 mm³ is likely to have a normal bleeding time while the patient with marrow aplasia will most likely have significant prolongation. There are no good data on how many units to transfuse and how often.

Most of us have settled on a six pack. But like beer this can also be reduced to 4 units and can be exceeded (fig. 4). Another problem is the patient in whom there is no platelet increment following transfusion whose defective

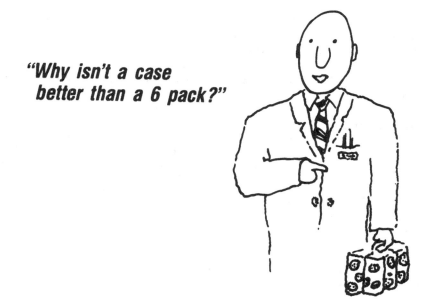

Figure 4.

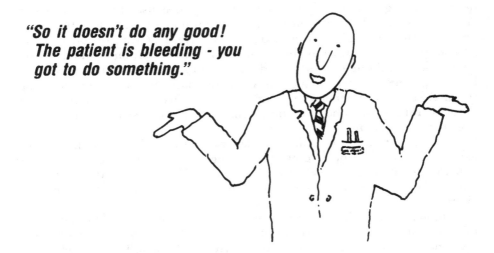

"So it doesn't do any good! The patient is bleeding - you got to do something."

Figure 5.

hemostasis is not corrected and for whom related or HLA compatible donors are not available (fig. 5). It is hard to stop platelet transfusions under these circumstances no matter how apparent it is that these transfusions are ineffective.

It is far more difficult for the hematologist – transfusion service director to be actively involved in judging what is needed at time of surgery. Only the surgeon and perhaps the anesthesiologist know what goes on at the time, in the operating room and only they can make decisions. Because of the delay in dilution of red cells by plasma, hemoglobin or hematocrit determinations have little meaning.

Table 1. Transfusion information of an orthopedic hospital.

	No. of opns	Total units trsfd	Mean units trsfd	SD	No. of opns w/o trans	Units min	Trsfd max
Lumbar decompression	6	4	0.67	1.21	4	0	3
Hip fusion	5	15	3.00	2.65	1	0	7
Laminectomy	5	7	1.40	1.67	2	0	4
Southwick osteotomy	5	6	1.20	0.84	1	0	2
Total shoulder replacement	4	13	3.25	5.25	2	0	11
Open reduction fracture hip	4	10	2.50	3.32	2	0	7
Rodding of femur and tibia	3	3	1.00	1.00	1	0	2

Perhaps the most effective approach to rational transfusion practice during surgery is to collect information on commonly performed operations and to establish norms. An example of this at an orthopedic hospital is shown in table 1.

For total hip replacement 3 units is the mean, shown with a standard deviation and range. The 'chief' uses 0.2 units, others average 6 or more.

On the assumption that less bloody surgery is better this kind of data serves as a very effective peer review. There is the connotation that less blood loss is associated with more careful hemostasis. Eventually it would be highly desirable to determine whether there is any correlation with surgical end results, or morbidity. There is some evidence that good hemostasis takes time, operations take longer, patients are under anesthesia for longer periods of time and there is longer wound exposure. How this affects post operative infection rate is not known.

Transfusion of plasma, plasma protein or colloid is another controversial area. We do not necessarily have to replace exactly what is lost. Collins [1], Moss [2], Virgilio [3,4] and others [5,6] have shown very clearly that resuscitation can be well accomplished administering larger quantities of crystalloid solutions. They were able to use Ringer's lactate or even saline very effectively in trauma victims in our misadventure in Viet Nam. Surprisingly pulmonary congestion was greatly reduced using salt solutions compared to when colloid was used. These data are still not fully accepted by the profession. In fact the main criticism is that data on young healthy soldiers can not be extrapolated to older sick patients. Virgilio's careful prospective study on patients mainly with aortic aneurysm refutes this argument [3].

His experience with a patient population of a mean age of 58 was similar to what was found in the young population in Viet Nam. Crystalloids given in a volume 3 – 8 times the blood loss is more effective than plasma or albumin at time of surgery. The lungs are less likely to be congested. Renal function after 24 hours is better in the crystalloid group than those receiving plasma proteins. The transfusion service director can make a major contribution by presenting this information to surgeons and anesthesiologists and to encourage them to try it because they may like it.

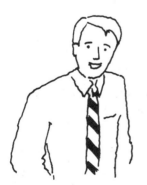

"Try it, you may like it."

Figure 6.

I have concentrated on the need to reduce transfusion to what is necessary. The other side of the coin is, of course, that it is our function to provide blood components, when needed, in a timely and safe manner. We have, therefore, developed much effort to simplifying compatibility testing and have been pioneers in depending on the serum screen to determine the method of crossmatch [7]. By ruling out the presence of unexpected antibodies in 94% of our patient population we have reduced the crossmatch to a simpler check on ABO compatibility. This permits us to quickly provide for unexpected needs during surgery. Our transfusion safety record is as good as any – two fatalities due to ABO incompatibility caused misidentification at the bedside, transfusing half a million units over 30 years.

A more serious problem we have encountered is graft vs host reaction in our severely immunosuppressed patient population. From this we had a number of deaths in the late 70s. This has, of course, been corrected by irradiation. Again the transfusion service director has a direct responsibility to educate and guide physicians that transfusion therapy is practiced properly and safer [8].

Conclusion

In order to provide more effective hemotherapy a case for the transfusion service director to be directly involved in monitoring and assuring the efficacy of transfusion has been presented. This includes the determination of whether any transfusion is really needed, what components are appropriate and the dosage and quantity to be transfused. This can be done in a collegial manner by acting as a strong creditable consultant, armed with data, facts and a good tract record.

References

1. Collins JA, Braitberg A, Butcher RH Jr. Changes in lung and body weight and lung water content in rats treated for hemorrhage with various fluids. Surgery 1973;73:401 – 11.
2. Moss GS, Gupta RK, Brinkman R et al. Changes in lung ultra-structure following heterologous and homologous serum albumin infusion in the treatment of hemorrhagic shock. Ann Surg 1979;189:236 – 42.
3. Virgilio RW, Rice CL, Smith DE et al. Crystalloid vs. colloid resuscitation: Is one better? Surgery 1979;85:129 – 39.
4. Virgilio RW, Smith DE, Zarins CK. Balanced electrolyte solutions: Experimental and clinical studies. Crit Care Med 1979;7:3,89.
5. Lucas CE, Ledgerwood AM, Higgins RF. Impaired salt and water excretion after albumin resuscitation for hypovolemic shock. Surgery 1979;86:544 – 9.
6. Mayer K. Crystalloids versus colloid. In: Silver R (ed). Blood, blood components and derivatives in transfusion therapy. A technical workshop. Washington, DC, AABB 1980:97 – 104.
7. Mayer K. Organization, functions, responsibilities and accountability of the hospital transfusion service and its medical director. Donor-recipient identification, pretransfusion testing and administration of blood and components. In: Mayer K (ed). Guidelines to transfusion practice. Washington, DC, AABB 1980:1 – 175.
8. Grindon AJ, Tomasulo PS, Bergin JJ, Klein HG, Miller JD, Mintz PD. The hospital transfusion committee. Guidelines for improving practice. JAMA 1985; 253:549 – 3.

DISCUSSION

Moderators: T.J. Greenwalt and M.R. Halie

J.A. van der Does: Dr. Schuurman, you had some two-by-two tables with graft survival by sex, blood groups, etc. I assume that this is a retrospective analysis. You had a Chi square analysis done on it and I am very curious to know how you come to taking one degree of freedom for comparison.

R.K.B. Schuurman (Leiden): The 4 two-by-two tables you refer to all had three degrees of freedom and none of them showed significance, thus precluding this statistical problem.

D.G. Woodfield (Auckland): Dr. Mayer has touched on a real problem that confronts transfusion services. We all realize the need for greater involvement on the clinical side. However, there are a number of factors mitigating that and one of these, I think, is very important. When considering Blood Transfusion Services, it is clear that many Services are understaffed on the medical side. Laboratory work is seductive and one is often involved heavily in this area. It seems to me that we must consider more clearly the speciality of transfusion medicine, to make it more acceptable academically, and to allow us to build up a highly specialized training programme suitable for young graduates, who can gain the respect of their clinical colleagues. When this is done, we might then be able to build up transfusion medicine into a more acceptable clinical speciality, with ramifications right throughout the medical area.

K. Mayer (New York): I certainly appreciate your comment and agree totally with you.

P.C. Das: Dr. Coffe showed the "Mission for Blood Banks". If I understand it correctly, it means that we should behave like King Solomon, be diplomats like Benjamin Franklin, entrepreneur like Henry Ford, with a touch of Einstein. A tremendous field is covered. The one thing missing, I thought: The blood banker of a couple of years ago was very enthusiastic about collecting pluripotent stem cells from peripheral blood. What happened to that?

C. Coffe (Besançon): You are referring to peripheral stem cell procurement. It is very difficult to know at what time it is good to take and to collect these stem cells.

T.J. Greenwalt: May I make a comment on that. Dr. Fliedner at Ulm probably wrote most of the papers on this subject. He has presented a model in using dextran sulphate to increase the peripheral stem cell level and actually succeeded in reconstituting two irradiated dogs with stem cells collected from the peripheral blood. There may be hope for this in the future. This has not been done in man of course, as we cannot use dextran sulphate in man.

M.R. Halie (Groningen): We have been doing some experiments on peripheral blood stem cells – whatever they may be. These peripheral blood stem cells, in our cultures and also in the literature, tend to behave different from bone marrow stem cells. Perhaps you could use them for the indications that you possibly have in mind, Dr. Das, but I think that there has to be some clarification as to what we have at hand.

T.J. Greenwalt: I am glad you said 'whatever they may be', because when people use the word 'stem cell', I just call them pluripotent cell.

C.Th. Smit Sibinga: Could I come back to Dr. Mayer's final remarks and try to outline one area which is of extreme importance to develop in the future – it should have been developed in the past, but we forgot about that entirely. What eventually happens at the bedside, after we have set the indications, after we have done all the compatibility testings, after we have gone over all the administrative points which need to be covered? The eventual safety and efficacy of the transfusion is the ultimate practice at the bedside. What we tend to forget is the way blood is administered to the patient. Most of these practices are done by our nurses; we trust them, we have great confidence in them, but we do not know what actually happens. Many times, I have come across problems when surgeons ask me: "What possibly are you giving us for platelets? They do not work at all. We do not find any increase in count whatsoever." You go back to the bedside and find a giving set which has been there for some days, through which an enormous amount of red cells has been transfused and the platelets are trapped in the debris in the filter. There is a mission for blood bankers and blood transfusionists in trying to develop that area specifically in the near future, because all our efforts will be wasted when this aspect is not being looked into more closely.